Updates in Intensive Care of OBGY Patients

Nissar Shaikh • Firdos Ummunnisa
Umm E Amara
Editors

Updates in Intensive Care of OBGY Patients

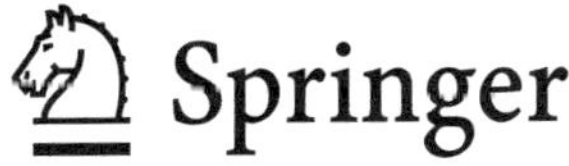

Editors
Nissar Shaikh
Surgical Intensive Care Unit
Hamad Medical Corporation
Doha, Qatar

Firdos Ummunnisa
Halima Al Tamimi OBGY Clinic
Doha, Qatar

Umm E Amara
Apollo Institute of Medical Sciences
Hyderabad, India

ISBN 978-981-99-9579-0 ISBN 978-981-99-9577-6 (eBook)
https://doi.org/10.1007/978-981-99-9577-6

This Springer imprint is published by the registered company Springer Nature Singapore Pte Ltd.
The registered company address is: 152 Beach Road, #21-01/04 Gateway East, Singapore 189721, Singapore

Paper in this product is recyclable.

Preface

Updates in Intensive Care of OBGY Patients is a book written by experienced as well as young talented writers with expertise in the field. It contains updated information about known diseases, peripartum cardiomyopathy, haemorrhage, microangiopathic haemolytic anaemia in pregnancy and hypertensive disorders of pregnancy as well as upcoming diseases such as the COVID infection in pregnancy and ovarian hyperstimulation syndrome. As gynaecological patients are increasing requiring intensive care therapy, due to increasing age and the number of comorbidities, we have covered their care updates as well in this book.

This book will serve as a source of information and knowledge, improving the care of pregnant and gynaecological patients. Acute care physicians, surgeons, anaesthesiologists, intensivists, obstetricians, and gynaecologists—both senior and junior—will find this book very helpful in the management of their patients. Paramedics and nurses also will find this book interesting in the care of their patients, as *Updates in Intensive Care of OBGY Patients* is written in a simplified and understandable language.

I am thankful to all chapter authors and co-editors for their patience and hard work. I am very much thankful and indebted to my wife Dr Firdos and daughters Dr Amara and Dr Nashrah for their constant support in bringing up this book.

Doha, Qatar — Nissar Shaikh
Doha, Qatar — Firdos Ummunnisa
Hyderabad, India — Umm E Amara

Contents

Peripartum Cardiomyopathy: An Update

Nissar Shaikh, Arshad Chanda, Umm E Amara, Umme Nashrah, Aisha Almotawa, Firdos Ummunnisa, Farookh Haider, and Mohamed Suliman

Abstract Peripartum cardiomyopathy (PPCM) is heart failure that develops in the last months of pregnancy or up to 5 months postpartum with left ventricular systolic dysfunction. Most common in Nigeria, which is related to micronutrient deficiency and high salt intake. The general risk for PPCM varies from hypertension to smoking. Pregnancy related-factors from advanced maternal age to preeclampsia. Etiological factors are genetic, autoimmune, malnutrition, inflammation, angiogenic imbalance due to hormonal changes.

Diagnosis is by the exclusion of frequent causes of heart failure, occurrence in the last months of pregnancy, or up to 5 months without any other cardiac disease. The echocardiogram will show a reduced left ventricular ejection fraction of less than 45%.

Treatment of PPCM in acute settings is oxygen supplementation, diuretics, vasodilators, and anticoagulation. If the patient presents in shock, they may have to resuscitate with vasopressors and inotropes. Long-term treatment includes lifestyle changes, diuretics, beta-blockers, anticoagulation, and heart transplants. Delivery of

N. Shaikh (✉) · A. Chanda
Surgical Intensive Care/Hamad Medical Corporation, Doha, Qatar
e-mail: smahcboob@hamad.qa

U. E Amara
Apollo Institute of Medical Sciences and Research, Hyderabad, India

U. Nashrah
Deccan College of Medical Sciences, Hyderabad, India

A. Almotawa
Women's Wellness and Research Center, Hamad Medical Corporation, Doha, Qatar

F. Ummunnisa
Dr. Halima Al Tamimi, Obstetrics and Gynecology Centre, Doha, Qatar

F. Haider · M. Suliman
Cardiology/Hamad Medical Corporation, Doha, Qatar

N. Shaikh et al. (eds.), *Updates in Intensive Care of OBGY Patients*,
https://doi.org/10.1007/978-981-99-9577-6_1

the fetus was not reported to improve PPCM. 50% of patients recover in 6 months, 25% have persistent symptoms, and 25% develop complications. Maternal mortality rates range from 4% to 11%.

Women with PPCM should be counseled for contraception and subsequent pregnancies. Those patients with recovered left ventricular ejection fraction seem to have minor changes with favorable maternal and fetal outcome.

Keywords Peripartum cardiomyopathy · African · Advanced age · Heart failure · Diuretics · Digoxin · Cathepsin D · Prolactin · Pregnancy · Re-pregnancy

1 Introduction

Peripartum cardiomyopathy (PPCM) occurs in pregnancy or up to 6 months postpartum. It is dilated cardiomyopathy in pregnant patients without any previous cardiac illness. It is a rare but cumbersome life-threatening clinical entity. It is challenging to differentiate peripartum cardiomyopathy from physiological changes in pregnancy, such as shortness of breath, tachypnea, and palpitation (Fig. 1). In lesser percentage of PPCM, patients recover from heart failure. It is important that the PPCM patient be aware of her re-pregnancy and subsequent recurrence of PPCM unless they recover from heart failure [1].

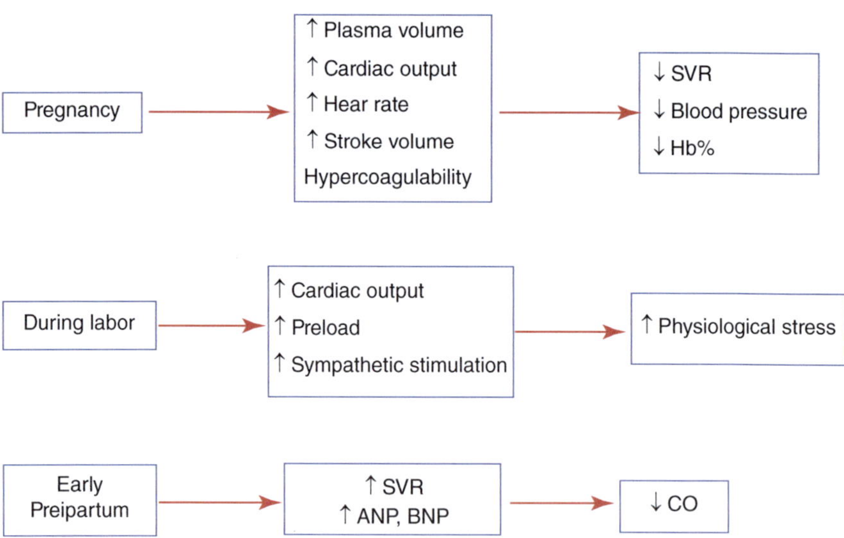

Fig. 1 Physiologic changes in pregnancy and peripartum

2 Epidemiology

The incidence of peripartum cardiomyopathy varies worldwide. PPCM is very common in Nigeria (995 per 100,000 live births) and Haiti (327 per 100,000 live births). There is a much lesser incidence in Japan (6 per 100,000 live births) and Denmark 10 per 100,000 live births. The higher incidence in Nigeria is reported due to custom of an eating kanwa, a dry lake salt, daily intake for 40 days postpartum, genetic predisposition, and selenium deficiency. Whereas in Haiti, PPCM is higher due to zinc deficiency and preeclampsia [2]. The rising incidence of PPCM in the USA may be related to increased maternal age [3].

3 Definition

Peripartum cardiomyopathy is heart failure that develops in the last months of pregnancy up to 5 months postpartum with left ventricular systolic dysfunction. The European Society of Cardiology defines PPCM as a heart failure that occurs toward the end of pregnancy or in the months following delivery, where no other cause of heart failure is found.

The diagnostic criteria for PPCM are:

1. Absence of pre-existing heart disease
2. Development of heart failure in the last months of pregnancy and up to 5 months postpartum
3. Idiopathic nature
4. Left ventricular end-diastolic dimension >2.7 cm/m, M-mode fractional shortening <30%, left ventricular ejection fraction <0.45 [3]

During pregnancy, there are various anatomic and physiological changes in the mother to support the mother and the fetus. Mainly there is increased plasma volume, heart rate, blood pressure, cardiac output, and dilutional anemia. They will also decrease systemic vascular resistance (SVR) and hemoglobin levels. Coagulation changes will be in a hypercoagulable state. During labor, the uterine contractions eject a large amount of blood into the circulation, raising cardiac output (CO) and preload. Anxiety and pain increase the sympathetic tone, thus raising cardiac output, blood pressure, and heart rate (Fig. 1).

In the initial 2 weeks postpartum, cardiac output, stroke volume, and heart rate return to normal. Atrial natriuretic peptide BNP (B-type natriuretic peptide) increases during postpartum, causing excessive diuresis. If all these hemodynamic changes are not reversed, the mother has a high risk of cardiovascular disease, mainly PPCM [4].

4 Risk Factors

Age is an important risk factor. Although PPCM can occur at any maternal age, more than 50% of cases are more than 30 years old.

The following are the risk factors for the development of PPCM:

1. Ethnicity:

   The occurrence of PPCM is significantly higher and black populations. It is reported that PPCM occurs 16 times more in the black race compared to the whites [5].
2. Hypertension, preeclampsia, and eclampsia:

   Hypertension and preeclampsia are strongly associated with PPCM. Hypertensive disorders were found in 37% of PPCM cases. Eclampsia is associated with PPCM with an odd ratio of 12.9 and much higher in multi-state hospital discharge cases in the USA [6].
3. Multiple gestations:

   The rate during pregnancy associated with PPCM is 90%.

   Detailed risk factors are described in Table 1.

Table 1 Detailed risk factors

General risk factors
• Hypertension • Diabetes mellitus • Obesity • Smoking • Substance abuse • Genetic factors • African Americans • Malnutrition (selenium and zinc deficiency)
Pregnancy-related risk factors
• Preeclampsia • Cesarean section • Multiparty • Twin pregnancy • Advanced maternal age • Prolonged tocolytic therapy
Further risk factors
• Environmental and lifestyle • Abnormal immune response • Abnormal adaptation to pregnancy changes

5 Pathophysiology

The etiology of PPCM is multifactorial, few of them are discussed in the following paragraph:Pregnancy causes significant hemodynamic changes. If these changes persist and do not return to normal, it causes an increase in the risk of PPCM and heart failure [7].Genetic factors for PPCM are described as PPCM cluster in families, which looks to be genes experiences with toxic environment during late pregnancy due to oxidative stress that can increase the risk of PPCM.The pro-inflammatory state proposed to play a role in the development of PPCM. The raised levels of pro-inflammatory markers, particularly interleukin-6 and TNF-alfa, are raised in PPCM patients.The autoimmune theory for PPCM describes that changes in the maternal immune system (immunosuppression) lead to maternal immune system exposure to the fetus cells, which generates an immune response leading to antibodies against certain cardiac tissue, leading to autoimmune myocardiomyopathy and PPCM.There are significant hormonal changes during pregnancy. There is an increased prolactin level in the late pregnancy and postpartum period. The animal models proved that there is knock out expression of STAT-3 in patients with PPCM. The enzyme which protects the myocardium from reactive oxygen species, reduction in STAT-3 leads to increased generation of peptidase known as Cathepsin D that breaks protein into angiostatic N-terminal 16-kDa prolactin fragments that promote apoptosis in the endothelial cells and cardiac myocytes (Fig. 2).

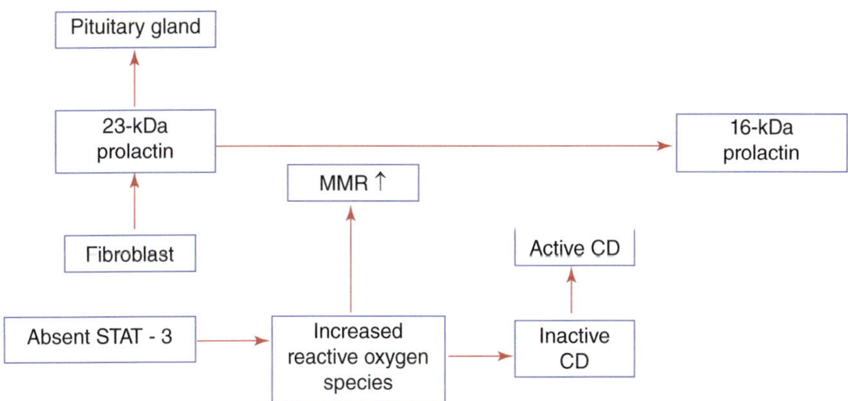

Cathepsin D - CD, maternal mortality rate -MMR, signal transducer and activator of transcription 3 (STAT3)

Fig. 2 Summary of PPCM pathophysiology

Autopsy findings in PPCM are pale, heavy, and dilated heart, with variable mural thrombi with patent coronaries and heart valves. The microscopic findings are interstitial edema, cellulitis swelling, fibrosis, and hypertrophy with abundant eosinophil.

6 Diagnosis

The majority of PPCM occurs in the postpartum period. PPCM presentation varies depending on the disease status. Common symptoms are nocturnal dyspnea, orthopnea, and pedal edema. One should have a high index of suspicion to diagnose PPCM. It is a diagnosis of exclusion and should be differentiated from physiological changes during pregnancy.The serum Pro-BNP is commonly elevated. The chest X-ray may reveal cardiomegaly or pulmonary edema. ECG findings are not specific, and it may show tachycardia, atrial fibrillation, or flutter and arrhythmia. POCUS (point-of-care ultrasound) might show multiple B-lines if the patient developed pulmonary edema. Echocardiography or POCUS showed markedly reduced left ventricular ejection fraction; less than 45% is diagnostic of PPCM.

7 Treatment

The management of PPCM is similar to heart failure, with additional therapy for arrhythmia management, anticoagulation, and mechanical support. With consideration of medication side effects for mother and fetus.

Optimizing volume status with a bolus between intra- and extravascular volume is essential. Initial therapy is diuresis, furosemide and hydrochlorothiazide are safe, there is no sufficient that about potassium-sparing diuretics.

ACE-I (angiotensin-converting enzyme inhibitor) and ARB (angiotensin II receptor blockers) are contraindicated during pregnancy but can be used postpartum avoiding breast-feeding. While in beta-blockers, Carvedilol has the advantage of reducing afterload. Again, breast-feeding is to be withheld in these patients.

Hydralazine is safe, but nitroprusside is contraindicated during pregnancy because of the concern of cyanide toxicity. Digoxin is safe during pregnancy and postpartum. It has both inotropic and chronotropic action. Anticoagulation can be either unfractionated or low molecular weight heparin depending on the mother's renal function.

If a PPCM patient is in shock, they may require inotropic support such as dobutamine and milrinone with additional vasopressors support. Patients with fulminant PPCM may require mechanical circulatory support by left ventricular assist device (LVAD) as a bridge for cardiac transplant or recovery.

Although there is no sufficient evidence that usefulness of bromocriptine, it is used increasingly, as it blocks the degeneration of cathepsin D. There is no published data about the delivery or elective cesarean section that can ameliorate PPCM or improve fetal outcome.

8 Morbidity and Mortality

Recovery from PPCM usually occurs within 6 months. Factors indicating good prognosis are small left ventricular dimension, left ventricular ejection fraction (LVEF) more than 35% and fractioning of shortening greater than 20%, normal troponins, no left ventricular thrombus, and African American ethnicity.

Poor prognosis indicators are QRS greater than 120 ms, delayed diagnosis, higher New York Heart Association grade, multiparity, and African descent. The common PPCM maternal complications are thromboembolism, arrhythmia, progressive heart failure, and the frequent fetal complication is fetal distress, stillbirth, lower Apgar score, and low birth weight [8].

The overall outcome of PPCM is improved in recent decades. As high as 71% of PPCM, patients recover with a left ventricular ejection fraction >50%. The maternal mortality in PPCM varies from 4% to 11%, and few studies mention 16% mortality in 7 years [9].

9 Re-pregnancy in PPCM

There is no guarantee that heart failure will not occur in the subsequent pregnancies in a patient with PPCM. Codsi et al. describe that patients with a history of PPCM who recover from LV function are at risk for a transient minor decrease in LV ejection fraction during further pregnancies with an obstetric and neonatal favorable outcome [10].

10 Conclusion

Peripartum cardiomyopathy is a rare but potentially fatal disease of pregnancy. It occurs in the last months of pregnancy up to 5 months postpartum most frequently in the postpartum. PPCM occurs all over the world but is more frequent in Nigeria and Haiti. There are various risk factors for PPCM, from African descent to multigravity. Diagnosis is reached by excluding other causes for heart failure and echocardiographic findings showing low left ventricular ejection fraction. Treatment is optimizing preload with diuresis, management of arrhythmia, and prevention of thromboembolism. Further pregnancies look safer in PPCM patients with recovered left ventricular function.

References

1. Shaikh N. An obstetric emergency called peripartum cardiomyopathy! J Emerg Trauma Shock. 2010;3(1):39–42.
2. Shaikh N, Ummunnisa F, Chanda A, Imran M, Ganaw A, Amara UE, et al. Peripartum cardiomyopathy: facts and figures. In: Inflammatory heart diseases. Intech Open; 2019. https://doi.org/10.5772/intechopen.85718.
3. Honigberg MC, Givertz MM. Peripartum cardiomyopathy. BMJ. 2019;364:k5287. https://doi.org/10.1136/bmj.k5287.
4. Mayama M, et al. Factors influencing brain natriuretic peptide levels in healthy pregnant women. Int J Cardiol. 2017;228:749–53.
5. Gentry MB, et al. African-American women have a higher risk for developing peripartum cardiomyopathy. J Am Coll Cardiol. 2010;55:654–9.
6. Kolte D, et al. Temporal trends in incidence and outcomes of peripartum cardiomyopathy in the united States: a nationwide population-based study. JAHA. 2014;3:e001056.
7. Mebazaa A, et al. Imbalanced angiogenesis in peripartum cardiomyopathy—diagnostic value of placenta growth factor. Circ J. 2017;81:1654–61.
8. Gunderson EP, et al. Epidemiology of peripartum cardiomyopathy: incidence, predictors, and outcomes. Obstet Gynecol. 2011;118:583–91.
9. Harper MA, Meyer RE, Berg CJ. Peripartum cardiomyopathy: population-based birth prevalence and 7-year mortality. Obstet Gynecol. 2012;120:1013–9.
10. Codsi E, Rose CH, Blauwet LA. Subsequent pregnancy outcomes in patients with peripartum cardiomyopathy. Obstet Gynecol. 2018;131(2):322–7.

Microangiopathic Hemolytic Anemia of Pregnancy: Facts and Figures

Seema Nahid, Fateen Shareef, Azha Fatima, Umm E Amara, Umme Nashrah, and Ifrah Fatima

Abstract Microangiopathic hemolytic anemia (MAHA) of pregnancy is a rare but severe pregnancy complication that is characterized by nonimmune intravascular hemolysis or destruction of red blood cells and the formation of small blood clots in the capillaries and small blood vessels of the body (microangiopathy) resulting in a wide variety of symptoms, some of which include weariness, weakness, shortness of breath, jaundice, and edema. This condition affects both the mother and the developing fetus. The primary aim is to differentiate primary thrombotic microangiopathy from other systemic illnesses that can present with microangiopathic hemolytic anemia (MAHA) and thrombocytopenia. We desire glorious motherhood and a healthy baby (George and Nester, N Engl J Med 371:654, 2014; Narayanan et al., Int J Hematol 96:122–124, 2012).

MAHA of pregnancy is often associated with other pregnancy-related conditions, such as preeclampsia, HELLP syndrome (hemolysis, elevated liver enzymes, and low platelet count), and pregnancy-associated TMA, especially thrombotic thrombocytopenic purpura (TTP) and complement-mediated hemolytic uremic syndrome (CM HUS). These conditions can cause similar symptoms and can be life-threatening if not promptly diagnosed and treated. Although there is clinical overlap, management varies significantly.

S. Nahid (✉)
Dr Hamad Medical Corporation, Doha, Qatar
e-mail: snahid@hamad.qa

F. Shareef · U. Nashrah
Deccan College of Medical Sciences, Hyderabad, Telangana, India

A. Fatima
Kamineni Academy of Medical Sciences and Research Centre, Hyderabad, Telangana, India

U. E Amara
Apollo Institute of Medical Sciences and Research, Hyderabad, Telangana, India

I. Fatima
University of Missouri-Kansas City, Kansas City, MO, USA

N. Shaikh et al. (eds.), *Updates in Intensive Care of OBGY Patients*,
https://doi.org/10.1007/978-981-99-9577-6_2

MAHA is caused by RBC fragmentation as they pass over platelet-rich thrombi in microcirculation. Thrombotic microangiopathies define small vessel changes, including endothelial cell swelling, vessel wall thickening, and platelet thrombi formation in the microvasculature. These changes obliterate the vessel lumen or microaneurysm, affecting the blood flow and resulting in single or multi-end-organ damage. MAHA in conjugation with thrombosis throughout microcirculation and consumptive thrombocytopenia occurs clinically in TMA. The goal is to limit irreversible end-organ damage.

Keywords Pregnancy · Thrombotic microangiopathies (TMA) · Preeclampsia (PET) · Hemolysis elevated liver enzymes, and low platelets (HELLP) Thrombotic thrombocytopenic purpura (TTP) · Complement-mediated hemolytic uremic syndrome (CM HUS) · Acute fatty liver of pregnancy (AFLP)

1 Introduction

Pregnancy and childbirth are times of celebration across the universe, but pregnant women can become suddenly sick and critically ill. Accepting illness in young and previously healthy women warrants intensive evaluation and management while waiting for the survival of at-risk infants. Physiological changes in the pregnancy groom's mother for adaptation of the fetus and challenges of delivery, however, may also introduce risk with significant morbidity and mortality. Pregnant women with underlying medical conditions or acquired disorders represent special concerns and challenges in diagnosis and management.

Thrombotic microangiopathy (TMA) is a pathological condition that affects the vasculature, specifically the arterioles and capillaries, and can lead to microvascular thrombosis. TMAs induce MAHA and thrombocytopenia, but MAHA is not always the underlying cause of TMAs. In pregnant women, thrombocytopenia may be associated with microangiopathic hemolytic anemia (MAHA), threatening maternal and fetal safety and emphasizing early diagnosis and intervention. The identification of certain systemic diseases requires additional diagnostic procedures (Fig. 1).

Primary TMA also includes TTP (hereditary or immune-mediated) and complement-mediated (hereditary or acquired) and other associated systemic disorders such as systemic infections, DIC, pregnancy-related, and systemic rheumatic diseases (e.g., SLE, SSc, APS) (Table 1, Fig. 2).

Thrombotic microangiopathies in pregnancy include heterogeneous disorders with similar pathological and clinical findings, commonly including four syndromes HELLP, thrombotic thrombocytopenic purpura (TTP), complement-mediated hemolytic uremic syndrome (HUS), acute fatty liver of pregnancy (AFP). Thrombotic microangiopathies may be pregnancy-related complications (HELLP/PET) or may be precipitated by disorders of pregnancy (TTP, CM HUS, AFLP).

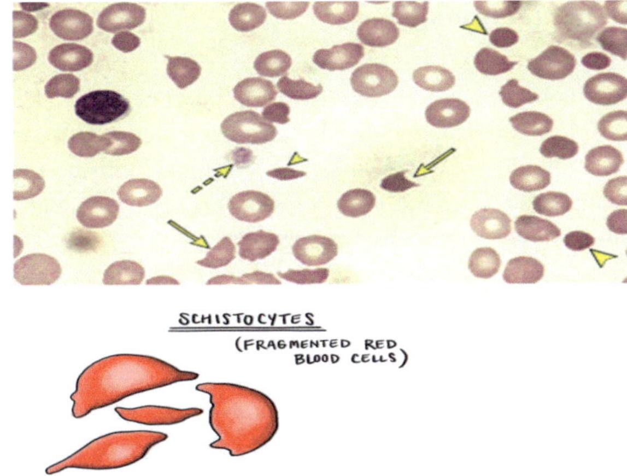

Fig. 1 Peripheral smear in MAHA showing the presence of schistocytes

Table 1 TMA in pregnancy with anemia and thrombocytopenia

Pregnancy-associated	Presenting/precipitating in pregnancy
Preeclampsia	TTP
Preeclampsia with severe features	CM HUS
HELLP	APLS
AFLP	Sepsis

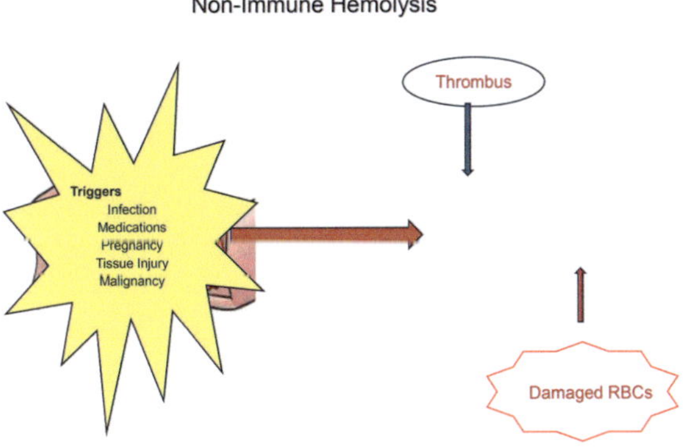

Fig. 2 Thrombus formation and Hemolysis in blood vessels

The complement system is central to the host innate immunity and interacts with coagulation factors and platelets. Complement regulatory proteins like complement factor H (CHF) and complement factor I (CFI) prevent excessive and inappropriate complement activation in the host cells. An acute inflammatory or prothrombotic stimulus may trigger clinical manifestations.

2 Epidemiology

The incidence of TTP and CM HUS previously quoted in pregnancy is 1 in 25,000, with true incidence higher because of increased awareness and better diagnostics. This unique group of high-risk conditions and the rarity of the disease in recent years emphasizes the need for an MDT approach and the need for management at multicentered good obstetric centers.

3 Etiopathology

TMA is characterized by small vessel changes, including swelling of endothelial cells and the subendothelial space, vessel wall thickening, and platelet microthrombi, typically in small arterioles and capillaries. These changes can obliterate the vessel lumen, especially in smaller vessels, and lead to hyaline occlusion and endothelial cell proliferation and/or vessel wall dilatation (e.g., microaneurysms) have been seen in the affected arterioles. Common pathological features are endothelial cell injury, microvascular thrombosis, and end-organ damage clinically present as thrombocytopenia, hemolytic anemia, and organ failure (Fig. 3). Renal pathological changes are found in the arterioles and the kidney's glomeruli.

The hematologic characteristic is microangiopathic hemolytic anemia MAHA is caused by mechanical RBC fragmentation that occurs as RBCs traverse platelet-rich thrombi in the microcirculation and thrombocytopenia due to platelet consumption in microthrombi throughout the microcirculation.

Defective complement regulation is responsible for complement-mediated TMA (CM-TMA). The alternative pathway protects self-cells from inappropriate complement-mediated attack and failure of normal control mechanisms to down-regulate the alternative pathway leads to endothelial damage. Specific complement regulatory proteins that protect self-cells from inappropriate complement activity include soluble complement factor H (CHF) and membrane cofactor protein (MCP). These factors promote the inactivation of the membrane-attack complex components. Loss of these protective factors may cause TMA.

Fig. 3 TMA components

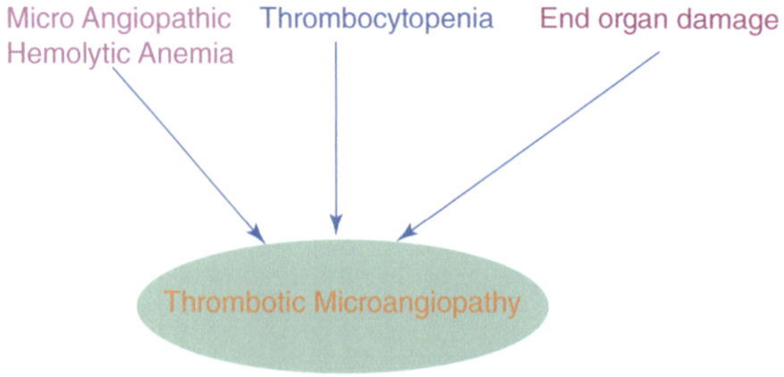

Risk factors—pregnancy is a well-established trigger and can be life-threatening with a significant clinical overlap in pregnancy. A high index of suspicion is vital to avoid severe consequences for the patient and pregnancy.

4 Diagnosis

Identification of associated MAHA and thrombocytopenia margins the differential diagnosis. Additional challenges in obstetric presentation with nonspecific and varied clinical symptoms can mimic or be mistaken for more common entities of pregnancy, like preeclampsia and HELLP. Full hematological screening is mandated.

Microangiopathic hemolytic anemia (MAHA) marked by prominent schistocytes, including helmet and triangular cells, on the peripheral blood smear and consumptive thrombocytopenia hallmarks the diagnosis (Fig. 1).

The number of schistocytes can vary in immune TTP and can be influenced by the duration of the disease. Two or more schistocytes per high power field (viewed by a 100× magnification oil immersion objective) in the appropriate clinical setting is suggestive of MAHA [1].

TTP should be suspected when a patient presents with microangiopathic hemolytic anemia (MAHA; hemoglobin almost always <10 g/dL) and severe thrombocytopenia (platelet count almost always <30,000/μL), with or without symptoms of organ involvement and in the absence of another obvious clinically etiology.

5 HELLP (Hemolysis, Elevated Liver Enzymes and Low Platelets)

HELLP is characterized by hemolysis, elevated liver enzymes and low platelets, and hypertension with or without proteinuria. The estimated incidence in pregnant women is between 0.5% and 0.9% of all pregnancies, and 10–20% of cases with preeclampsia commonly only occur in the third trimester although 30% can present postpartum. Among patients with severe preeclampsia/eclampsia, 1–2% have microangiopathic hemolysis and thus can be considered to have HELLP. It can present as an obstetric complication or be misdiagnosed due to the variable nature of the presentation. Diagnosis can be challenging as symptoms of HELLP can mimic idiopathic thrombocytopenic purpura, thrombotic thrombocytopenic purpura, HUC, AFP, and DIC.

The overall maternal mortality rate in HELLP syndrome is 1%, with a high range of 0–24.4% depending on the severity of the disease and perinatal mortality rate between 7% and 34%, with prematurity contributing to the main cause.

The pathophysiology of MAHA secondary to HELLP is due to the fragmentation of red blood cells as they pass through small blood vessels with endothelial damage and microthrombi. These changes are more marked in the liver, with fibrin deposits obstructing hepatic blood flow, leading to periportal necrosis, infarcts, and hemorrhage.

MAHA associated with thrombocytopenia is secondary to activation of the coagulation system and microthrombus formation in circulation, attributed mainly to platelet consumption. DIC may complicate severe cases.

Various classifications have been suggested according to clinical presentation and severity of the disease. Pregnant/postpartum patients who have some of the typical laboratory abnormalities but do not meet all the laboratory criteria described below are considered to have partial HELLP [2]. These patients may progress to meet all criteria.

6 Complete

- MAHA
- Thrombocytopenia
- LFT
- LDH

Partial—one or two of above

Classifications by laboratory criteria and severity of thrombocytopenia (Table 2).

Table 2 Tabulated summary of the fetal and maternal risks and considerations for the various imaging modalities and contrast studies

Tennessee classification [3]	Mississippi classification
Diagnostic laboratory criteria for diagnosis of HELLP require the presence of the following criteria: • Hemolysis, established by at least two of the following: • Peripheral smear with schistocytes and burr cells • Serum bilirubin ≥1.2 mg/dL (20.52 μmol/L) • Low serum haptoglobin (≤25 mg/dL) or lactate dehydrogenase (LDH) ≥2 times the upper level of normal (based on laboratory-specific reference ranges) • Severe anemia unrelated to blood loss • Elevated liver enzymes: • Aspartate aminotransferase (AST) or alanine aminotransferase (ALT) ≥two times the upper level of normal (based on laboratory-specific reference ranges) • Low platelets: <100,000 cells/μL	Based on the severity of thrombocytopenia, HELLP is subclassified as follows • Class 1—Platelet count ≤50,000 cells/μL plus LDH >600 IU/L and AST or ALT ≥70 IU/L • Class 2—Platelet count >50,000 but ≤100,000 cells/μL plus LDH >600 IU/L and AST or ALT ≥70 IU/L • Class 3—Platelet count >100,000 but ≤150,000 cells/μL plus LDH >600 IU/L and AST or ALT ≥40 IU/L

7 Clinical Presentation Criteria

Clinically presents as new onset hypertension after 20 weeks gestation with coexisting of one or more of either proteinuria or maternal organ dysfunction including hepatic, renal, hematological, neural, or uteroplacental dysfunction. Clinically may present with nausea, vomiting, epigastric tenderness, and right upper quadrant pain caused by obstructed blood flow in hepatic sinusoids and necrosis. Laboratory tests are done to establish/exclude the diagnosis of HELLP because pain may precede (4–6 h) several hours before hematological abnormalities. Common laboratory tests are CBC, PS, liver, and renal function test, LDH, and coagulation profile.

The hallmark of hemolytic anemia is the presence of schistocytes, triangular cells, and burr cells on peripheral smears, and thrombocytopenia is a characteristic feature. The time of presentation, the severity of hemolysis (mild in HELLP), and the degree of thrombocytopenia may suggest the diagnosis [4].

HELLP can overlap symptoms with preeclampsia with severe features in its more serious form, which can complicate pregnancy. The frequent differential diagnoses include pregnancy-related hemolytic uremic syndrome, acute fatty liver of pregnancy, and thrombotic thrombocytopenic purpura. In HELLP, angiopathy and liver dysfunction are marked. Initial management involves evaluation and stabilization in unstable patients, and fetal assessment is done because of the possibility of serious maternal complications that may develop rapidly [5]. Definitive management of PET/HELLP is pregnancy termination with clinical improvement in 48–72 h. Obstetric factors and gestational age guide the mode of delivery HELLP should be managed at a tertiary care center with appropriate maternal and neonatal intensive care levels [6].

The maternal outcome is generally good, and the risk of maternal morbidity correlates with the increasing severity of maternal symptoms and laboratory abnormalities; however, serious complications such as abruption, acute kidney injury, subcapsular liver hematoma or hepatic rupture, pulmonary edema, ARDS, hemorrhage, retinal detachment, and death may occur.

8 Thrombotic Thrombocytopenic Purpura

Thrombotic thrombocytopenic purpura is caused by severe deficiency of ADAMTS13 (A Disintegrin and Metalloprotease with a Thrombospondin type 1 motif, member 13) metalloprotease enzyme activity required for the cleavage of Von Willebrand factor (VWF) also called as von Willebrand factor (VWF) cleaving protease ADAMTS13 is synthesized in hepatic stellate cells and also by endothelial cells. It breaks down large molecules of VWF into small units preventing the accumulation of larger units [7, 8] (Fig. 4).

When protease ADAMTA13 activity is reduced, it leads to incomplete cleavage and accumulation of large multimers of VWF on the endothelial surface, where

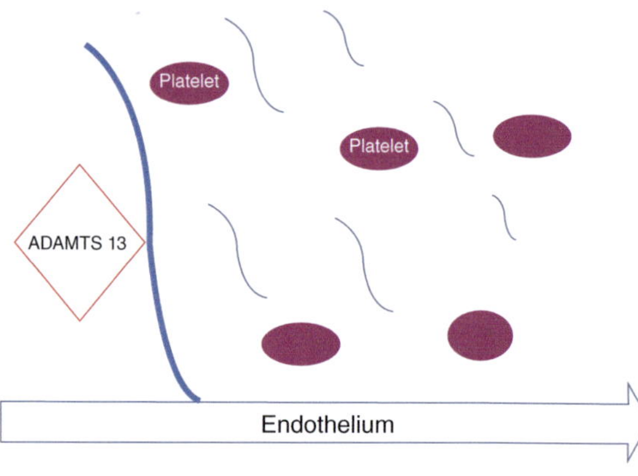

Fig. 4 ADAMTS13 physiological activity

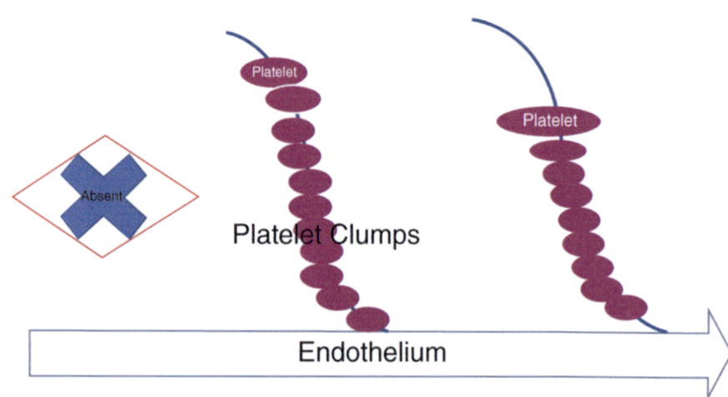

Fig. 5 Absent ADAMTS13

spontaneous platelet aggregation occurs in the high-shear microvasculature and thrombus formation get activated, promoting microvascular thrombosis resulting in blocking a blood vessel and end-organ damage [9, 10] (Fig. 5).

In the general population, congenital TTP is rare, with a prevalence of less than 1 per million, whereas immune TTP is approximately 6 per million, according to UK data. Immune TTP is approximately 30-fold more common than hereditary TTP however, when TTP occurs during the first pregnancy; hereditary TTP must be considered.

Pregnancy is a prothrombotic condition with additionally reduced ADAMTS13 activity during the third trimester of pregnancy, reaching its lowest levels between 36 and 40 weeks of gestation and during the early puerperium. Commonly presents in the late trimester, with 10–25% associated with pregnancy carrying significant maternal and fetal mortality when untreated.

The major cause of ADAMTS13 deficiency

- Congenital/inherited—gene mutation
- Immune-mediated/acquired—autoantibodies

Individuals with congenital TTP due to inherited congenital ADAMTS13 enzyme deficiency may not exhibit any signs or symptoms of TTP until they are exposed to triggers such as an infection or pregnancy. The PLASMIC score can assess risk and

ADAMTS13 activity test [11]. The assessment of ADAMTS13 activity can be performed on either plasma or serum. Normal >60% suggest an etiology other than TTP [12, 13].

9 Immune-Mediated Thrombotic Thrombocytopenic Purpura (TTP)

Immune-mediated thrombotic thrombocytopenic purpura (TTP) is a primary thrombotic microangiopathy (TMA) caused by severe ADAMTS13 deficiency (typically, activity <10%) due to inhibitory autoantibodies against ADAMTS13; therefore, the enzyme ADAMTS13 is rendered inactive or is cleared from the body. Risk factors for the development of antibodies are not defined clearly.

It affects approximately three out of 1 million adults, the female gender is a risk factor, and the incidence is higher among individuals of African descent. The frequency of immune TTP may be increased in pregnancy, where it may be misdiagnosed as preeclampsia with severe features or HELLP syndrome.

The clinical manifestations of this condition include severe microangiopathic hemolytic anemia (MAHA) and thrombocytopenia in a previously healthy individual (Fig. 6). The onset of symptoms can be gradual, from the onset of headache in pregnancy to a wide range of symptoms, including mild weakness, disorientation, gastrointestinal issues, heart impairment, or impaired kidney function before overt clinical diagnosis. Neurologic manifestations can range from moderate, such as a headache and temporary confusion, to severe, including tonic-clonic seizures, stroke, and/or coma. They can also be a combination of these symptoms or focal abnormalities, transitory aphasia, or vision impairment.

Diagnosis of congenital/inherited TTP is pointed when ADAMTS13 activity <10% with negative antibody assay and identification of the pathogenic gene, while

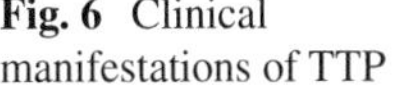

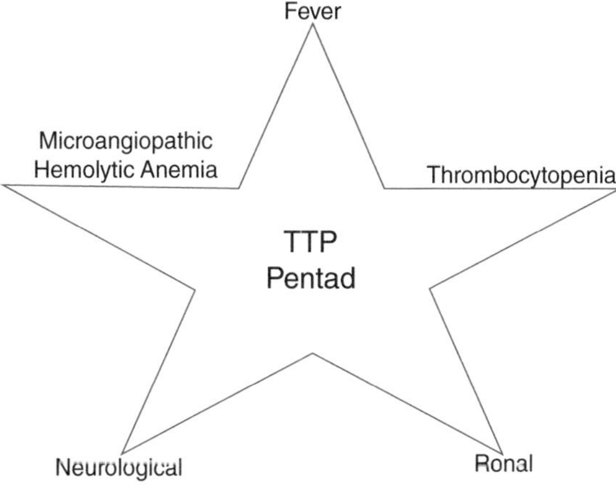

Fig. 6 Clinical manifestations of TTP

immune TTP is confirmed by ADAMTS13 activity less than 10% in the presence of IgG antibodies to ADAMTS13. Results are often unavailable immediately, vary according to the assay methods used, and may be impacted by transfusions, TPE, or bilirubin levels higher than 20 mg/dL.

A potentially lifesaving therapy should not be delayed while waiting for a confirming test if a presumptive diagnosis of immunological TTP is made based on clinical symptoms and laboratory testing with platelet count, peripheral blood smear, serum chemistries, and creatinine and quantified by PLASMIC scores. A presumptive diagnosis of MAHA with thrombocytopenia with appropriate clinical presentation is an indication to initiate therapeutic plasma exchange (TPE) and other therapies.

The mainstay of treatment is plasma therapy. In congenital TTP, plasma infusion repletes ADAMTS13 levels, whereas for immune TTP, plasma exchange combined with immunosuppression removes causative antibodies and replenishes ADAMTS13.

10 Triggering Factors

Pregnancy is a well-established trigger in 5 % of cases and can be life-threatening with a significant clinical overlap in pregnancy. A high index of suspicion is important to avoid severe consequences for the patient and pregnancy [8, 14].

Physiological changes in pregnancy lead to elevated VWF and associated reduction in ADAMTS13 activity to reduce the risk of excessive bleeding around delivery. However, individuals with congenital TTP can lead to critically low-level ADAMTS13 and overt clinical features of TTP. In pregnant women with induced alterations in the immune system, antibody-mediated TTP may be triggered.

Untreated TTP commonly presents with increased fetal losses due to underlying microvascular thrombosis, placental ischemia, and infarction.

The large increase in the number of pregnant women with the first presentation of TTP who had late-onset congenital TTP highlights the importance of prompt diagnosis and management for improved maternal and fetal outcomes.

11 Management TTP Presenting in Pregnancy

The therapeutic aim is to normalize platelet count and ADAMTS13 activity by eradicating autoantibody. Confirmation of congenital TTP by very low ADAMTS13 antibody levels pins the diagnosis and is further confirmed by genetic testing while plasma therapy remains the mainstay of treatment until platelet count normalizes. Congenital TTP responds briskly to plasma infusion therapy which replenishes ADAMTS13 activity. Platelet transfusions are avoided throughout the disease course.

Immune-mediated TTP is confirmed by ADAMTS13 antibodies and effectively managed by plasma exchange to eliminate antibodies. Plasma therapy is continued in the antenatal and postnatal periods. Further immunosuppression with corticosteroids is also required.

Closed maternal and fetal monitoring is required with regular obstetric input for fetal growth scanning and uterine artery Doppler monitoring. Time management is crucial for improved maternal and fetal outcomes. The delivery time is dictated by fetal factors or progressive maternal clinical symptoms for emergency cesarean section. The risk of thromboprophylaxis is minimized to ensure adequate placental blood flow (low-dose aspirin and prophylactic low molecular weight heparin).

Pregnancy may continue until 36–37 weeks gestation, provided there are no maternal or fetal adverse effects. Clinical remission may be temporary when plasma therapy is stopped, with ADAMTS13 activity returning to <10% by 2 weeks.

12 Management Pregnancy in Known TTP

Closed monitoring of ADAMTS13 activity through pregnancy and 6 weeks postpartum period is essential for the risk of relapse and progression of the disease process. The risk of relapse is highest with a low ADAMTS13 enzyme level (<10%) or in the absence of treatment in previously diagnosed TTP.

Plasma therapy is initiated at the confirmation of pregnancy at 10 mL/kg every 2 weeks and may be increased with the advancement of pregnancy. Thromboprophylaxis with aspirin or low molecular weight heparin is considered to maintain the adequacy of placental blood flow with regular obstetric input for ultrasound scanning and uterine artery Doppler monitoring. Prognostic markers for escalation of treatment are falling platelet and rising LDH [15].

13 CM HUS—Complement-Mediated Hemolytic Uremic Syndrome

The hemolytic uremic syndrome is classified as

- Toxin mediated—T HUS
- Complement mediated—CM HUS

Complement mediate HUS, also known as atypical HUS, is a rare condition with an incidence of 1–2 per million population carrying significant maternal and fetal mortality. 24th September is recognized as CM HUS awareness day [16].

The complement system is part of innate and adaptive immunity. A major function of the complement system is to guard and promote a pro-inflammatory response, altering the host response. Although it plays an adaptive immune response eliminating damaged cells, tissue regeneration, and angiogenesis.

The classical, alternative, and lectin pathways are three major complement cascade systems. All three pathways result in a pro-inflammatory response deposition of large amounts of C3 on the target cell (opsonization) and membrane perturbation, including lysis by the membrane-attack complex (MAC). Each of the complement pathways is triggered distinctly. The alternative pathway protects self-cells from inappropriate complement-mediated attack, and failure of normal control mechanisms to downregulate the alternative pathway may lead to endothelial damage. It serves as an independent immune system.

Specific complement regulatory proteins responsible for protecting self-cells from inappropriate complement activity include soluble factors such as complement factor H (CFH) and membrane-bound factors such as membrane cofactor protein (MCP), decay accelerating factor (DAF), and thrombomodulin (TM) [17]. These factors promote the inactivation of membrane-attack complex components. CFH and TM act as cofactors in the proteolytic inactivation of C3b by complement factor I (CFI). Loss of these protective factors may cause TMA by a variety of mechanisms.

Defective complement regulation is responsible for complement-mediated TMA (CM-TMA). CM HUS is a hereditary deficiency of regulatory proteins that normally regulate alternate pathways of complement (complement factor H CHF) or hereditary abnormality of proteins that accelerate the activation of the pathway (CFB, C3), leading to uncontrolled excessive activation of complement activity on vascular endothelium and kidney cells. Endothelial cells express receptors for complement and are susceptible to complement attack and injury. Renal cells are sensitive to complement activation, explaining the predominance of acute kidney injury. A deficiency of complement factor H (CFH) or complement factor I (CFI) can also be acquired, caused by an autoantibody that inhibits CFH or CFI activity [18, 19].

CM HUS is the inherited pathogenic variants in complement genes or acquired autoantibodies against certain complement proteins. Complement-mediated Thrombotic Microangiopathy (CM-TMA), which affects individuals, is caused by complement dysregulation. Autoantibodies to factors in the alternative complement pathway and heterozygosity for a pathogenic mutation in a gene encoding one of these components can be observed in patients with this condition [20, 21].

Clinical presents as a triad of MAHA with thrombocytopenia and renal end-organ impairment. Symptoms may vary from headache or thrombocytopenia before overt clinical presentation. Commonly present during the postpartum period. Hematological screening is requested. Unfortunately, there is no single specific test for diagnosis.

The probability of complement-mediated TMA requires the exclusion of other causes of MAHA and thrombocytopenia associated with severe acute kidney injury.

The diagnostic role of testing for complement dysregulation by measuring complement proteins (e.g., C3 and C4, CH50), antibodies to complement proteins, or complement gene mutations may be helpful markers, but not specific nor sensitive. Decreased levels of complement factors or the presence of anti-complement factor H (CFH) antibodies may help suggest a complement-mediated TMA; however, normal complement levels do not eliminate the possibility of a complement-mediated TMA.

14 Management

Management with monoclonal antibody blocks activated terminal complement pathway in the majority of cases, the optimal duration of treatment may be judged clinically after full recovery or complete remission, overweighing the risk of relapse versus the risk of long-term immunosuppression.

Literature is limited, comprising cohorts and retrospective case series. Its empirical use in patients with advanced renal failure may prevent end-stage kidney disease and reverse acute kidney injury.

15 Pregnancy as a Trigger

Pregnancy accounts for 21% of cases in the female population in the French registry.

Normal pregnancy protects the fetus from damage by complement activation. Still, in susceptible individuals with the tendency of complement dysregulation, pregnancy could trigger acute episodes of CM HUS, having adverse effects on the fetus. Pregnancy trigger activates an inflammatory response in genetically susceptible individuals with complement pathway activation or dysregulation.

16 Management of CM HUS in Pregnancy

It is the diagnosis of exclusion and, therefore, reasonable to initiate complement inhibitor therapy as early as possible (preferably within 24–48 h) to limit preventable renal damage. Suggested data using eculizumab in paroxysmal nocturnal hemoglobinuria is safe in pregnancy and not excreted in breast milk. An increase in dose or frequency may be required in pregnancy with an increased volume of distribution and increased C5 synthesis. Monitoring the degree of complement blockade with the multi-disciplinary review is required with a special obstetric review for time and mode of delivery [22, 23].

17 Management of Pregnancy in Known CM HUS

Women diagnosed with CM HUS require periconceptional counseling about the risk of recurrence and relapse in future pregnancies and the long-term consequences of chronic kidney disease. Women who conceive while on eculizumab were counseled about the risk versus benefits of continuing or stopping complement inhibitor therapy. Various approaches have been defined late to initiation of complement therapy in early pregnancy in women with adverse obstetric history (fetal loss).

However, a wait and watch policy to start therapy with the first sign of relapse can be adopted, which is not evidence-based [24, 25]. Regular hematological and clinical monitoring with obstetric fetal growth scans and uterine artery Doppler is obligatory at a specialized center for improved maternal and fetal outcomes.

18 Acute Fatty Liver of Pregnancy (AFLP)

Acute fatty liver is a medical emergency that occurs during pregnancy and is defined by maternal liver dysfunction and/or failure that can lead to maternal and fetal complications.

It is an uncommon complication of late pregnancy or presented in the postpartum period affecting 1 in 7000 to 20,000 deliveries [26] with maternal mortality rates ranging from 5% to 20%. Increased risk of perinatal mortality rate in AFLP can range from 20% to 60%, depending on the severity of the condition, gestational age at diagnosis, and the availability of appropriate medical care.

Most fetal and neonatal deaths are secondary to maternal decompensation and/or preterm birth. Maternal acidosis is associated with reduced uterine blood flow, which can result in fetal hypoxia and, ultimately, fetal asphyxia. In LCHAD deficiency, the unoxidized fatty acids are transferred to the mother through the placenta rather than accumulating in the fetus, and thus are not a direct cause of fetal demise and are not the primary cause of fetal mortality [27].

Potential risk factors for AFLP are fetal long-chain 3-hydroxy acyl CoA dehydrogenase deficiency, multiple gestations, primigravid, prior history of AFLP, and pregnancy carrying male fetus [28].

In normal pregnancy, free fatty acids normally increase, particularly in late gestation, to fuel fetoplacental growth and development. However, abnormalities in the metabolism of fatty acids that occur during pregnancy appear to play a role. It is the unoxidized fatty acids transferred by the placenta to the mother. When maternal-fetal fatty acid metabolism is defective, intermediate products of metabolism can accumulate in maternal blood and hepatocytes, with deleterious effects on maternal hepatocytes [29].

An enzyme deficiency associated with AFLP is fetal long-chain 3-hydroxy acyl CoA dehydrogenase (LCHAD) deficiency that results in fetal fatty oxidation defects. It is the defective fatty acid metabolism during pregnancy linked to gene mutation mitochondrial beta-oxidation and fetal long-chain 3-hydroxy acyl CoA dehydrogenase (LCHAD) deficiency resulting in unmetabolized hepatotoxic long-chain fatty acid metabolites produced by the fetus or placenta are transferred to maternal circulation, the probable reason for the toxic effects and maternal hepatic dysfunction.

Initially it may present with nonspecific nausea and vomiting, anorexia, and right quadrant pain, blurring the diagnosis, and has the potential to progress for coagulation impairment, jaundice, hypoglycemia, encephalopathy, and hepatic failure. A presumptive diagnosis of AFLP is usually clinically based on nonspecific symptoms (nausea, vomiting, abdominal pain, malaise, and/or anorexia) in a pregnant woman

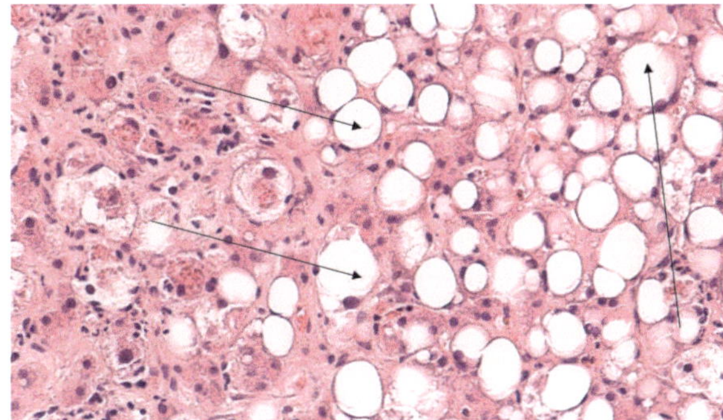

Fig. 7 AFLP hepatocytes [32]. There are swollen vacuolated hepatocytes containing micro vesicular fat droplets with centrally located nuclei. Uptodate

with significant hepatic dysfunction in the second half pregnancy after other potential causes of these findings have been excluded. There is a large clinical overlap between AFLP, HELLP syndrome, and severe preeclampsia with severe features, adding to the complexity of diagnosis, and it is sometimes difficult to differentiate between them [30, 31].

Apparent hematological findings include low platelet count, prolonged PT and low fibrinogen levels, low antithrombin levels, and associated coagulopathy due to reduced blood clotting factors by the liver than consumption. Impending signs of liver failure are associated with significantly raised aminotransferase levels in the liver, 5–10 times the upper limit of normal. Elevated hepatic functions are associated with full blood count, liver function test, renal function, coagulation profile, and cross-matched blood are advocated for diagnosis. Multi-organ involvement, especially concurrent renal failure, strengthens the diagnosis of AFLP [32].

Diagnostic imaging and ultrasound have limitations due to low sensitivity and specificity. When the diagnosis is opaque, a liver biopsy is the gold standard if coagulopathy status permits (Fig. 7).

The common cause of maternal death is hemorrhage and sepsis, and hepatorenal syndrome.

In addition, non-pregnancy-related causes of abnormal liver chemistries need to be assessed, such as hepatitis (i.e., hepatitis B virus, herpes simplex virus, hepatitis E virus, autoimmune), gallstone disease, Budd-Chiari syndrome, and acetaminophen or other drug-induced liver injuries.

19 Management

Multi-disciplinary team approach assessing multi-organ dysfunction and severity of hepatic dysfunction at specialized centers with obstetric input, hepatology experts, intensivists, and anesthesiologist improves outcomes. Intensive monitoring of the progress of the disease process with supportive care and prompt delivery of the fetus, regardless of gestational age, reduces morbidity and mortality.

A systemic approach to nourish fetoplacental growth includes early delivery, maintaining fluid balance, and controlling bleeding diathesis with fresh frozen plasma, cryoprecipitate, and platelets in critical care settings recommended. Rapid reversal of clinical condition is expected following delivery. Mothers need to be stabilized with special attention to coagulopathy and plan delivery according to the rate and degree of maternal/fetal decompensation.

Future pregnancies in women with a history of AFLP should be closely monitored and undergo genetic testing, as the risk of recurrence is high in subsequent pregnancies. They should be advised to seek early medical attention if they develop any signs or symptoms of AFLP (e.g., malaise, new onset nausea, vomiting, headache, upper abdominal pain, jaundice) in addition to routine prenatal care.

These parturients are managed by both feto-maternal specialists and its dedicated centers. Treatment is otherwise largely supportive of maternal stabilization and liver dysfunction recovery goals.

20 Conclusion

Important causes of TMA in pregnancy are TTP and CM HUS. A high index of suspicion by physicians emphasizes the need for early diagnosis and management for improved maternal and fetal outcomes. Diagnosis may be challenging due to clinical overlap. Diagnostic assay of ADAMTS13 activity <10% confirms the diagnosis of TTP. The first line of treatment is plasma infusion in congenital TTP and plasma exchange in acquired or immune-mediated TTP (Fig. 8).

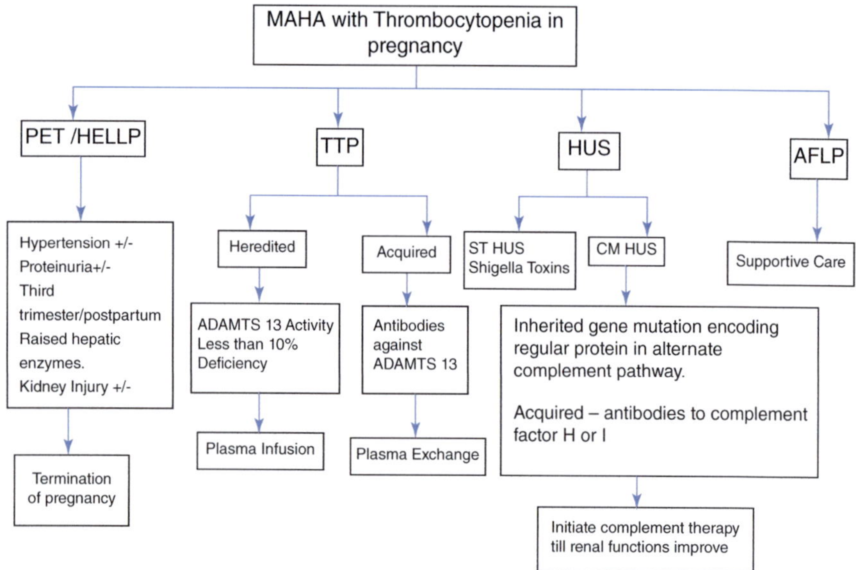

Fig. 8 Classification and management

CM HUS is a diagnosis of exclusion and early diagnosis, and prompt initiation of appropriate complement inhibition therapy prevents end-stage renal impairment and optimizes outcomes.

The risk of recurrence and relapse is high in a subsequent pregnancy in TTP and CM HUS. Timely diagnosis, monitoring, and therapy have superior maternal and fetal outcomes.

AFLP results in enzyme deficiency associated with fetal fatty acid oxidation defects. Unmetabolized long-chain fatty acids produced by the fetus or placenta are toxic to the maternal liver when it enters maternal circulation. Maternal acidosis reduces uteroplacental perfusion and may affect fetal well-being. Predicting the risk process for future pregnancy is difficult; however, genetic counseling of the newborn and parents is offered. Early diagnosis, prompt therapy, and critical care maximizes a good outcome.

References

1. Thomas MR, Robinson S, Scully MA. How we manage thrombotic microangiopathies in pregnancy. Br J Haematol. 2016;173(6):821–30.
2. Audibert F, Friedman SA, Frangieh AY, Sibai BM. Clinical utility of strict diagnostic criteria for the HELLP (hemolysis, elevated liver enzymes, and low platelets) syndrome. Am J Obstet Gynecol. 1996;175:460.
3. Ditisheim A, Sibai BM. Diagnosis and management of HELLP syndrome complicated by liver hematoma. Clin Obstet Gynecol. 2017;60:190.
4. Martin JN Jr, Rose CH, Briery CM. Understanding and managing HELLP syndrome: the integral role of aggressive glucocorticoids for mother and child. Am J Obstet Gynecol. 2006;195:914.
5. Martin JN Jr, Rinehart BK, May WL, et al. The spectrum of severe preeclampsia: comparative analysis by HELLP (hemolysis, elevated liver enzyme levels, and low platelet count) syndrome classification. Am J Obstet Gynecol. 1999;180:1373.
6. Catanzarite VA, Steinberg SM, Mosley CA, et al. Severe preeclampsia with fulminant and extreme elevation of aspartate aminotransferase and lactate dehydrogenase levels: high risk for maternal death. Am J Perinatol. 1995;12:310.
7. Furlan M, Robles R, Solenthaler M, Wassmer M, Sandoz P, Lammle B. Deficient activity of von Willebrand factor–cleaving protease in chronic relapsing thrombotic thrombocytopenic purpura. Blood. 1997;89:3097–103.
8. Tsai HM, Lian EC. Antibodies to von Willebrand factor–cleaving protease in acute thrombotic thrombocytopenic purpura. N Engl J Med. 1998;339:1585–94.
9. Mannucci PM, Canciani MT, Forza I, Lussana F, Lattuada A, Rossi E. Changes in health and disease of the metalloprotease that cleaves von Willebrand factor. Blood. 2001;98:2730–5.
10. Sanchez-Luceros A, Farias CE, Amaral MM, Kempfer AC, Votta R, Marchese C, et al. von Willebrand factor–cleaving protease (ADAMTS13) activity in normal non-pregnant women, pregnant and post-delivery women. Thromb Haemost. 2004;92:1320–6.
11. Jamme M, Rondeau E. The PLASMIC score for thrombotic thrombocytopenic purpura. Lancet Haematol. 2017;4:e148.
12. Routh JK, Koenig SC. Severe vitamin B12 deficiency mimicking thrombotic thrombocytopenic purpura. Blood. 2014;124:1844.
13. Noël N, Maigné G, Tertian G, et al. Hemolysis and schistocytosis in the emergency department: consider pseudothrombotic microangiopathy related to vitamin B12 deficiency. QJM. 2013;106:1017.

14. Scully M, Yarranton H, Liesner R, Cavenagh J, Hunt B, Benjamin S, et al. Regional UK TTP registry: correlation with laboratory ADAMTS 13 analysis and clinical features. Br J Haematol. 2008;142:819–26.
15. Fujimura Y, Matsumoto M, Kokame K, Isonishi A, Soejima K, Akiyama N, et al. Pregnancy-induced thrombocytopenia and TTP, and the risk of fetal death, in Upshaw-Schulman syndrome: a series of 15 pregnancies in 9 genotyped patients. Br J Haematol. 2009;144:742–54.
16. Noris M, Remuzzi G. Atypical hemolytic-uremic syndrome. N Engl J Med. 2009;361:1676–87.
17. Berger BE. The alternative pathway of complement and the evolving clinical-pathophysiological spectrum of atypical hemolytic uremic syndrome. Am J Med Sci. 2016;352:177–90.
18. Jokiranta TS. HUS and atypical HUS. Blood. 2017;129:2847–56.
19. Bresin E, Rurali E, Caprioli J, Sanchez-Corral P, Fremeaux-Bacchi V, Rodriguez de Cordoba S, et al. Combined complement gene mutations in atypical hemolytic uremic syndrome influence clinical phenotype. J Am Soc Nephrol. 2013;24:475–86.
20. Dragon-Durey MA, Loirat C, Cloarec S, Macher MA, Blouin J, Nivet H, et al. Anti-factor H autoantibodies associated with atypical hemolytic uremic syndrome. J Am Soc Nephrol. 2005;16:555–63.
21. Noris M, Caprioli J, Bresin E, Mossali C, Pianetti G, Gamba S, et al. Relative role of genetic complement abnormalities in sporadic and familial aHUS and their impact on clinical phenotype. Clin J Am Soc Nephrol. 2010;5:1844–59.
22. Gruppo RA, Rother RP. Eculizumab for congenital atypical hemolytic-uremic syndrome. N Engl J Med. 2009;360:544–6.
23. Legendre CM, Licht C, Muus P, Greenbaum LA, Babu S, Bedrosian C, et al. Terminal complement inhibitor eculizumab in atypical hemolytic-uremic syndrome. N Engl J Med. 2013;368:2169–81.
24. Walle JV, Delmas Y, Ardissino G, Wang J, Kincaid JF, Haller H. Improved renal recovery in patients with atypical hemolytic uremic syndrome following rapid initiation of eculizumab treatment. J Nephrol. 2017;30:127–34.
25. Macia M, de Alvaro Moreno F, Dutt T, Fehrman I, Hadaya K, Gasteyger C, et al. Current evidence on the discontinuation of eculizumab in patients with atypical haemolytic uraemic syndrome. Clin Kidney J. 2017;10:310–9.
26. Tran TT, Ahn J, Reau NS. ACG clinical guideline: liver disease and pregnancy. Am J Gastroenterol. 2016;111:176.
27. Nelson DB, Yost NP, Cunningham FG. Acute fatty liver of pregnancy: clinical outcomes and expected duration of recovery. Am J Obstet Gynecol. 2013;209:456.e1.
28. Joueidi Y, Peoc'h K, Le Lous M, et al. Maternal and neonatal outcomes and prognostic factors in acute fatty liver of pregnancy. Eur J Obstet Gynecol Reprod Biol. 2020;252:198.
29. Browning MF, Levy HL, Wilkins-Haug LE, et al. Fetal fatty acid oxidation defects and maternal liver disease in pregnancy. Obstet Gynecol. 2006;107:115.
30. Vigil-De Gracia P. Acute fatty liver and HELLP syndrome: two distinct pregnancy disorders. Int J Gynaecol Obstet. 2001;73:215.
31. Casey LC, Fontana RJ, Aday A, et al. Acute liver failure (ALF) in pregnancy: how much is pregnancy related? Hepatology. 2020;72:1366.
32. Lie G, Eleti S, Chan D, et al. Imaging the acute abdomen in pregnancy: a radiological decision-making tool and the role of MRI. Clin Radiol. 2022;77:639.

Sepsis and Septic Shock in the Peripartum Period

Adnan A. Saadeddin, Umm E Amara, Umme Nashrah, Bothina Ali AlMulla, Firdos Ummunnisa, and Nissar Shaikh

Abstract Maternal sepsis is a life-threatening condition that can develop during pregnancy, delivery, or the postpartum period. It is one of the most significant causes of maternal mortality worldwide and is the third most common cause of maternal death, accounting for 10.7% of all maternal deaths. It is characterized by an abnormal inflammatory response to a pathogen that can result in the excessive release of cytokines and mediators leading to many pathophysiological changes that ultimately cause septic shock. Early identification and treatment of sepsis are essential to prevent maternal and fetal morbidity and mortality. The initial management involves rapid activation of a sepsis rapid response team, stabilization of the patient, and history-taking and physical examination. Laboratory investigations aid in evaluating alternative diagnoses and identifying organ dysfunctions. Antibiotic therapy should be initiated as soon as possible and adjusted accordingly based on culture results. Common antibiotic regimens for maternal sepsis based on the suspected etiology are also discussed. This chapter provides an overview of epidemiology, etiology, pathophysiology, and the management of peripartum sepsis.

Keywords Sepsis · Septic shock · Maternal sepsis · Peripartum sepsis · Obstetric emergency · Surviving Sepsis Campaign · Lactate level · Blood cultures · Antibiotics · Vasopressors · Chorioamnionitis · Endometritis · Hypotension · Organ dysfunction

---

A. A. Saadeddin · N. Shaikh (✉)
Surgical Intensive Care/Hamad Medical Corporation, Doha, Qatar
e-mail: smaheboob@hamad.qa

U. E Amara
Apollo Institute of Medical Sciences and Research, Hyderabad, India

U. Nashrah
Deccan College of Medical Sciences, Hyderabad, India

B. A. AlMulla
Women's Wellness and Research Center, Hamad Medical Corporation, Doha, Qatar

F. Ummunnisa
Dr. Halima Al Tamimi, Obstetrics and Gynecology Centre, Doha, Qatar

N. Shaikh et al. (eds.), *Updates in Intensive Care of OBGY Patients*,
https://doi.org/10.1007/978-981-99-9577-6_3

1 Introduction

Peripartum infection is defined by the World Health Organization (WHO) as a bacterial infection of the genital tract or its surrounding tissues occurring at any time between the onset of rupture of membranes or labor and up to 42nd day postpartum in which two or more of the following are present: pelvic pain thrombosis (septic), fever, abnormal vaginal discharge (foul odor discharge), or delay in uterine involution [1].

In this chapter, we will discuss epidemiology, risk factors, etiology, pathophysiology, and management of peripartum sepsis.

2 Epidemiology

According to the World Health Organization (WHO), the incidence of peripartum sepsis alone in live births is 4.4%, equating to 5.7 million cases per year. This burden is greater in low- and middle-income countries compared to high-income countries [2]. Sepsis is one of the most significant causes of maternal mortality worldwide and is the third most common cause of maternal death, accounting for 10.7% of all maternal deaths [3]. However, due to advancements in diagnosis and management, maternal deaths due to sepsis have decreased.

A new study has shown that maternal sepsis has declined globally over the last three decades. The study found that after accounting for population growth and aging, the number of cases of maternal sepsis and infection decreased, with the highest burden of the disease found in low and low-middle human development index areas. The study's authors suggest that the economic level, education level, and health worker awareness are all factors in the incidence of maternal sepsis and recommend more investment, better access to prophylactic antibiotics and innovation in early diagnosis and targeted management [4].

A Group A Streptococcus infection can cause streptococcal septic shock syndrome during the peripartum period, which can be fatal. Sepsis from group A streptococcus can lead to high maternal mortality rates, ranging from 40% to 60% in developed nations [5].

3 Risk Factors

Several risk factors have been identified that increase the likelihood of developing peripartum sepsis. A population-based study in the United States found that smoking is a risk factor for peripartum sepsis. Additionally, an association was found between maternal sepsis and diabetes mellitus, cardiovascular disease, eclampsia, preterm birth, hysterectomy, puerperal infection, postpartum hemorrhage, blood transfusion, and chorioamnionitis [6]. Another study in the United States found that certain conditions also increase the risk of severe sepsis, such as congestive heart failure, chronic liver disease, chronic renal disease, systemic lupus erythematous, and rescue cerclage placement [7]. In a UK national case-control study, researchers found that women who were Black, Asian, Hispanic, had only high school education or lower, had public/no-insurance, had a cesarean section, delivered in hospitals with fewer than 1000 births per year, were primiparous, had multiple birth, diabetes, or chronic hypertension had significantly increased odds of progressing to sepsis. Preeclampsia and postpartum hemorrhage were also found to be significantly associated with progression to sepsis. For every risk factor, the risk of uncomplicated sepsis increased by 25% and the risk of progression to septic shock increased by 57% [8]. The use of artificial reproduction techniques also appears to increase the risk of developing sepsis [9].

The risk factors for maternal death from sepsis differ between developed and developing countries and are summarized in Tables 1 and 2 [10].

The incidence of postpartum infection is five times higher in women who underwent cesarean section (CS) compared to those who underwent vaginal birth. Wound infection at the surgical site is the most frequently encountered form of CS-related postpartum infection, while urinary tract infection can also be a potential source. It

Table 1 Risk factors for maternal death from sepsis identified in developed countries

Emergency caesarian section
Prolonged rupture of membrane
Retained products of conception
Premature labor
History of pelvic or other infection
Interventions, e.g., cerclage, multiple vaginal examinations
Low income
Obesity
Diabetes
Anemia
Recent sore throat or upper respiratory tract infection in family
Winter months
Migrants from developing countries

Table 2 Risk factors for maternal death from sepsis identified in developing countries

Poverty
Young age
First pregnancy
Anemia
Home delivery without trained birth assistant
Specified traditional birth assistant practices
Failure to recognize severity
Distance from healthcare facilities
Lack of medical resources

should be noted that the risk of postpartum infection is higher in cases of emergency CS compared to elective CS [11].

Chorioamnionitis is an inflammation of the fetal membranes and amniotic fluid and can result from prolonged rupture of membranes. Other factors that increase the risk of intra-amniotic infection include a young maternal age, prolonged labor, nulliparity, multiple vaginal examinations, meconium-stained amniotic fluid, internal monitoring, group B streptococcus colonization, and bacterial vaginosis. This type of infection is often polymicrobial in nature and results from an ascending infection from the lower genital tract [9, 12].

4 Etiology

Table 3 lists the common causes of peripartum sepsis. Identifying the cause of maternal sepsis helps guide the management and control and source of infection. Table 4 lists the microbial organisms involved in maternal sepsis.

Chorioamnionitis, also known as intra-amniotic infection, is a condition characterized by an acute inflammatory response in the chorion, amnion, and placenta. The presence of risk factors such as young maternal age, prolonged labor, nulliparity, prolonged rupture of membranes, frequent vaginal exams, meconium-stained amniotic fluid, internal monitoring, group B streptococcus colonization, and bacterial vaginosis can increase the likelihood of chorioamnionitis [12].

Endometritis is a condition characterized by the inflammation of the endometrial lining, myometrium, and parametrium due to bacterial infection. The mode of delivery

Table 3 Bacterial infections associated with septic shock in the obstetric patient [13]

Obstetric
Chorioamnionitis
Postpartum endometritis (more common after cesarean section)
Septic abortion
Septic pelvic thrombophlebitis
Cesarean wound infection
Episiotomy infections
Nonobstetric
Appendicitis
Cholecystitis urinary tract infections
Pyelonephritis (perinephric abscess, renal calculi)
Pneumonia
HIV
Malaria
Invasive procedures
Necrotizing fasciitis
Infected cerclage
Postchorionic villus sampling/amniocentesis (septic abortion)
Miscellaneous
Toxic shock syndrome

Table 4 Organisms involved with maternal sepsis [12]

Gram-positive cocci	**Gram-negative rods**
Pneumococcus	*Escherichia coli*
Streptococcus A and B	*Haemophilus influenza*
Enterococcus faecalis	*Klebsiella*
Staphylococcus aureus	*Enterobacter* spp.
	Proteus spp.
Gram-positive rods	*Pseudomonas* spp.
Listeria monocytogenes	*Serratia* spp.
Anaerobes	**Miscellaneous**
Bacteroides spp.	Fungal species
Prevotella	**Viral organisms**
Clostridium perfringens	Herpes and varicella
Fusobacterium spp.	HIV
Peptococcus	Influenza A and B
Peptostreptococcus	

is the most significant risk factor, with other factors such as labor and ruptured membranes also contributing to its onset. The infection is believed to arise from the ascent of bacteria from the lower genital tract during the labor process, which then colonizes the decidua and amniotic fluid. However, clinical manifestation of the infection is not observed until after delivery. The causative agents of endometritis are typically polymicrobial in nature and consist of a mixture of anaerobic and aerobic bacteria.

Pregnancy is associated with a higher incidence of acute pyelonephritis which may lead to sepsis and septic shock. This is due to the relative obstruction of the urinary tract caused by changes in pregnancy physiology such as dilation of the ureters, decreased protective peristalsis, and mechanical compression of the urinary system by the uterus.

Surgical Site Infections (SSIs) are prevalent sources of infections and can be categorized into superficial or deep based on the extent of involvement of the abdominal wall. The use of prophylactic antibiotics prior to cesarean deliveries has diminished the incidence of postoperative infections, however, wound morbidity remains a significant issue, with an SSI rate of 2–6% after cesarean sections.

5 Pathophysiology

The pathophysiology of sepsis is yet to be fully understood. The host response to pathogens is a complex variable process [14]. The host's inflammatory response is a regulated balance of pro-inflammatory and anti-inflammatory mechanisms, which allows for the elimination of pathogens while minimizing potential harm to the host. When the pro-inflammatory response is exaggerated, this balance is threatened and an abnormal inflammatory response may occur, resulting in sepsis [15, 16].

It is still not clear why local inflammatory processes may lead to a generalized response leading to sepsis. Response to infection can vary greatly due to a combination of factors including genetics and environment, age and sex, comorbidities, nutrition, medication use, and the pathogen load and virulence [16]. Genetic factors play a crucial role in the susceptibility and outcome of infections [17, 18].

The dysregulated inflammatory response leads to a systemic release of cytokines, mediators, and pathogen-related molecules, resulting in activation of coagulation and complement cascades. This leads to the initiation of disseminated microvascular thrombosis and consumption of clotting factors, which is a characteristic of disseminated intravascular coagulation (DIC) [19].

6 Systemic Effects of Sepsis

Septic cardiomyopathy is a condition characterized by ventricular dysfunction and arrhythmias during sepsis. The pathogenesis of septic cardiomyopathy is thought to involve a complex interplay of endothelial, metabolic, and immune response abnormalities [20].

Lung injury can occur due to increased permeability of alveolar and capillary endothelium caused by cytokine-mediated mechanisms and leads to noncardiogenic pulmonary edema which impairs oxygenation and ventilation.

Sepsis-related acute kidney injury is characterized by several pathophysiological changes including changes in hemodynamics, endothelial dysfunction, inflammation of the renal parenchyma, and obstruction of tubules with necrotic cells and debris.

Hematological manifestations of sepsis can include anemia, leukocytosis, neutropenia, thrombocytopenia, and disseminated intravascular coagulation (DIC). Thrombocytopenia is caused by inhibition of thrombopoiesis and immunologic platelet damage, while anemia is secondary to inflammation, shortened red blood cell survival, and hemolysis in the setting of DIC. Liver failure can occur due to hemodynamic, cellular, molecular, and immunologic changes leading to parenchymal hypoxia. Hyperglycemia is also common in septic patients and is believed to be caused by stress-induced elevation of hormones and cytokines, which results in combined insulin resistance [21].

Sepsis-associated encephalopathy occurs as a result of metabolic changes and disruptions in cellular signaling pathways that lead to blood–brain barrier dysfunction, which subsequently increases leukocyte infiltration, exposure to toxic substances, and cytokines transport into the brain parenchyma [22].

7 Management

7.1 Diagnostic Challenge

Early recognition and prompt treatment are crucial for reducing maternal morbidity and mortality. However, the symptoms of peripartum sepsis can be non-specific and may mimic other obstetric conditions, making it challenging to diagnose. It is important for healthcare providers to have a high index of suspicion and consider all relevant clinical and laboratory information when evaluating a patient for peripartum sepsis.

Furthermore, the unique physiological adaptations of pregnancy can result in a more subtle presentation of sepsis. Pregnancy is characterized by hyperdynamic circulation, marked by an increase in blood volume, which can result in decreased blood pressure and an increase in heart rate. Tachypnea, a common symptom of sepsis, can be mistaken for the physiological tachypnea that occurs during pregnancy. These similarities can lead to confusion when utilizing sepsis criteria systems qSOFA for diagnosis [23]. Altered mentation is rare in pregnant women, even in the setting of severe disease, and can be considered a more specific sign of end-organ injury and sepsis in the presence of infection.

7.2 Early Recognition

Timely recognition of peripartum sepsis is essential in preventing further deterioration and possible death. Regular recording of vital signs, such as temperature, pulse rate, blood pressure, and respiratory rate, should be done, and should be repeated at an appropriate frequency to detect trends in the hemodynamic status of the patient.

Sepsis should be considered in any patient suspected to have an infection who develops evidence of end-organ dysfunction including confusion, hypoxia, hypotension, coagulopathy, oliguria, ileus, hyperglycemia, and elevation in liver function tests. Serial bedside evaluation is desirable to detect trends in vital signs and clinical status and to more rapidly assess and reassess for signs of sepsis. Once suspected, cultures should be obtained, and antibiotics started within 1 h. Initial fluid resuscitation and administration of broad-spectrum antibiotics should not be delayed.

Sequential (Sepsis-related) Organ Failure Assessment (SOFA) score is used to identify the presence of organ dysfunction (Table 5). However, SOFA score utility in early identification of sepsis is limited.

Using early warning systems to survey patients for possible sepsis is intuitive. The latest update in Surviving Sepsis campaign guidelines does not recommend

Table 5 Clinically relevant criteria to identify high-risk peripartum patients in sepsis

Body temperature	<35 or >38 °C
Systolic blood pressure	<90 or >160 mmHg
Diastolic blood pressure	<45 or >100 mmHg
Heart rate	<50 or >120 beats/min
Respiratory rate	<10 or >30 breaths/min
Oxygen saturation (SpO_2) on room air	<95%
Alterations in consciousness	Agitation, or confusion
Urine output	<35 mL

using SIRS or qSOFA scores for screening for sepsis. In the context of peripartum sepsis, the utility of these scores is further compromised for the reasons mentioned previously [19]. Although there are many early warning systems used in peripartum women in different countries and centers around the world, there is no widely accepted screening tool that consistently facilitates rapid diagnosis of sepsis in pregnancy. Some of these systems including the modified early obstetric warning score (MEOWS), maternal early recognition criteria (MERC), maternity SIRS (mSIRS), maternal early warning system (MEWS), SOS (Sepsis in Obstetrics Score), omqSOFA (obstetric modified quick SOFA), and maternal early warning trigger (MEWT) [24–27].

However, most of these systems are designed mainly to identify patients who are at high risk, utilizing a limited number of clinically relevant criteria. These criteria include [28]:

Recently, the Targeted Real-Time Early Warning System (TREWS), an artificial intelligence screening tool, has been evaluated as a potential bedside tool for early recognition of sepsis. Studies found that this tool may reduce mortality by 3.3% [29, 30]. However, its utility is limited by the low specificity. Additionally, this tool has not been evaluated in the context of peripartum sepsis.

7.3 *Initial Investigations*

Obtaining microbiologic cultures (e.g., blood, urine, sputum, indwelling lines, expected sites/source of infection) before starting antibiotics is strongly encouraged as long as it does not result in a significant delay in initiation of antibiotic therapy [31, 32]. SOFA and qSOFA scores will help in knowing organ dysfunction Tables 6 and 7, respectively, serum lactate is part of Hour-1 Surviving Sepsis Campaign Bundle of Care Table 8 and should be measured in the first hour of suspecting sepsis. Although serum lactate alone doesn't rule in or out the diagnosis of sepsis, the likelihood of sepsis is increased with elevated lactate levels and decreased with normal lactate levels. Additionally, lactate can be used to follow the resuscitative efforts. Other markers that can be used include procalcitonin and C-Reactive Protein (CRP) and recleaning imaging studies.

Table 6 Sequential [sepsis-related] organ failure assessment score

	Score				
System	0	1	2	3	4
Respiration					
PaO_2/FiO_2, mmHg	≥400	<400	<300	<200 with respiratory support	<100 with respiratory support
Coagulation					
Platelets, $\times 10^3/\mu L$	≥150	<150	<100	<50	<20
Liver					
Bilirubin, mg/dL	<1.2	1.2–1.9	2.0–5.9	6.0–11.9	>12.0
Cardiovascular	MAP ≥70 mmHg	MAP <70 mmHg	Dopamine <5 or dobutamine (any dose)[a]	Dopamine 5.1–15 or epinephrine ≤0.1 or norepinephrine ≤0.1[a]	Dopamine >15 or epinephrine >0.1 or norepinephrine >0.1
Central nervous system					
Glasgow coma scale	15	13–14	10–12	6–9	<6
Renal					
Creatinine, mg/dL	<1.2	1.2–1.9	2.0–3.4	3.5–4.9	>5.0
Urine output, mL/day				<500	<200

Table 7 qSOFA (quick SOFA) criteria

Respiratory rate ≥22/min
Altered mentation
Systolic blood pressure ≥100 mmHg

Table 8 Maternal early warning criteria [33]

Systolic BP (mmHg)	<90 or >160
Diastolic BP (mmHg)	>100 mmHg
Heart rate (beats/min)	<50 or >120
Respiratory rate (breaths/min)	<10 or >30
Oxygen saturation on room air, at sea level, %	<95
Oliguria, mL/h for 2 h	<35

Maternal agitation, confusion, or unresponsiveness
Patient with preeclampsia reporting a non-remitting headache or shortness of breath
BP blood pressure

7.4 Initial Management

The implementation of a standardized pathway for the activation of a sepsis rapid response team, coupled with timely arrival at the bedside of the patient, can enhance the appropriate treatment and resource utilization in cases of maternal deterioration.

Peripartum sepsis should be considered an obstetric emergency. Timely management of sepsis is essential to improve patient outcomes. Surviving Sepsis Campaign (SSC) guidelines are intended to provide guidance for the clinician caring for adult patients with sepsis or septic shock in the hospital setting [31].

Stabilization should be prioritized according to the ABCDE. Once stabilized, history-taking and physical examinations should be performed [34].

During maternal resuscitation, a paramount consideration should be given to the fetus. To achieve optimal fetal blood flow, the patient should be positioned in the left decubitus position to alleviate aortocaval compression. The objective of the therapeutic intervention is to preserve the oxygenation and circulation of vital organs, including the placenta, and to detect and address any potential infection. Oxygen supplementation should be administered to attain a saturation level of at least 94% [35].

Studies have shown that initiating antimicrobial therapy within the first hour of sepsis identification significantly decreases mortality, with an increase in mortality by 7.6% with each hour delay in initiating antimicrobial therapy [32]. In line with this, the SSC guidelines strongly recommend administering antimicrobials within 1 h for all patients suspected to have sepsis and have signs of shock, and immediately if sepsis is highly likely Table 9.

Other laboratory investigations include complete blood count, electrolytes, coagulation profile, and renal and liver function tests. These investigations aid evaluating for alternative diagnoses, identify organ dysfunctions, and prompt additional management.

When choosing an initial antibiotic, it is crucial to consider the likely source of infection, patient characteristics, and local guidelines. The initial choice should be wide spectrum, and once culture results are available, the antibiotic can be adjusted

Table 9 Hour-1 surviving sepsis campaign bundle of care [36]

Measure lactate level. Remeasure if initial lactate is >2 mmol/L
Obtain blood cultures prior to administration of antibiotics
Administer broad-spectrum antibiotics
Begin rapid administration of 30 mL/kg crystalloid for hypotension or lactate 24 mmol/L
Apply vasopressors if patient is hypotensive during or after fluid resuscitation to maintain MAP ≥65 mmHg

accordingly. The involvement of an infectious disease specialist may help adjusting the antibiotic regimen [37, 38].

In cases where sepsis is suspected but without shock, a rapid assessment should be conducted to determine within 3 h whether antibiotics should be administered. The duration of antimicrobial treatment typically ranges from 7 to 10 days. The common antibiotic regimens for maternal sepsis are listed in Table 10 by etiology [34].

ICU admission—Patients should be admitted to the intensive care unit (ICU)/HDU as early as possible depending upon clinical condition. Delayed admissions

Table 10 Common antibiotic regimens for maternal sepsis by suspected etiology

Suspected source	Initial antibiotic selection	Alternative antibiotic selection
Chorioamnionitis	Ampicillin 2 g IV every 6 h Plus gentamicin 1.5 mg/kg IV, then 1 mg/kg IV every 8 h Plus clindamycin 900 mg IV every 8 h or metronidazole (if cesarean delivery is anticipated)	Vancomycin 15 mg/kg IV, then dose by pharmacy Plus piperacillin-tazobactam 4.5 g IV every 6 h
Endometritis, endomyometritis	Gentamicin 1.5 mg/kg IV, then 1 mg/kg IV every 8 h Plus clindamycin 900 mg IV every 8 h or metronidazole (if cesarean delivery is performed)	Ceftriaxone 1–2 g IV daily Plus metronidazole 500 mg IV every 8 h
UTI	Ampicillin 2 g IV every 6 h Plus gentamicin 1.5 mg/kg IV, then 1 mg/kg IV every 8 h	Ceftriaxone 1–2 g IV daily or piperacillin-tazobactam 4.5 g IV every 6 h ± Gentamicin 1.5 mg/kg IV, then 1 mg/kg IV every 8 h
Intra-abdominal abscess, abdominal infections	Single agent: piperacillin/tazobactam 4.5 g IV every 6 h Combined agents: ceftriaxone plus metronidazole or clindamycin	Carbapenem 1 g IV or IM single daily dose
Appendicitis	Cefoxitin 2 g IV every 6–8 h Plus, clindamycin 900 mg IV every 8 h	Cefoxitin 2 g IV every 6–8 h Plus metronidazole 500 mg IV every 8 h
Skin and soft tissue infection	Vancomycin 15 mg/kg IV, then dose by pharmacy Plus, piperacillin/tazobactam 4.5 g IV every 6 h If group A streptococcus (or *Clostridium perfringens*): penicillin G 2–3 million units/day IM or IV given in divided doses every 4–6 h Plus clindamycin 900 mg IV every 8 h or vancomycin 15 mg/kg IV, then dose by pharmacy	Cefotaxime 2 g IV every 6 h Plus metronidazole 500 mg IV every 6 h

from the emergency department to the ICU can lead to decreased compliance with sepsis bundles and increased mortality, ventilator duration, and length of stay in the ICU and hospital [39]. However, timely transfer to an ICU may not always be possible, particularly in limited resources centers where ICU bed availability can be limited. In this case, regular assessment, evaluation, and appropriate treatment should not be delayed, independent of patient location.

Fluids—SSC Guidelines recommend initiating appropriate resuscitation within 3 h of recognizing sepsis or septic shock with a minimum of 30 mL/kg of IV crystalloids in initial fluid resuscitation [40].

Fluid administration beyond the initial resuscitation should be guided by careful assessment of intravascular volume status and organ perfusion, and dynamic measures have been shown to be more accurate at predicting fluid responsiveness than static techniques. Dynamic measures include passive leg raising combined with cardiac output (CO) measurement, fluid challenges against stroke volume (SV), systolic pressure or pulse pressure, and increases of SV in response to changes in intrathoracic pressure. Alternative measures such as temperature of the extremities, skin mottling and capillary refill time (CRT) can be used to evaluate the effectiveness and safety of volume administration when advanced hemodynamic monitoring is not available. These measures have been validated and shown to be reliable indicators of tissue perfusion [31].

Blood pressure should be monitored by invasive means (arterial line) because non-invasive cuff methods can be inaccurate, particularly in shock states. Vasopressors should ideally be administered through central venous access due to concerns of extravasation, but this can be time consuming and may not be available in under-resourced settings. Because of the increased mortality associated with delaying vasopressors in patients with septic shock, administration of vasopressors should not be delayed if central venous access is not available, and a peripheral administration can be started until the central venous access is established [41].

Target MAP—The initial mean arterial pressure target should be 65 mmHg [42].

Hemodynamic management—In cases fluid resuscitation is not enough to maintain a mean arterial pressure at 65 mmHg or higher, the initiation of vasopressor therapy is recommended. The Surviving Sepsis Campaign (SSC) advocates for using norepinephrine as the initial vasopressor agent of choice. If the mean arterial pressure remains uncontrolled, the addition of vasopressin should be considered [32, 34, 43].

IV steroids—The role of IV steroids in sepsis is controversial. A recent meta-analysis showed that in adult patients diagnosed with septic shock and treated with low doses of corticosteroids, there was no significant effect on both short-term and long-term mortality [44]. The Surviving Sepsis Campaign issued a weak recommendation to administer intravenous corticosteroids in patients requiring vasopressors. The commonly used corticosteroid is hydrocortisone, which is administered in a dose of 50 mg IV every 6 h, when the patient is receiving norepinephrine at a rate of $\geq$0.25 mcg/kg/min for a minimum of 4 h [31].

8 Prevention

Providing maternity care requires the implementation of strict infection prevention and control protocols. This involves the promotion of hand hygiene and the utilization of clean and sterile products, as well as equipment. Aseptic surgical practices must also be strictly adhered to in order to minimize the risk of infection. Additionally, continuous clinical monitoring of women during labor and the postpartum period is crucial for the early detection of any signs of infection.

In the case of vaginal delivery, routine antibiotic prophylaxis is recommended for women who have experienced preterm prelabor rupture of membranes or those who have sustained third- or fourth-degree perineal tears. Antibiotic prophylaxis is also advised for women undergoing operative vaginal birth. For women undergoing elective or emergency cesarean section, routine antibiotic prophylaxis is recommended prior to skin incision. This can be achieved through the administration of a single dose of first-generation cephalosporin or penicillin. Intrapartum antibiotic administration is recommended for women who are colonized with Group B Streptococcus (GBS) in order to prevent early neonatal GBS infection. This helps to maintain the health and well-being of both the mother and her newborn [1].

9 Conclusion

Peripartum infection is a bacterial infection of the genital tract occurring between the onset of labor and 42nd day postpartum, while sepsis is a life-threatening organ dysfunction caused by a dysregulated host response to infection. The incidence of peripartum sepsis is high in low- and middle-income countries, and it is the third most common cause of maternal death.

Several risk factors have been identified that increase the likelihood of developing peripartum sepsis, including smoking, maternal sepsis, and certain conditions such as congestive heart failure, chronic liver disease, and chronic renal disease. The incidence of postpartum infection is also higher in women who underwent cesarean section, and other factors that increase the risk of intra-amniotic infection include young maternal age, prolonged labor, and group B streptococcus colonization. Poverty, lack of medical resources, and traditional birth assistant practices contribute to the development of peripartum sepsis in low-income countries.

Sepsis is caused by an abnormal inflammatory that results in "the dysregulated response leads to systemic effects such as septic cardiomyopathy, lung injury, and acute kidney injury."

Peripartum sepsis can be difficult to diagnose due to non-specific symptoms, and the unique physiological adaptations of pregnancy. Early recognition is important to prevent further deterioration, and regular recording of vital signs, obtaining microbiologic cultures, and using early warning systems are some of the ways to aid in early identification. Various screening tools have been evaluated as potential bedside tools, but their utility is limited by low specificity, and most are designed to identify patients at high risk using a limited number of clinically relevant criteria.

The timely management of sepsis is essential to improve patient outcomes, and studies have shown that initiating antimicrobial therapy within the first hour of sepsis identification significantly decreases mortality. Laboratory investigations aid in evaluation, and the initial choice of antibiotic should be wide spectrum with an adjustment made once culture results are available. The involvement of an infectious disease specialist may be beneficial. The Surviving Sepsis Campaign guidelines recommend administering antimicrobials within 1 h for all patients suspected to have sepsis and have signs of shock, and immediately if sepsis is highly likely.

References

1. WHO recommendations for prevention and treatment of maternal peripartum infections [cited 2023 Jan 28]. Available from: https://www.who.int/publications/i/item/9789241549363.
2. Greer O, Shah NM, Johnson MR. Maternal sepsis update: current management and controversies. Obstet Gynaecol. 2020;22(1):45–55.
3. Say L, Chou D, Gemmill A, Tunçalp Ö, Moller AB, Daniels J, et al. Global causes of maternal death: a WHO systematic analysis. Lancet Glob Health. 2014;2(6):e323–33.
4. Chen L, Wang Q, Gao Y, Zhang J, Cheng S, Chen H, et al. The global burden and trends of maternal sepsis and other maternal infections in 204 countries and territories from 1990 to 2019. BMC Infect Dis. 2021;21(1):1074.
5. Cortez Granados S, Batsch J, Lui A, Hessman J, Gloyeske N, Panchal A. A rare case of group a streptococcal toxic-shock syndrome in a postpartum adolescent leading to multi-organ failure. Clin Case Reports. 2020;8(5):793–7.
6. Al-Ostad G, Kezouh A, Spence AR, Abenhaim HA. Incidence and risk factors of sepsis mortality in labor, delivery and after birth: population-based study in the USA. J Obstet Gynaecol Res. 2015;41(8):1201–6.
7. Bauer ME, Bateman BT, Bauer ST, Shanks AM, Mhyre JM. Maternal sepsis mortality and morbidity during hospitalization for delivery: temporal trends and independent associations for severe sepsis. Anesth Analg. 2013;117(4):944–50.
8. Acosta CD, Knight M, Lee HC, Kurinczuk JJ, Gould JB, Lyndon A. The continuum of maternal sepsis severity: incidence and risk factors in a population-based cohort study. PLoS One. 2013;8(7):e67175.
9. Kramer HMC, Schutte JM, Zwart JJ, Schuitemaker NWE, Steegers EAP, van Roosmalen J. Maternal mortality and severe morbidity from sepsis in The Netherlands. Acta Obstet Gynecol Scand. 2009;88(6):647–53.
10. Sriskandan S. Severe peripartum sepsis. J R Coll Physicians Edinb. 2011;41(4):339–46.
11. Leth RA, Møller JK, Thomsen RW, Uldbjerg N, Nørgaard M. Risk of selected postpartum infections after cesarean section compared with vaginal birth: a five-year cohort study of 32,468 women. Acta Obstet Gynecol Scand. 2009;88(9):976–83.
12. Morgan J, Roberts S. Maternal sepsis. Obstet Gynecol Clin N Am. 2013;40(1):69–87.
13. Guinn DA, Abel DE, Tomlinson MW. Early goal directed therapy for sepsis during pregnancy. Obstet Gynecol Clin N Am. 2007;34(3):459–79, xi.
14. Cinel I, Dellinger RP. Advances in pathogenesis and management of sepsis. Curr Opin Infect Dis. 2007;20(4):345–52.
15. Arina P, Singer M. Pathophysiology of sepsis. Curr Opin Anaesthesiol. 2021;34(2):77–84.
16. Kawai T, Akira S. The role of pattern-recognition receptors in innate immunity: update on Toll-like receptors. Nat Immunol. 2010;11(5):373–84.

17. Boyd JH, Russell JA, Fjell CD. The meta-genome of sepsis: host genetics, pathogens and the acute immune response. J Innate Immun. 2014;6(3):272–83.
18. Ince C, Mayeux PR, Nguyen T, Gomez H, Kellum JA, Ospina-Tascón GA, et al. The endothelium in sepsis. Shock. 2016;45(3):259–70.
19. Jarczak D, Kluge S, Nierhaus A. Sepsis—pathophysiology and therapeutic concepts. Front Med (Lausanne). 2021;8:628302.
20. Carbone F, Liberale L, Preda A, Schindler TH, Montecucco F. Septic cardiomyopathy: from pathophysiology to the clinical setting. Cell. 2022;11(18):2833.
21. Font MD, Thyagarajan B, Khanna AK. Sepsis and septic shock—basics of diagnosis, pathophysiology and clinical decision making. Med Clin North Am. 2020;104(4):573–85.
22. Iacobone E, Bailly-Salin J, Polito A, Friedman D, Stevens RD, Sharshar T. Sepsis-associated encephalopathy and its differential diagnosis. Crit Care Med. 2009;37(10 Suppl):S331–6.
23. Ali A, Lamont RF. Recent advances in the diagnosis and management of sepsis in pregnancy. F1000Res. 2019;8:1546.
24. Shafik S, Mallick S, Fogel J, Tetrokalashvili M, Hsu CD. The utility of systemic inflammatory response syndrome (SIRS) for diagnosing sepsis in the immediate postpartum period. J Infect Public Health. 2019;12(6):799–802.
25. Abutheraa N, Grant J, Mullen AB. Sepsis scoring systems and use of the sepsis six care bundle in maternity hospitals. BMC Pregnancy Childbirth. 2021;21(1):524.
26. Blumenthal EA, Hooshvar N, McQuade M, McNulty J. A validation study of maternal early warning systems: a retrospective cohort study. Am J Perinatol. 2019;36(11):1106–14.
27. Burlinson CEG, Sirounis D, Walley KR, Chau A. Sepsis in pregnancy and the puerperium. Int J Obstet Anesth. 2018;36:96–107.
28. Friedman AM, Campbell ML, Kline CR, Wiesner S, D'Alton ME, Shields LE. Implementing obstetric early warning systems. AJP Rep. 2018;8(2):e79–84.
29. Adams R, Henry KE, Sridharan A, Soleimani H, Zhan A, Rawat N, et al. Prospective, multi-site study of patient outcomes after implementation of the TREWS machine learning-based early warning system for sepsis. Nat Med. 2022;28(7):1455–60.
30. Henry KE, Adams R, Parent C, Soleimani H, Sridharan A, Johnson L, et al. Factors driving provider adoption of the TREWS machine learning-based early warning system and its effects on sepsis treatment timing. Nat Med. 2022;28(7):1447–54.
31. Evans L, Rhodes A, Alhazzani W, Antonelli M, Coopersmith CM, French C, et al. Surviving sepsis campaign: international guidelines for management of sepsis and septic shock 2021. Intensive Care Med. 2021;47(11):1181–247.
32. Scheer CS, Fuchs C, Gründling M, Vollmer M, Bast J, Bohnert JA, et al. Impact of antibiotic administration on blood culture positivity at the beginning of sepsis: a prospective clinical cohort study. Clin Microbiol Infect. 2019;25(3):326–31.
33. Mhyre JM, D'Oria R, Hameed AB, Lappen JR, Holley SL, Hunter SK, et al. The maternal early warning criteria: a proposal from the national partnership for maternal safety. Obstet Gynecol. 2014;124(4):782–6.
34. de Assis V, Halscott T. Top 10 pearls for the recognition, evaluation, and management of maternal sepsis. Obstet Gynecol. 2021;138(2):289–304.
35. Jain V, Arora A, Jain K. Sepsis in the parturient. Indian J Crit Care Med. 2021;25(Suppl 3):S267–72.
36. The surviving sepsis campaign bundle: 2018 update [cited 2023 Feb 2]. Available from: https://pubmed.ncbi.nlm.nih.gov/29675566/.
37. Kumar A, Roberts D, Wood KE, Light B, Parrillo JE, Sharma S, et al. Duration of hypotension before initiation of effective antimicrobial therapy is the critical determinant of survival in human septic shock. Crit Care Med. 2006;34(6):1589–96.
38. Seymour CW, Gesten F, Prescott HC, Friedrich ME, Iwashyna TJ, Phillips GS, et al. Time to treatment and mortality during mandated emergency care for sepsis. N Engl J Med. 2017;376(23):2235–44.
39. Mohr NM, Wessman BT, Bassin B, Elie-Turenne MC, Ellender T, Emlet LL, et al. Boarding of critically ill patients in the emergency department. Crit Care Med. 2020;48(8):1180–7.

40. Rochwerg B, Alhazzani W, Sindi A, Heels-Ansdell D, Thabane L, Fox-Robichaud A, et al. Fluid resuscitation in sepsis: a systematic review and network meta-analysis. Ann Intern Med. 2014;161(5):347–55.
41. Loubani OM, Green RS. A systematic review of extravasation and local tissue injury from administration of vasopressors through peripheral intravenous catheters and central venous catheters. J Crit Care. 2015;30(3):653.e9–17.
42. Lamontagne F, Richards-Belle A, Thomas K, Harrison DA, Sadique MZ, Grieve RD, et al. Effect of reduced exposure to vasopressors on 90-day mortality in older critically ill patients with vasodilatory hypotension: a randomized clinical trial. JAMA. 2020;323(10):938–49.
43. Comparative haemodynamic effects of dopamine and dobutamine in septic shock [cited 2023 Jan 24]. Available from: https://pubmed.ncbi.nlm.nih.gov/500939/.
44. Rygård SL, Butler E, Granholm A, Møller MH, Cohen J, Finfer S, et al. Low-dose corticosteroids for adult patients with septic shock: a systematic review with meta-analysis and trial sequential analysis. Intensive Care Med. 2018;44(7):1003–16.

Preeclampsia: Updates in Diagnosis and Management—ICU Perspective

Hiafa Shaikh, Nada S. M. Elamin, Ebtehag Elfadil Ahmed, Shameena Ajmal, Arshad Chanda, and Nissar Shaikh

Abstract Preeclampsia is a multisystem disorder that can arise in pregnancy and result in grave consequences if not managed appropriately. Although advances in medicine have vastly helped mitigate the effects of the complications that can potentially result from the development of preeclampsia, it can still be challenging to recognize them in a timely manner and effectively manage the complications that may arise. Fetal wellbeing also must be considered in addition to maternal condition as part of management of preeclampsia and its potential sequelae. Preeclampsia can be complicated by HELLP (Hemolysis, Elevated Liver enzymes and Low Platelets) syndrome; stroke; posterior reversible encephalopathy syndrome (PRES); peripartum cardiomyopathy (PPCM); maternal morbidity; acute kidney injury (AKI); pulmonary edema; reversible cerebral vasoconstriction syndrome (RCVS) which requires intensive care therapy. This chapter details the management of preeclampsia as well as its potential complications from an intensive care perspective.

Keywords Preeclampsia · Eclampsia · Cardiovascular disease · Pregnancy · HELLP (Hemolysis, Elevated Liver enzymes and Low Platelets) syndrome · Stroke · Posterior reversible encephalopathy syndrome (PRES) · Peripartum cardiomyopathy (PPCM) · Maternal morbidity · Acute kidney injury (AKI) · Pulmonary edema · Reversible cerebral vasoconstriction syndrome (RCVS)

H. Shaikh · N. S. M. Elamin · E. E. Ahmed · S. Ajmal
Women's Wellness and Research Centre, Hamad Medical Corporation, Doha, Qatar

A. Chanda (✉) · N. Shaikh
Surgical Intensive Care, Hamad Medical Corporation, Doha, Qatar
e-mail: achanda@hamad.qa

N. Shaikh et al. (eds.), *Updates in Intensive Care of OBGY Patients*,
https://doi.org/10.1007/978-981-99-9577-6_4

1 Introduction

First descriptions of preeclampsia and eclampsia date back to 400 BC and concentrated on headaches and convulsions, characterizing central nervous system symptoms and signs [1]. Understandably, clinical findings such as proteinuria and high blood pressure (BP) were not described until the 1800s. From ancient times up until the nineteenth century, physicians focused on understanding the underlying cause of eclamptic seizures and improving treatment using a variety of measures available at the time such as bloodletting, use of opiates, warm baths, and hastening delivery. The introduction of magnesium sulfate for seizure prevention in the twentieth century was a turning point and remains the therapeutic approach that is currently recognized as standard of care [2].

Severe preeclampsia and eclampsia can present as grave and life-threatening conditions requiring intensive care (Table 1). Preeclampsia is estimated to complicate 2–8% of pregnancies globally [3]. Maternal mortality in developed countries is much lower than in developing countries; nevertheless, hypertensive disorders can attribute to around 16% of maternal deaths [4]. Hypertensive disorders contributed to almost 26% of maternal deaths in Latin America and the Caribbean, whereas in Africa and Asia this number is 9% [5]. Most of the hypertension-related maternal deaths occur intrapartum or in the immediate postpartum due to avoidable and treatable causes [6]. Preeclampsia and its complications are of increasing importance due to a number of factors contributing to its rising incidence; the United States reported an increase in the rate of preeclampsia by 25% between 1987 and 2004 [7]. Furthermore, women giving birth in 2003 were found to have a 6.7-fold increased risk of developing severe preeclampsia in comparison to women giving birth in 1980 [8].

Preeclampsia is also a significant contributor to the rising cost of healthcare; one study reported the estimated cost of preeclampsia in the United States in 2012 in the first 12 months following delivery was $2.18 billion (comprising $1.03 billion for women and $1.15 billion for infants); this cost was disproportionately borne by preterm births [9].

Recognizing preeclampsia and its associated complications in a timely manner and instituting prompt treatment through a multidisciplinary team in an ICU setting is of vital importance; this can potentially prevent complications and reduce

Table 1 Definitions of hypertensive disorders in pregnancy

Pre-existing (chronic) hypertension	Hypertension that develops before 20 weeks' gestation (in the absence of a hydatiform mole) OR persistent hypertension beyond 6 weeks postpartum
Gestational hypertension	Hypertension developing for the first time at ≥20+0 weeks' gestation in a previously normotensive non-proteinuric woman
Preeclampsia	Gestational hypertension with the presence of one or more of the following: – New-onset proteinuria – Involvement of organ systems

morbidity and mortality [10]. Preeclampsia must be differentiated form other hypertensive conditions in pregnancy like HELLP syndrome, etc. (Table 2).

Box 1 Diagnostic Criteria for Preeclampsia

Blood pressure (BP)

- Systolic BP of ≥140 mmHg or diastolic BP of ≥90 mmHg on two occasions at least 4 h apart after 20 weeks of gestation in a previously normotensive woman
- Systolic BP of ≥160 mmHg or diastolic BP of ≥110 mmHg (severe hypertension can be confirmed within minutes to facilitate timely antihypertensive therapy)

and

Proteinuria

- ≥300 mg per 24 h urine collection
- Protein/creatinine ratio of ≥0.3
- Dipstick reading of 2+ (used only if other quantitative methods not available)

or in the absence of proteinuria, new-onset hypertension along with the new-onset of any of the following:

- Thrombocytopenia (platelet count less than 100×10^9/L)
- Renal insufficiency (serum creatinine concentrations >1.1 mg/dL or doubling of the serum creatinine concentration in the absence of other renal disease)
- Impaired liver function (elevated serum liver transaminases to twice the normal concentration)
- Pulmonary edema

New-onset headache that does not improve with medication and is not accounted for by alternative diagnoses or visual symptoms

Table 2 Differentiating HELLP syndrome from other clinical conditions (adapted from Sibai BM. Imitators of severe preeclampsia [11])

Clinical and biochemical feature	HELLP syndrome	AFLP	TTP	HUS
Urine findings	Proteinuria and evidence of hemolysis	Occasional proteinuria with conjugated bilirubin	Proteinuria with blood	Proteinuria
Thrombocytopenia	Present	Present	Present	Present
Hemolysis (%)	50–100	15–20	100	100
Anemia	Sometimes	No	Yes	Yes

(continued)

Table 2 (continued)

Clinical and biochemical feature	HELLP syndrome	AFLP	TTP	HUS
DIC	<20	50–100	Uncommon	Uncommon
Elevated transaminases	High	High	Usually mild	Usually mild
Elevated bilirubin	Sometimes	Always	Always	Always
Elevated ammonia	Rare	Sometimes	No	No
Impaired renal function (%)	50	90–100	30	100
Hypoglycemia	No	Common	No	No

Box 2 Preeclampsia with Severe Features

- Systolic BP of ≥160 mmHg or diastolic BP of ≥110 mmHg on two occasions at least 4 h apart (unless antihypertensive therapy is initiated before this time)
- Thrombocytopenia (platelet count <100 × 10^9/L)
- Impaired liver function (in the absence of other cause) as indicated by abnormally elevated liver enzymes of more than twice the upper limit of normal levels, or by severe persistent right upper quadrant or epigastric pain that is unresponsive to medications
- Renal insufficiency (serum creatinine concentration >1.1 mg/dL or a doubling of the serum creatinine concentration in the absence of other renal disease)
- Pulmonary edema
- New-onset headache without other cause that is unresponsive to medication
- Visual disturbances
- Eclampsia

2 Pathophysiology

Eclampsia is thought to be caused by hypertensive encephalopathy or ischemia from vasoconstriction. Women with eclampsia have been shown to have evidence of neuroinflammation and an injured blood–brain barrier [12].

Arterial ischemic stroke (AIS) can occur when occlusion of a cerebral artery leads to infarction of the central nervous system. This can occur in women with preeclampsia by multiple mechanisms. Severe vasospasm can cause hypoperfusion resulting in AIS [13]. Peripartum cardiomyopathy resulting as a complication of preeclampsia can lead to cardioembolic AIS which can also provoke in situ thrombosis in cerebral vessels. Cervical artery dissections have been reported in patients with preeclampsia which cause AIS through occlusion of the cervical vessel or distal embolization of clot from the false lumen at the site of the dissection (Fig. 1).

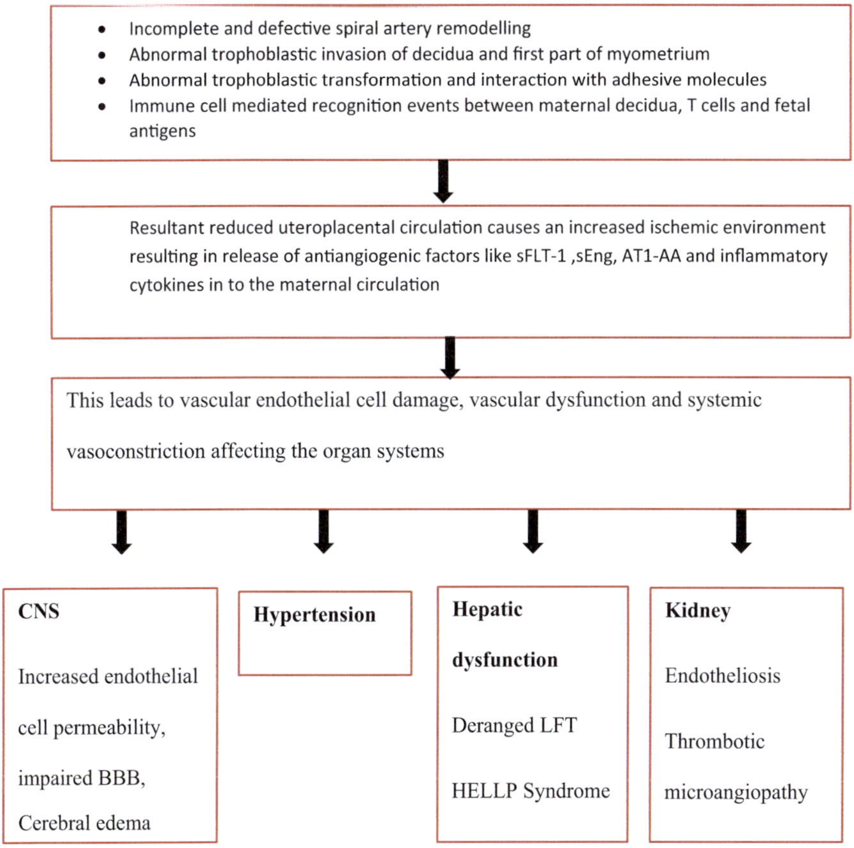

- Incomplete and defective spiral artery remodelling
- Abnormal trophoblastic invasion of decidua and first part of myometrium
- Abnormal trophoblastic transformation and interaction with adhesive molecules
- Immune cell mediated recognition events between maternal decidua, T cells and fetal antigens

↓

Resultant reduced uteroplacental circulation causes an increased ischemic environment resulting in release of antiangiogenic factors like sFLT-1 ,sEng, AT1-AA and inflammatory cytokines in to the maternal circulation

↓

This leads to vascular endothelial cell damage, vascular dysfunction and systemic vasoconstriction affecting the organ systems

↓

CNS

Increased endothelial cell permeability, impaired BBB, Cerebral edema

Hypertension

Hepatic dysfunction

Deranged LFT

HELLP Syndrome

Kidney

Endotheliosis

Thrombotic microangiopathy

Fig. 1 Pathophysiology of preeclampsia

Hemorrhagic stroke can occur spontaneously or secondary to rupture of vascular lesions such as aneurysms, arteriovenous malformations (AVMs), or Moya Moya vasculopathy [15, 16].

The vascular pathophysiology of ICH in preeclampsia may be due to arteriolar dysfunction, with compromised autoregulation that is unable to compensate for acute hypertension that could be aggravated by preeclampsia-related coagulopathy. However, few studies have demonstrated radiological or pathological details of primary hemorrhagic strokes seen in preeclampsia [17, 18].

The mechanism underlying PRES remains unclear but the most widely accepted hypothesis is that severe hypertension causes breakdown of the blood–brain barrier causing impaired cerebral autoregulation and vasogenic edema. Typically, PRES is reversible, but lesions can evolve to irreversible damage and encephalomalacia [19].

Cases of women who develop both RCVS and PRES have been reported, which suggests that the two are interrelated and may share underlying pathophysiologic mechanisms [20].

The kidneys undergo remarkable changes as part of the normal physiological adaptation to pregnancy. In comparison to non-pregnant state, the effective plasma flow rate increases by up to 80%, and the GFR increases by 40–60%. However in preeclampsia, both GFR and renal plasma flow is significantly reduced by 30–40% [21]. This is caused by the damage of endothelial cells of the glomerulus by the hypoxia-induced stress mediators released from the placenta. There is also increased protein loss due to the resulting cellular and filtration apparatus damage. The anti-angiogenic mediators released from the ischemic placenta in women with preeclampsia affect the kidney as part of the disease process, causing deterioration in kidney function before proteinuria [22]. This pathological process is said to predate the onset of symptoms by weeks. Elevated serum uric acid levels in preeclampsia result from decreased renal clearance rather than tissue breakdown from hypoxia. Hyperuricemia, more than 90th centile of typical pregnancy values, is the earliest change in renal function, followed by proteinuria.

3 Management of Preeclampsia

The management of severe preeclampsia involves prompt recognition and diagnosis of the condition, adequate control of the elevated BP, timely recognition of possible organ system involvement, and their efficient management accordingly.

The criteria for the diagnosis of preeclampsia as per the American College of Obstetricians and Gynecologists (ACOG) in the ACOG Practice Bulletin Number 222 are listed in Box 1 [5], and the diagnostic features of severe preeclampsia are listed in Box 2 [5]. The antihypertensive medications used in the management of preeclampsia are listed in Table 3. In addition to antihypertensive agents, other medications also play a vital role in the management of preeclampsia and are listed in Table 4.

The adverse conditions that can occur with severe preeclampsia and the organ system involvement with their corresponding management will be discussed in the following sections (see Table 5).

Table 3 Antihypertensive agents used for control of BP in pregnancy [5]

Drug	Dose	Comments	Onset of action
Labetalol	10–20 mg IV, then 20–80 mg every 10–30 min to a maximum cumulative dosage of 300 mg A continuous IV infusion of 1–2 mg/min can be used instead of intermittent therapy or started after 20 mg IV dose	Requires use of programmable infusion pump and continuous noninvasive monitoring of blood pressure and heart rate Tachycardia is less common with fewer adverse effects Avoid in women with asthma, pre-existing myocardial disease, decompensated cardiac function, and heart block and bradycardia	1–2 min

Table 3 (continued)

Drug	Dose	Comments	Onset of action
Hydralazine	5 mg IV or IM, then 5–10 mg IV every 20–40 min to a maximum cumulative dosage of 20 mg; or constant infusion of 0.5–10 mg/h	Higher or frequent dosage is associated with maternal hypotension, headaches, and abnormal fetal heart rate tracings; may be more common than other agents	10–20 min
Nifedipine (immediate release)	10–20 mg orally, repeat in 20 min if needed; then 10–20 mg every 2–6 h; maximum daily dose is 180 mg	May observe reflex tachycardia and headaches. May be associated with precipitous drops in BP in some women, with associated fetal heart rate decelerations for which emergency cesarean delivery may be indicated As such, this regimen is not typically used as a first-line option and is usually reserved only for women without IV access. If used, FHR should be monitored while administering short-acting nifedipine	5–10 min

Table 4 Other drugs used in preeclampsia [5]

Drug	Dosage	Special consideration
Magnesium sulfate	Loading dose: 4 g IV over 5 min, followed by an infusion of 1 g/h maintained for 24 h Recurrent seizures should be treated with a further dose 2–4 g given over 5 min	Monitor for signs of toxicity by clinical assessment Deep tendon reflexes Respiratory rate Urine output Are usually checked at close intervals In women with compromised renal function, serum magnesium levels should be checked every 4–6 h in addition to clinical assessment [19]
Betamethasone	12 mg IM, 2 doses 24 h apart or 12 h apart based on severity	Indication: <34 weeks Delaying delivery for optimal corticosteroid exposure may not always be advisable
Nitrates	Glyceryl trinitrate intravenous infusion 5–10 μg/min	First line in acute pulmonary edema

Diuretics: Not routinely recommended due to potential risk of altered uteroplacental flow/possible teratogenicity. Only a few controlled studies of diuretic use during pregnancy, and for each individual diuretic; data are therefore limited. Decision to use in pregnancy is clinical, based on the benefits of effectively treating the maternal condition versus the possible risks to the fetus [23]

Table 5 Maternal and fetal complications in severe preeclampsia [23]

Maternal complications	– Eclampsia – Stroke – Pulmonary edema – Adult respiratory distress syndrome – HELLP syndrome with/without liver damage – Acute renal failure – Placental abruption with/without disseminated intravascular coagulopathy – Long-term cardiovascular, central nervous system and renal morbidity – Death
Fetal complications	– Fetal growth restriction – Oligohydramnios – Hypoxia-acidosis – Preterm delivery – Death – Long-term morbidity • Neurological deficit • Cerebral palsy • Cardiovascular disease

4 Central Nervous System

4.1 Eclampsia

Eclampsia is defined as a convulsive episode characterized by new-onset tonic-clonic, focal, or multifocal seizures occurring in the setting of preeclampsia in the absence other conditions like epilepsy, intracranial hemorrhage, cerebral arterial ischemia/infarction, or drug abuse. Eclamptic convulsions are an acute complication of preeclampsia and are one of the most distressing neurological manifestations of preeclampsia. Eclampsia is considered as an obstetric emergency and is still a significant cause of maternal mortality in the developing countries. It is a common reason for requiring intensive care therapy, and its management entails a multidisciplinary approach with the involvement of different medical specialties such as obstetricians, pediatricians, anesthetists, and intensivists.

The most important goal of the treatment of severe preeclampsia besides treating high BP is the prevention of eclampsia. Magnesium sulfate remains the drug of choice for the prevention and treatment of eclampsia and has shown results in reducing maternal mortality and morbidity. The mechanism of action of magnesium sulfate is not fully understood but animal studies suggest that it may decrease neuroinflammation and protect the function of the blood–brain barrier. It is given in the form of an intravenous bolus dose followed by an intravenous infusion (Table 4), with precaution for women with impaired renal function.

In the event of an eclamptic fit, appropriate seizure management should be promptly instituted such as calling for help, measures to prevent maternal injury such as padding side rails, placement of the patient in lateral decubitus position, prevention of aspiration, and administration of supplemental oxygen. Magnesium sulfate should then be started immediately if not already done so. The purpose of magnesium sulfate is not to arrest the seizure but to prevent recurrence of convulsions as the initial seizure is usually self-limiting. Around 10% of women will have a second seizure after starting magnesium sulfate infusion, in which case an additional 2 g of magnesium sulfate can be given along with the ongoing magnesium sulfate infusion. If repeat magnesium bolus fails to control the seizure, lorazepam, midazolam, diazepam, or other status epilepticus treatment modalities to be administered. Simultaneously, hypertension should be addressed with the appropriate antihypertensive medications. Once the seizure has subsided and the patient has been stabilized, delivery must be planned as soon as it is practical. For women requiring cesarean delivery, the infusion should ideally begin before surgery and continue for 24 h following completion of the surgery. The infusion should continue for 24 h after delivery for women who deliver vaginally. Magnesium sulfate infusion should be continued for at least 24 h after the last seizure if occurring in the postnatal period [24].

Fetal heart rate decelerations or bradycardia are commonly noted during eclamptic seizure. Maternal hypoxia following the seizure may lead to fetal heart rate tracing abnormalities such as recurrent decelerations, tachycardia, or reduced variability; however, one should proceed with delivery only once maternal hemodynamic stabilization has been achieved. Maternal resuscitation is usually followed by normalization of the fetal tracing. Eclampsia is not considered on its own as an indication for cesarean delivery; however, it is more likely the earlier the gestational age and the more unfavorable the cervical conditions [25].

Maternal complications that can result from eclampsia include ischemic cerebrovascular accidents, intracerebral hemorrhage, placental abruption, DIC, and acute renal failure. Aspiration pneumonia and cardiopulmonary arrest occur in as many as 5% of women [26]. Temporary neurological abnormalities such as cortical blindness, focal motor deficits, and coma may occur, and these are likely caused by a transient cerebral insult such as hypoxia, ischemia, or edema.

4.2 Stroke

Extreme elevations in BP can lead to cerebrovascular accident; however, a very rapid decline in BP will compromise the uteroplacental blood flow causing fetal distress. Hence, a slower decrease to achieve a BP in the mild hypertension range is more appropriate. Guidelines released by the American Heart Association and the American Stroke Association focus on stroke prevention in women recommend documenting preeclampsia as a risk factor for both compromise the uteroplacental blood flow and stroke [27].

4.3 Posterior Reversible Encephalopathy Syndrome

Posterior reversible encephalopathy syndrome (PRES) is marked by headache, altered mental status, seizures, visual disturbances, and extensive white-matter changes. One of its distinctive features is the reversibility of the clinical and radiological abnormalities after suitable treatment and removal of the triggering factor. It is possible for patients with preeclampsia to develop PRES even without developing eclampsia, with mild elevation in BP, serum LDH, and serum uric acid levels [26].

CT scanning is generally the first form of imaging for diagnosing PRES with low sensitive but a good diagnostic modality in urgent situation. MRI scan helps to confirm the diagnosis of PRES as well as show its extent. Imaging findings of PRES include almost symmetrical hemispheric vasogenic edema involving subcortical white matter, frequently extending to the overlying cortex. PRES may rarely involve the spinal cord. Intraparenchymal or subarachnoid hemorrhages are found in 10–25% of cases [28].

The acute management is generally supportive, such as hydration and correction of electrolyte disturbances and removing or reversing the suspected cause. The BP of patients with acute hypertension should be gradually reduced by no more than 20–25% in the initial few hours in order to circumvent the risk of cerebral, coronary, and renal ischemia [26] to achieve a target mean arterial pressure between 105 and 125 mmHg. Nitroglycerine is not recommended in the presence of PRES as it may worsen cerebral edema. Patients in whom cerebral edema has caused raised intracranial pressure may need neurosurgical intervention.

Cases of suspected PRES warrant transfer of the patient to an intensive care setting, as up to 70% of patients will ultimately require intensive care and 35%–40% require mechanical ventilation for 3–7 days. Development of encephalopathy, seizures, ventilatory depression, and the need for invasive BP monitoring are among indications for transfer to an intensive care unit. Early delivery should be considered for patients in these patients. Patients with significant renal failure require prompt dialysis. Management of PRES-associated seizures without status epilepticus is with antiseizure medications decided on an individual basis. Development of status epilepticus needs emergency management with benzodiazepines, as well as loading doses of sodium valproate, levetiracetam, or phenytoin. Resolution of the acute phase of PRES is an indication for weaning and stopping these medications.

Malignant PRES is diagnosed based on a Glasgow Coma Scale (GCS) score of less than 8 along with clinical decline despite standard medical management for elevated intracranial pressure, in the presence of radiological evidence of edema or intracerebral hemorrhage exerting mass effect such as effacement of basal cisterns, transtentorial, tonsillar, or uncal herniation. Malignant PRES requires aggressive supportive care comprising mechanical ventilation, transfusion of blood products to reverse coagulopathy, corticosteroids for those with autoimmune disorders, and intracranial pressure monitoring in patients with GCS of less than 8. Patients with acute obstructive hydrocephalus may need an external ventricular drain [27].

4.4 Reversible Cerebral Vasoconstriction Syndrome

Reversible cerebral vasoconstriction syndrome (RCVS) shares clinical and radiographic features with PRES. It is a monophasic disorder that is usually characterized by thunderclap headache. It can be complicated by seizure, ischemic or hemorrhagic stroke, brain edema, and subarachnoid hemorrhage. Angiography usually shows bilateral, diffuse, and ultimately reversible cerebral vasoconstriction of the intracerebral arteries. RCVS can occur in the postpartum period [28].

5 Renal System

Preeclampsia is the leading cause of pregnancy-related acute kidney injury (AKI) and is associated with increased rates of maternal mortality and fetal loss. Approximately 2% of women with preeclampsia with severe features and 15% of women with HELLP syndrome will develop AKI [29]. Renal insufficiency is one of the severe features of preeclampsia necessitating admission to intensive care unit.

Clinical manifestations of renal pathology in preeclampsia include proteinuria, proteinuria with nephrotic syndrome and AKI.

5.1 Acute Kidney Injury

Renal insufficiency in preeclampsia is defined as a serum creatinine level ≥1.1 mg/dL or a value doubling in the absence of renal disease. Hypertensive disorders, especially preeclampsia and HELLP syndrome, are considered the most common causes of pregnancy-related AKI. Acute renal failures is seen in 1–2% of patients with preeclampsia and 7.4% of patients with HELLP syndrome. A retrospective cohort study showed an increased incidence of acute renal failure in pregnant women with preeclampsia and the authors suggested that this could be attributed to certain management aspects specifically fluids, antihypertensives, and drug use that may have led to hypovolemia, renal hypoperfusion, and nephrotoxicity [30].

5.2 Nephrotic Syndrome

Nephrotic syndrome complicates 0.32% of pregnancies, with preeclampsia contributing up to 0.19% (i.e., >50% of cases), making it the leading cause of nephrotic syndrome in pregnancy. A thorough assessment of the patient is needed to exclude other differential diagnoses such as lupus nephritis, which may present de novo in pregnancy. Occasionally, a renal biopsy may be needed to make this distinction. The use of renal biopsy in pregnancy is controversial and performing one may be considered reasonable if it results in a potential change in therapeutic management. The risk of various complications with a renal biopsy is higher during pregnancy compared to the postpartum period (7% versus 1%). Nephrotic syndrome is a hypercoagulable state and those with severe proteinuria (Urine Protein: Creatinine ratio (uPCR) >300 mg/mmol or Albumin: Creatinine Ratio (ACR) >250 mg/mmol) should be started on thromboprophylaxis with low molecular weight heparin antenatally and continued postpartum unless there is a specific contraindication [31].

5.3 Specific Considerations in the Management of Patients with Renal Dysfunction in Preeclampsia

Management aspects to be considered in these cases include adequate blood pressure control, eclampsia prevention, fluid balance, and possibly dialysis along with close monitoring of the fetus. Nephrotoxic drugs should be avoided. Complications like hyperkalemia, and metabolic acidosis, should be promptly addressed along with judicious fluid management, aiming to avoid tissue hypoperfusion and maintain adequate uteroplacental circulation for fetal wellbeing while avoiding volume overload and pulmonary edema.

5.4 When to Consider Delivery in Renal Impairment?

Deteriorating renal function diagnosed by serum creatinine levels of more than 1 mg/dL, blood urea nitrogen of 13 mg/dL, or the development of oliguria (urine output less than 500 mL/day) are indications for immediate delivery to prevent further damage to the kidneys. Renal function in pregnancy is assessed using serum creatinine concentrations as estimated GFR (eGFR) is not valid for use in pregnancy. The onset of heavy proteinuria (defined as >3 g/24 h) is not an indication for immediate delivery in all pregnancies. In such cases, careful monitoring of the fetus and mother is vital as deterioration can occur rapidly [32].

5.5 Managing Hypertension and Eclampsia Prevention in Renal Impairment

Magnesium sulfate is the drug of choice for eclampsia treatment and prevention [33]. It is excreted by the kidneys. Women with renal insufficiency should be given a standard loading dose of 4 g since their volume of distribution is not affected. The maintenance dose in these women should be reduced and tailored to the serum creatinine levels. Strict monitoring for any signs of magnesium toxicity is vital to prevent related complications. Magnesium toxicity is unlikely with the usual regimens and levels do not need to be routinely measured. However in women with compromised renal function, serum magnesium levels should be checked every 4–6 h as an adjunct to clinical assessment.

5.6 Fluid Management

As already mentioned, women with preeclampsia are more prone to develop pulmonary edema. Therefore, judicious use of fluids with strict input output chart is vital in the management as iatrogenic fluid administration is a major preventable cause of pulmonary edema.

The current guidelines advise a restrictive approach in the fluid management in patients with preeclampsia. Fluid is administered for maintaining water and electrolyte balance or for replacement of lost intravascular volume [34] (Table 6).

Maintenance therapy is commonly given slowly over 24 h and may be calculated to match the urinary output combined with stool and insensible loss. It is usually administered at a rate of 80 mL/h in uncomplicated women who are fasting for several hours in labor. In patients with renal insufficiency, it is crucial to readjust the maintenance fluid delivery rate, taking into account the volume of fluid used to infuse other intravenous medications (which includes antihypertensives, magnesium sulfate, oxytocin, and anesthesia medications). In these situations where, risk of complications are low due to the slow administration, hemodynamic monitoring may be requires depending on the clinical situation.

Women with preeclampsia are more prone to develop shock from hemorrhage due to abruptio placentae, operative blood loss, and rupture of subcapsular liver hematoma. Replacement therapy in such patients is administered according to an estimated deficit and is usually transfused rapidly. Comorbidity due to renal failure complicates intravenous fluid administration as the kidneys may not respond to diuretic therapy making over-transfusion an inevitable cause of pulmonary edema. Hemodynamic monitoring in these cases may prevent iatrogenic complications [35].

5.7 *Renal Replacement Therapy*

Indications to initiate renal replacement therapy are metabolic acidosis, presence of uremic symptoms, refractory hyperkalemia, and volume overload. Dialysis in pregnant women should be planned and done carefully with minimal hemodynamic fluctuations to avoid adverse effects on fetal wellbeing by reduced uteroplacental perfusion. Hence in pregnancy, longer and more frequent sessions are preferred aiming to keep serum urea levels <45–60 mg/dL. HELLP syndrome accounts for 40% of all cases of pregnancy-related AKI and up to 60% of severe cases. 30–50% of these patients will require dialysis temporarily.

Table 6 Intravenous fluid indications in preeclampsia

Maintenance 60–80 mL/h	Clinical observation for observation Calculate the drug administration volume
Replacement Aim for systolic BP >90	Consider noninvasive hemodynamic monitoring and arterial line insertion if uncontrolled blood pressure or severe hemorrhage
Oliguria 300 mL fluid challenge Aim for urine output ≥100 mL/4 h	Not routinely indicated consider repeating the fluid challenge if persistent oliguria

Metabolic acidosis is usually corrected with sodium bicarbonate keeping in mind that a 4 mEq/L decrease in bicarbonate concentration is common in a healthy pregnant woman, and thus avoiding over correction.

Hyperkalemia is a life-threatening complication. Approaches to lowering serum potassium should start with decreasing the intake of potassium in diet or tube feeds. Use of potassium-binding resins to facilitate exchange of potassium across the gut lumen in pregnancy has not been adequately studied. As it is meant to act locally in the gastrointestinal tract, no fetal harm is essentially anticipated. Insulin, dextrose solutions, and beta agonists can be used to promote intracellular shifts in potassium and hence reduce serum levels. Hyperkalemia refractory to these management strategies should be then treated with hemodialysis [36].

5.8 Delivery

Box 3 Indications for Immediate Delivery
Maternal

- Gestational age above 34 weeks
- Patient declining expectant management
- Uncontrolled severe range blood pressure (persistent systolic blood pressure 160 mmHg or more or diastolic blood pressure 110 mmHg or more) not responsive to maximum antihypertensive medications
- Suspected placental abruption or preterm labor
- Pulmonary edema
- Eclampsia or encephalopathy
- Persistent headache, refractory to treatment
- Persistent epigastric pain or right upper pain unresponsive to repeated analgesia
- Stroke
- HELLP syndrome
- New or worsening renal dysfunction (serum creatinine greater than 1.1 mg/dL or twice baseline) or persistent oliguria despite therapy

Fetal

- Gestational age above 34 weeks
- Fetal death
- Lethal fetal anomaly
- Extreme prematurity (less than 24 weeks)
- Abnormal fetal testing
- Persistent reversed end diastolic flow in the umbilical artery Doppler
- Persistent oligohydramnios

Rupture of membranes

Historically, the definite cure for severe preeclampsia has been early delivery knowing that the course of the disease is a progressive leading to detrimental maternal and fetal complications. However, there are many reasons for immediate delivery, expectant management can still be offered in some situations. Box 3 illustrates indications for immediate delivery after maternal stabilization. However, in special circumstances and with precautions in inpatient setting, delay for 24–48 h to administer steroids can be safely offered to the patient after detailed counseling [37].

Several studies have investigated the role of expectant management in severe preeclampsia at gestational ages below 28 weeks where fetal morbidity and mortality are the highest. Most of these studies have reported prolongation of pregnancy by 7–10 days and improvement in neonatal outcome without affecting the maternal outcome. Belghiti et al. [38] and Bombrys et al. [39] have concluded that expectant management should not be offered below 24 weeks of gestation or if there is severe intrauterine growth restriction below 26 weeks.

Vigilant fetal and maternal surveillance is recommended during expectant management. The maternal surveillance should be in a tertiary care hospital with daily multidisciplinary review of symptoms and signs as well as laboratory tests that may indicate worsening of the disease and need of intervention. The fetal surveillance includes nonstress test, biophysical profile, and ultrasound scan for fluid and Doppler as well as growth scan every 2 weeks. Persistent oligohydramnios or reversed end diastolic flow in umbilical artery Doppler should be considered as indications to terminate expectant management after delivery of steroids. Ending expectant management can be considered in the absence of fetal growth in 2 weeks [23].

5.9 *Mode of Delivery*

Vaginal delivery can be offered to women with severe preeclampsia as long as there are no other indications for cesarean section. However, the likelihood for cesarean delivery is inversely proportion to the gestational age. At 28 weeks, it is 97%, 65% at gestational age 28–32 weeks, 32% at 34–36 weeks, and 28% at gestational age above 37+0 weeks. Some studies have compared induction of labor versus cesarean section in patients with severe preeclampsia remote from term. They found no additional risks on low-birth-weight infants. Hence, the option of mode of delivery should be individualized bearing in mind the organs involved, the progression of the disease and fetal condition. In special circumstances like eclampsia at or near term, vaginal delivery is considered a safer option in comparison to cesarean section since it is associated with less hemodynamic instability [23].

Neuraxial analgesia and anesthesia are recommended during delivery as long as there is no coagulopathy or significant thrombocytopenia [40]. Special care should be taken in women who may require general anesthesia while taking magnesium sulfate as it prolongs the duration of nondepolarizing muscle relaxants. However, magnesium sulfate should not be stopped during the procedure as these women are at increased risk of developing eclampsia especially with the induction of anesthesia.

6 Postpartum and Beyond

Patients with severe preeclampsia need to receive meticulous care after delivery. These patients need their blood pressure monitored and antihypertensive therapy initiated/continued if the blood pressure is above 150 mmHg systolic or 100 mmHg diastolic in two occasions 4–6 h apart. Strict fluid input and output monitoring should be continued as these patients tend to receive large amount fluids during labor, for example, magnesium sulfate, antihypertensive, and oxytocin infusions. Due to fluid shift, risk of pulmonary edema must be considered. The blood pressure usually starts to decrease 48 h after delivery. Patients with severe preeclampsia need at least 3 days of inpatient observation.

Many studies have linked preeclampsia with an increased risk of future cardiovascular and cerebrovascular diseases. The risk is even higher with severe preeclampsia in comparison to mild preeclampsia (mild: RR, 2: 95% CI 1.83–2.19; severe: RR, 5.36: 95% CI, 3.96–7.27, $p < 0.0001$) and with early onset disease [41]. Hence, this group of patients need long-term routine follow-up at primary care level.

The risk of recurrence of severe preeclampsia in future pregnancies is almost 50% [5]. These patients may benefit from lifestyle modification, weight control, early booking, and initiation of low-dose aspirin towards the end of first trimester in subsequent pregnancies [42].

7 Levels of Care in Severe Preeclampsia

Severe preeclampsia needs multidisciplinary input that mandates early involvement of anesthetists and sometimes an intensivist or other specialized physician. Advanced obstetrics units need to adopt levels of care 0–3 terminology rather than high dependency or intensive care units to improve communication among team members (Box 4). Decision regarding level of care should be individualized and discussed among the team.

Box 4 Admission Criteria and Decision for Level of Care

Admission criteria for level 1 care:

- Step down from higher level of care
- Need for additional monitoring or clinical input, for example, observation more than 4 hourly, fluid input/output, pulse oximetry, magnesium sulfate
- Any concern regarding physical condition

Admission criteria for level 2 care:

- Need for monitoring that cannot be delivered in level 1
- Need for respiratory support, for example, respiratory rate >25/min, noninvasive ventilation or CPAP

- Patients with hemodynamic instability, for example, on intravenous antihypertensive infusions or patients with arterial line blood pressure monitoring
- Glasgow coma score less than 14
- Need for hemofiltration

Admission criteria for level 3 care:

- Need for advanced respiratory support, for example, IPPV.
- Need for monitoring or support of two or more organs.

8 Pulmonary Edema

Pulmonary edema is a rare disease in pregnancy (0.6–0.7%). Despite that, it is a recognized complication of preeclampsia. It is considered a leading cause of death in women with preeclampsia [32, 33] and a common cause of admission to the intensive care unit [42]. It has been reported that pulmonary edema may occur in around 3% of preeclampsia patients, and around 70% of cases occur postpartum [43].

Cough, dyspnea, and orthopnea are the cardinal symptoms of acute pulmonary edema, especially when combined with the signs of tachycardia, tachypnea, decreased oxygen saturation, wheezing, and cardiac gallop rhythm are the diagnostic features of pulmonary edema.

8.1 The Management of Hypertensive Acute Pulmonary Edema in Pregnancy

From a clinical point of view, acute pulmonary edema can be classified into hypertensive pulmonary edema and pulmonary edema without hypertension.

The important pillars of care and management for the patient with acute pulmonary edema are to follow the ABC airway and breathing circulation by clearing the obstruction if any and administering oxygen, upright position, positive airway pressure, nitrates, frusemide, morphine, and inotropes. These goals are to reduce left ventricular preload and afterload.

Noninvasive ventilation as well as avoidance of aortocaval compression should be tried first, as they will improve oxygenation through positive airway pressure that increases the inspired oxygen concentration, displace the fluids from the alveoli, and decrease the need for intubation [44].

Diuretics like frusemide can be used in cases of fluid overload in the management of acute pulmonary edema but should not be used with patients with intercellular volume depletion. Morphine can be used for vasodilation and to relieve the feeling of dyspnea by decreasing the preload and reducing sympathetic nervous activity. It does not improve pulmonary edema or cardiac output; instead, it acts as an anxiolytic and helps reduce the patient's respiratory effort [45].

8.2 *Peripartum Cardiomyopathy (PPCM) and Preeclampsia*

Since the 1990s, peripartum cardiomyopathy has been defined as a rare disease with unknown etiology that is characterized by acute idiopathic left heart failure in the last month of pregnancy or up to 5 months after delivery and is characterized by left ventricular dysfunction in the absence of any history of previous cardiac disease [46]. It is not uncommon to easily miss the diagnosis of PPCM. Despite the growing knowledge about its pathophysiology and its risk factors, it still needs a high index of suspicion for its diagnosis that the main cause of morbidity and mortality with PPCM is a failure or delay in its diagnosis.

A careful history and examination with a high clinical sense of suspicion are crucial in the diagnosis of PPCM, as it is a diagnosis of exclusion. Risk factors include African-Asian ethnicity, advanced maternal age, multiparity, multiple gestations, preeclampsia, low levels of selenium, prolonged use of tocolytics, and viral infection. The symptoms of shortness of breath, especially orthopnea, nocturnal dyspnea, the inability to lie flat, and needing more than two pillows at night, even in the presence of high blood pressure, should ring the bell for the differential diagnosis of cardiac diseases [47].

8.3 *Management of PPCM*

The management of PPCM is almost identical to the management of heart failure for any other reason; the basic goal is to reduce preload and afterload, reduce vasoconstriction, and improve contractility. Multidisciplinary team management and critical care admission for advanced cardiac support are needed for pregnant and parturient women who have been diagnosed with cardiogenic shock, respiratory failure, or hemodynamic instability. A timely start of the anti-failure medication is associated with a good prognosis and outcome. Angiotensin-converting enzyme (ACE) inhibitors, angiotensin receptor blockers (ARBs), mineralocorticoid receptor blockers (MRBs), ivabradine, vasodilators (nitrates and hydralazine), digoxin, and diuretics are examples of oral heart failure medications. ACE inhibitors, ARBs, MRBs, and ivabradine are contraindicated in pregnancy and should be used with caution during breastfeeding [48].

9 Conclusion

Severe preeclampsia remains one of the commonest reasons for maternal admissions to intensive care units and a major cause of significant maternal and perinatal morbidity and mortality. Early recognition and optimum management by a multidisciplinary team augment both maternal and fetal improved outcomes. Appropriate use of antihypertensive medications for blood pressure more than 160/110 mmHg, antiseizure therapy and prophylaxis with magnesium sulfate, adequate fluid management and respiratory support when needed, correction of coagulopathy if indicated in patients with HELLP syndrome, fetal surveillance and timely delivery are the corner stones for better outcome. The long-term cardiovascular risks for patients who develop severe preeclampsia must not be overlooked and a documented follow-up plan is of paramount importance.

References

1. Bell M. A historical overview of preeclampsia-eclampsia. J Obstet Gynecol Neonatal Nurs. 2010;39:510–8.
2. Shawwa K, McDonnell N, Garovic V. Pregnancy, preeclampsia, and brain three thousand years of progress. Hypertension. 2018;72(6):1263–5.
3. Steegers E, von Dadelszen P, Duvekot J, Pijnenborg R. Pre-eclampsia. Lancet. 2010;2010(376):631–44.
4. Khan K, Wojdyla D, Gülmezoglu A, Van Look P. WHO analysis of causes of maternal death: a systematic review. Lancet. 2006;367:1066–74.
5. Gestational hypertension and preeclampsia: ACOG Practice Bulletin, Number 222. Obstet Gynecol. 2020;135(6):e237–60.
6. Kassebaum N, Bertozzi-Villa A, Coggeshall M, et al. Global, regional, and national levels and causes of maternal mortality during 1990-2013: a systematic analysis for the Global Burden of Disease Study 2013. Lancet. 2014;384:980–1004.
7. Wallis A, Saftlas A, Hsia J, et al. Secular trends in the rates of preeclampsia, eclampsia, and gestational hypertension, United States, 1987-2004. Am J Hypertens. 2008;21:521–6.
8. Ananth C, Keyes K, Wapner R. Pre-eclampsia rates in the United States, 1980-2010: age-period-cohort analysis. BMJ. 2013;347:f6564.
9. Stevens W, Shih T, Incerti D, Ton T, Lee H, Peneva D, et al. Short-term costs of preeclampsia to the United States health care system. Am J Obstet Gynecol. 2017;217:237–48.e16.
10. Lam M, Dierking E. Intensive care unit issues in eclampsia and HELLP syndrome. Int J Crit Illn Inj Sci. 2017;7(3):136–41.
11. Sibai BM. Imitators of severe preeclampsia. Obstet Gynecol. 2007;109(4):956–66.
12. Bergman L, Hastie R, Zetterberg H, Blennow K, Schell S, Langenegger E, et al. Evidence of neuroinflammation and blood–brain barrier disruption in women with preeclampsia and eclampsia. Cell. 2021;10:3045.
13. Fugate J, Wijdicks E, Parisi J, Kallmes D, Flemming K, Giraldo E, et al. Fulminant postpartum cerebral vasoconstriction syndrome. Arch Neurol. 2012;69:111–7.
14. Euser A, Bullinger L, Cipolla M. Magnesium sulphate treatment decreases blood-brain barrier permeability during acute hypertension in pregnant rats. Exp Physiol. 2007;93:254–61.
15. Sharma A, Whitesell R, Moran K. Imaging pattern of intracranial hemorrhage in the setting of posterior reversible encephalopathy syndrome. Neuroradiology. 2010;52:855–63.
16. Williams B, Mancia G, Spiering W, et al. 2018 ESC/ESH guidelines for the management of arterial hypertension: the task force for the management of arterial hypertension. J Hypertens. 2018;36:1953–2041.
17. Li R, Mitchell P, Dowling R, et al. Is hypertension predictive of clinical recurrence in posterior reversible encephalopathy syndrome? J Clin Neurosci. 2013;20:248–52.
18. Miller E. Preeclampsia and cerebrovascular disease. Hypertension. 2019;74(1):5–13.
19. Hinduja A, Habetz K, Rania S, et al. Predictors of intensive care unit utilization in patients with posterior reversible encephalopathy syndrome. Acta Neurol Belg. 2017;117:201–6.
20. Casey S, Sampaio R, Michel E, et al. Posterior reversible encephalopathy syndrome: utility of fluid-attenuated inversion recovery MR imaging in the detection of cortical and subcortical lesions. AJNR Am J Neuroradiol. 2000;21:1199–206.

21. Karumanchi SA, Maynard SE, Stillman IE, Epstein FH, Sukhatme VP. Preeclampsia: a renal perspective. Kidney Int. 2005;67(6):2101–13.
22. Sani HM, Vahed SZ, Ardalan M. Preeclampsia: a close look at renal dysfunction. Biomed Pharmacother. 2019;109:408–16.
23. Heazell A, Norwitz E, Kenny L, Baker P. Hypertension in pregnancy. In: Sebai BM, Norwitz E, editors. Management of severe preeclampsia. Cambridge University Press; 2010. p. 134.
24. Pottecher T, Luton D, Zupan V, Collet M. Multidisciplinary management of severe preeclampsia (PE) experts' guidelines. In Ann Fr Anesth Réan. 2009;28:275–81.
25. Catherine C, Yanta C, Saand A, et al. Pearls & Oysters: the dangers of PRES: an atypical case with life-threatening presentation. Neurology. 2019;92:e282–5.
26. Wolff V, Ducros A. Reversible cerebral vasoconstriction syndrome without typical thunderclap headache. Headache. 2016;56:674–87.
27. Ducros A. Reversible cerebral vasoconstriction syndrome. Lancet Neurol. 2012;11:906–17.
28. Razmana A, Bakhadirov K, Batra A, Feske S. Cerebrovascular complications of pregnancy and the postpartum period. Curr Cardiol Rep. 2014;16:532.
29. Wallace AS, Aline MP. Renal and cardiovascular repercussions in preeclampsia and their impact on fluid management: a literature review. Braz J Anesthesiol. 2021;71(4):421–8. https://doi.org/10.1016/j.bjane.2021.02.052.
30. Mehrabadi A, Liu S, Bartholomew S, et al. Hypertensive disorders of pregnancy and the recent increase in obstetric acute renal failure in Canada: population based retrospective cohort study. BMJ. 2014;349:g4731.
31. Udupa V, Keepanasseril A, Vijayan N, Basu D, Negi VS. Early onset preeclampsia with nephrotic range proteinuria as the initial manifestation of lupus nephritis: report of three cases. Sultan Qaboos Univ Med J. 2019;19(1):e73–6.
32. Özkara A, Kaya AE, Başbuğ A, Ökten SB, Doğan O, Çağlar M, et al. Proteinuria in preeclampsia: is it important? Ginekol Pol. 2018;89(5):256–61.
33. NICE Guideline (NG133). Hypertension in pregnancy: diagnosis and management. Published Jun 2019. Accessed 12 Mar 2020.
34. von Schmidt auf Altenstadt JF, Hukkelhoven CWPM, van Roosmalen J, Bloemenkamp KWM. Pre-eclampsia increases the risk of postpartum haemorrhage: a Nationwide cohort study in the Netherlands. PLoS One. 2013;8(12):e81959. https://doi.org/10.1371/journal.pone.0081959.
35. Fadi F, Caroline V, Veronique FB. Obstetric nephrology: AKI and thrombotic microangiopathies in pregnancy. CJASN. 2012;7(12):2100–6. https://doi.org/10.2215/CJN.13121211.
36. Ahmed SMG, Kily LJM, Valappil SS, Ajmal S, Elfil H, Elamin NS, Konje JC. Renal dysfunction in pre-eclampsia: etiology, pathogenesis, diagnosis and perioperative management: a narrative review. EJMED. 2022;4(5):11–9 [cited 2022 Dec 10]. Available from: https://www.ej-med.org/index.php/ejmed/article/view/1463.
37. Balogun O, Sibai B. Counseling management and outcome in women with severe preeclampsia at 23-28 weeks gestation. Clin Obstet Gynecol. 2017;60:183–9.
38. Belghiti J, Kayem G, Tsatsaris V, et al. Benefits and risks of expectant management of severe preeclampsia at less than 26 weeks gestation: the impact of gestational age and severe fetal growth restriction. Am J Obstet Gynecol. 2011;205:465.
39. Bombrys AE, Barton JR, Nowaki EA, et al. Expectant management of severe preeclampsia at less than 27 weeks gestation: maternal and perinatal outcomes according to gestational age by weeks at onset of expectant management. Am J Obstet Gynecol. 2008;199:247.
40. Heazell A, Norwitz E, Kenny L, Baker P. Hypertension in pregnancy. In: Cliff J, Heazell A, editors. Anesthesia in preeclampsia. Cambridge University Press; 2010. p. 159–74.
41. McDonald SD, Malinowski A, Zhou Q, Yusuf S, Devereaux PJ. Cardiovascular sequelae of preeclampsia/eclampsia: a systematic review and meta-analyses. Am Heart J. 2008;156:918.
42. Sriram S, Robertson MS. Critically ill obstetric patients in Australia: a retrospective audit of 8 years' experience in a tertiary intensive care unit. Crit Care Resusc. 2008;10:120–4.

43. Sibai BM, Mabie BC, Harvey CJ, Gonzalez AR. Pulmonary edema in severe preeclampsia-eclampsia: analysis of thirty-seven consecutive cases. Am J Obstet Gynecol. 1987;156:1174–9.
44. Mas A, Masip J. Noninvasive ventilation in acute respiratory failure. Int J Chron Obstruct Pulmon Dis. 2014;9:837–52.
45. da Silva WA, Pinheiro AM, Lima PH, Malbouisson LMS. Renal and cardiovascular repercussions in preeclampsia and their impact on fluid management: a literature review. Braz J Anesthesiol. 2021;71(4):421–8.
46. Bauersachs J, König T, van der Meer P, Petrie MC, Hilfiker-Kleiner D, Mbakwem A, Hamdan R, Jackson AM, Forsyth P, de Boer RA, Mueller C, Lyon AR, Lund LH, Piepoli MF, Heymans S, Chioncel O, Anker SD, Ponikowski P, Seferovic PM, Johnson MR, Mebazaa A, Sliwa K. Pathophysiology, diagnosis and management of peripartum cardiomyopathy: a position statement from the Heart Failure Association of the European Society of Cardiology Study Group on peripartum cardiomyopathy. Eur J Heart Fail. 2019;21(7):827–43.
47. Hilfiker-Kleiner D, Haghikia A, Nonhoff J, Bauersachs J. Peripartum cardiomyopathy: current management and future perspectives. Eur Heart J. 2015;36(18):1090–7.
48. Savarese G, Edner M, Dahlström U, Perrone-Filardi P, Hage C, Cosentino F, Lund LH. Comparative associations between angiotensin-converting enzyme inhibitors, angiotensin receptor blockers and their combination, and outcomes in patients with heart failure and reduced ejection fraction. Int J Cardiol. 2015;199:415–23.

Peripartum Pulmonary Embolism: From Diagnoses to Management

Firdos Ummunnisa, Umme Nashrah, Umm E Amara, Aalami Zeba, Arshad Chanda, and Nissar Shaikh

Abstract Pulmonary embolism (PE) is a life-threatening clinical condition during pregnancy and peripartum. There is a significant increase in the risk of PE postpartum. There are various risk factors for PE in pregnant patients. The most absolute risk factor is hereditary thrombophilia. The pathophysiology of PE is venodilatation, increase in venous volume, and venous stasis along with endothelial damage or injury during pregnancy and postpartum period due to hormonal and hematological changes. For the probability scoring for PE, the clinical criteria are not well-defined in pregnancy. Echocardiogram may show right-sided heart changes. The diagnostic tool most frequently used is CTPA (computed tomographic pulmonary angiography) as it is easily available and may give an alternative diagnosis. If there is no PE, lower limb deep venous thrombosis (DVT) can be easily diagnosed with ultrasound Doppler.

Pending diagnosis of DVT/PE, the anticoagulation should be started early, once more, it is critical to prevent missing or delayed diagnoses. The low molecular weight heparin during pregnancy and unfractionated heparin in the postpartum period are the anticoagulant agents of choice, as they are reversible and have no fetal effects of low molecular weight heparin and are safe. Warfarin is not used due to its teratogenic effect. The new oral anticoagulants are not frequently used as safety is yet to be proved. If the patient is in shock with PE, thrombolysis, throm-

F. Ummunnisa (✉)
Halima Al-Tamimi OBGY Center, Doha, Qatar

U. Nashrah
Deccan College of Medical Sciences, Hyderabad, India

U. E Amara
Apollo Institute of Medical Sciences and Research, Hyderabad, India

A. Zeba
OBGY:Al Khor Hospital/Hamad Medical Corporation, Doha, Qatar

A. Chanda · N. Shaikh
Surgical Intensive Care/Hamad Medical Corporation, Doha, Qatar

N. Shaikh et al. (eds.), *Updates in Intensive Care of OBGY Patients*,
https://doi.org/10.1007/978-981-99-9577-6_5

bectomy, or ECMO therapy can be done. PE can be prevented up to some extent with LMWH during pregnancy and thrombophilia patients and the use of elastic stockings and early mobility in low-risk patients.

Keywords Pregnancy · Prepartum · Pulmonary embolism · Deep venous thrombosis · Thrombophilia · Fever dilatation · Venous stasis · Endothelial injury · Heparin

1 Background

Virchow in 1856 demonstrated the relation between DVT (deep venous thrombosis) and PE (pulmonary embolism); later on in 1920, a consensus was published regarding the factors contributing to thrombosis mainly hypercoagulability, blood stasis, and endothelial injury [1].

Thromboembolism is one of the leading causes of maternal mortality and according to confidential enquiries from the United Kingdom, more than 50% of the time, these patients receive substandard care [1]. All acute care physicians, anesthesiologists, obstetricians, and gynecologists, intensive care and other paramedical staff taking care of these patient should be well aware of thromboembolism in general and pulmonary embolism, in particular, to accurately diagnose and manage it.

Diagnosis and treatment of pulmonary embolism (PE) are complex, we have to arrive to the diagnosis accurately using various diagnostic tools, and at the same time should be aware of and minimize the adverse effects on the mother and the fetus. Regarding the treatment, the anticoagulation is the corner stone and one has to be aware of its effects on during peripartum period and effect on the fetus has to be highlighted. This chapter will be reviewed under the following subheadings.

2 Epidemiology

The risk of venous thromboembolism occurrence and pulmonary embolism is increased during the postpartum period compared to the pre- and intrapartum. Due to physiological changes in the maternal coagulation cascade during pregnancy and peripartum period, it causes hypercoagulability to conserve the blood loss. The risk of peripartum pulmonary embolism (PPE) is increased by 20 times in the postpartum period [2]. The incidence of venous thromboembolism during pregnancy is described to be 5–12 per 100,000 pregnancies whereas pulmonary embolism is less reported with an incidence of 1.59 per 100,000 deliveries. The DVT seems to be more common on the left side due to the anatomical crossing of the right common iliac artery over the left common iliac vein [2].

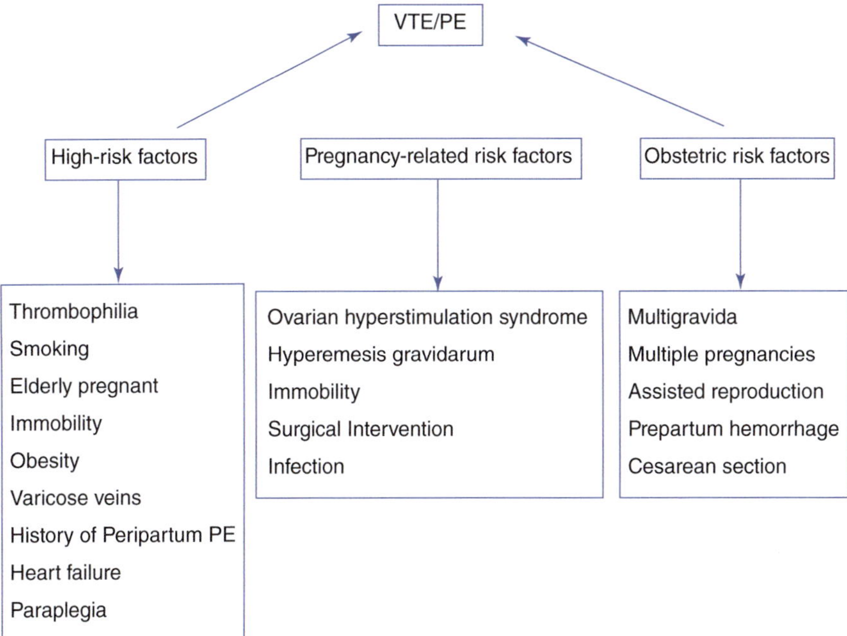

Fig. 1 Risk factors for peripartum PE

3 Risk Factors

There are various risk factors for VTE and PPE during pregnancy and postpartum; they are divided into high risk, transient risk, and obstetrical risk. High-risk factors thrombophilia (acquired or congenital), history of VTE, obesity, smoking, and pregnancy in elderly. The transient risk factors include ovarian hyperstimulation syndrome, hyperemesis gravidarum, immobility, and infections. Whereas the obstetrical risk factors for VTE and PPE include multigravida, assisted reproduction, surgical intervention, and peripartum hemorrhage [3]. Details of peripartum PE are described in Fig. 1.

4 Pathophysiology

The physiological, hormonal, and biochemical changes of pregnancy generate a favorable environment for the VTE. By fulfilling all three criteria of thromboembolism, which are all discussed in the following subheadings.

4.1 Venous Stasis

Throughout pregnancy, there is progesterone-induced vasodilatation, renal vasodilatation, there is increased GFR, and total blood volume. There is an increase in the diameter of the femoral, saphenous, and popliteal veins. These dilated veins with increased venous pressure, lead to vascular distention and venous stasis, and lower limb edema. Unlike in the general population, VTE in pregnancy seems to start in the pelvic area, as the right common iliac artery pulsation from crossing over the left iliac veins causes pulsatile compression of the veins, this causes frequent left pelvic veins VTE as it is reported up to 90% of VTE occurring in the left side during pregnancy [4].

4.2 Vascular Injury and Dysfunction

Apart from normal and surgical delivery of the fetus causing endothelial injury, another main reason for vascular injury during pregnancy and postpartum is circulating cytokines and growth factor that breaks down the vascular endothelial morphology, causing vascular dysfunction and injury by degradation or removing the cell junction protein. Additional injury to veins occurs with increased blood volume and diameter causing sheering stress on the vasculature, thus potentially damaging the vessels [5].

4.3 Hypercoagulability

Blood becomes hypercoagulable during pregnancy due to increasing procoagulant factors V, VII, VIII, IX, X, XII, and von Willebrand factor with a decrease in anticoagulant factors. There is a ten-fold increase in factor VIII, fibrinogen rises by two-fold during pregnancy, and peripartum period. Protein S level is decreased with a decrease in fibrinolysis [6].

Congenital or inherited thrombophilia is one of the important risk factors for VTE and PPE, about 40% of these patients develop VTE. The inherited thrombophilia includes factor V Leiden, prothrombin A-mutants, antithrombin, protein S and C deficiencies [7] (Table 1).

Table 1 Inherited thrombophilia and described risk of VTE [7]

Factor V Leiden	3–40% VTE risk
Prothrombin A mutation	3–17% VTE risk
Antithrombin deficiency	25-fold increased risk of VTE
Protein C deficiency	6–7% increased risk of VTE

Other general risk factors for VTE and PPE reliant to geographic areas are also common risk factors for VTE and PPE.

Deep venous emboli are detected and dislodged into the pulmonary circulation. Thus, these emboli cause pulmonary vascular occlusion, impairing the gas exchange. The larger the emboli, there will be a wedge in the main pulmonary arteries, and the smaller emboli mainly occlude the peripheral pulmonary arteries causing pulmonary infarctions. All these emboli cause obstruction to the blood in the pulmonary circulation, thus contributing to ventilation-perfusion mismatch and increased pulmonary vascular resistance, and pulmonary pressure which leads to increased right ventricular pressure, impairment, and failure ultimately causing cardiac arrest [8].

5 Diagnosis

It is of utmost importance to diagnose or rule out pulmonary embolism or VTE in the peripartum to avoid morbidity and mortality. The common clinical manifestations are shortness of breath, chest pain, and leg pain and swelling.

ECG may show right-sided changes, and arterial blood gas (ABG) commonly shows respiratory alkalosis. D-dimer is commonly used to rule out PE, it is not useful during pregnancy and peripartum. As they are physiologically raised during pregnancy and weeks after in the postpartum period.

The probability tests are not validated in pregnancy and postpartum for the diagnoses of PE. Although negative and sensitive predicted values of Well's criteria were shown to have excellent correlations peripartum period, but this retrospective design combined D-dimer, and had a small power to its disadvantages [9].

Following imaging studies are done in those PPE patients:

5.1 Chest X-Ray

Pregnant patients can have chest X-rays after covering the abdomen with a shield. Oligemic lung fields or wedge-shaped opacity may be suggestive of PE.

5.2 Bilateral Lower Limb Sonography

Bilateral lower limb compression sonography is an easily available, portable machine without radiation and diagnoses DVT with accuracy. If it is positive and showed thrombosis, then immediate anticoagulation needs to be started.

5.3 Ventilation-Perfusion Scan

The low- and high-probability scans are diagnostics. High-probability scans are reported to be up to 90% sensitive. Lung collapse and consolidation will decrease the accuracy of the VQ scanning.

5.4 Single Photon Emission CT Ventilation (SPECT VQ)

SPECT VQ is superior to plain VQ scan scintigraphy and CTPA with improved sensitivity of diagnosis.

5.5 Digital Subtraction Angiography

DSA is a historical gold standard for the diagnosis of PE. Nowadays, rarely used due to lesser sensitivity and higher false positivity.

5.6 Computed Tomographic Pulmonary Angiography (CTPA)

CTPA is increasingly used for the diagnosis of PE as it is sensitive as well as specific for PE, it not only rules out PE but also gives an alternative diagnosis. Only the concern is missing small thrombi in pulmonary circulations. Patients with acute kidney injury, allergic to contrast CTPA is a relative contrast indication.

5.7 Magnetic Resonance Pulmonary Angiography (MRPA)

It has higher sensitivity and specificity in diagnosing PE reported up to 92% and 100%, respectively. It is not validated in pregnancy and needs further studies. It is time consuming and not available in some centers.

5.8 Echocardiography

2D ECHO may show typical McConnell sign in patients with PE, and it is also helpful in ruling out other cardiac abnormalities or pathologies.

6 Treatment

Treatment of pulmonary embolism during pregnancy depends on the timing of the PE and hemodynamic stability. For pregnant patients with severe hypotension and hemodynamic derangements, treatment options are thrombolysis, thrombectomy, and extracorporeal membrane oxygenation (ECMO).

1. Thrombolysis is considered if there are no contraindications for it. Tissue plasminogen activator is still the drug of choice for thrombolysis. In case series of thrombolysis for PE in pregnant patients with shock, main complications were bleeding 8% and no intracranial hemorrhage were reported.
2. The second line of therapy in pregnant patients with PE and hemodynamic instability is ECMO, there are case reports of the successful use of ECMO in pregnant patients with massive PE [10].
3. Surgical thrombectomy is another alternative to the above-mentioned procedures in pregnant patients with hemodynamic instability. However, the data is limited, in a case series of 8 patients, there was no maternal death, with 37.5% fetal mortality and 50% preterm deliveries [11].

Peripartum PE; Management of PE in this period, we have to weigh the risk and benefits, and it's common to use unfractionated heparin with blood and blood products standby, and fractionated heparin as a choice as it can be easily reversible.

During pregnancy, low molecular weight heparin (LMWH) is the anticoagulant of choice due to the advantage of better bioavailability, lower bleeding risk, lower rates of HIT (heparin-induced thrombocytopenia), and osteopenia.

Warfarin is contraindicated due to its teratogenicity. To know about the use of direct oral anticoagulation (DOAC) and newer oral anticoagulation (NOAC), still further studies are needed on their safety during pregnancy.

7 Prevention

Pharmacological prophylaxis (commonly) with LMWH is recommended in pregnancy with absolute risk such as inherited thrombophilia. Postpartum thromboprophylaxis is recommended in patients with thrombophilia, a family history of DVT, obesity, and the patients with more than two risk factors for DVT. Patients with low risk for DVT or PE should use elastic compression stockings and should be mobilized early.

8 Conclusion

Pulmonary embolism is a life-threatening clinical entity in pregnancy. There are various risk factors, the common one is inherited thrombophilia. Commonly DVT leads to PE and can cause right heart failure and cardiac arrest. CTPA remained the commonest radiological technique for the diagnosis of PE. Low molecular weight heparin is the anticoagulation of choice during pregnancy due to obvious advantages. Early mobilization, the use of elastic stockings, and pharmacological thrombo-prophylaxis may help in the prevention of PE.

References

1. Cantwell R, et al. Saving mothers' lives: reviewing maternal deaths to make motherhood safer: 2006-2008. BJOG Int J Obstet Gynaecol. 2011;118:1–203.
2. Simcox LE, Ormesher L, Tower C, Greer IA. Pulmonary thrombo-embolism in pregnancy: diagnosis and management. Breathe. 2015;11:282–9.
3. Alsayegh F, et al. Venous thromboembolism risk and adequacy of prophylaxis in high risk pregnancy in the Arabian Gulf. Curr Vasc Pharmacol. 2016;14:368–73.
4. Greer IA. Thrombosis in pregnancy: maternal and fetal issues. Lancet. 1999;353:1258–65.
5. Boeldt DS, Bird IM. Vascular adaptation in pregnancy and endothelial dysfunction in pre-eclampsia. J Endocrinol. 2017;232:R27–44.
6. Bremme KA. Haemostatic changes in pregnancy. Best Pract Res Clin Haematol. 2003;16:153–68.
7. American College of Obstetricians and Gynecologists' Committee on Practice Bulletins–Obstetrics. ACOG Practice Bulletin No. 197: inherited thrombophilias in pregnancy. Obstet Gynecol. 2018;132:e18–34.
8. Shaikh N, Ummunnisa F, Aboobacker N, Gazali M, Kokash O. Open J Obstet Gynecol. 2013;3:158–64.
9. Cutts BA, et al. The utility of the Wells clinical prediction model and ventilation-perfusion scanning for pulmonary embolism diagnosis in pregnancy. Blood Coagul Fibrinolysis. 2014;25:375–8.
10. Bataillard A, et al. Extracorporeal life support for massive pulmonary embolism during pregnancy. Perfusion. 2016;31:169–71.
11. te Raa GD, Ribbert LSM, Snijder RJ, Biesma DH. Treatment options in massive pulmonary embolism during pregnancy; a case-report and review of literature. Thromb Res. 2009;124:1–5.

Peripartum Hemorrhage: Recent Updates in Management

Arabo Ibrahim Bayo, Isaac Babarinsa, Tukur Ado Jido, Sawsan Al Obaidly, and Mohamed A. M. Shahata

Abstract Peripartum hemorrhage, which can occur during pregnancy, labor, or delivery, is an all-inclusive term for bleeding that can happen from 24+0 weeks of gestation to 12 weeks after birth. It is a serious obstetric emergency that affects the entire world and is linked to both mother and fetal morbidity and mortality. It continues to be difficult to treat and to be a significant financial burden. One to ten percentage of deliveries are being complicated by peripartum hemorrhage, and it is the sixth most common cause of maternal mortality in the UK between 2015 and 2017, accounting for 8% of all maternal deaths. Postpartum hemorrhage can be categorized into primary and secondary categories. The 4Ts (Tone, Trauma, Tissue, and Thrombin) are typically used to describe the etiopathogenesis of primary PPH. Over 70% of primary PPH cases had inadequate uterine contractions or uterine atony as a contributing factor. Clinical detection of bleeding severity necessitates alertness and a high degree of suspicion. It is a preventable cause of maternal death and improvements in pharmacology, anesthesia, blood transfusion/hematological support, and innovative surgical methods have dramatically reduced mortality. Rotational thrombelastometry (ROTEM) testing has recently been proven to be a quicker way to diagnose coagulopathy in those who are bleeding. Early resuscitation to prevent hypovolemic shock, to achieve hemodynamic stability, and other specialized strategies as well as identification and management therapy of the underlying cause(s) of the hemorrhage are crucial in controlling peripartum hemor-

A. I. Bayo (✉)
Women's Wellness and Research Center, Hamad Medical Corporation, Doha, Qatar

College of Medicine, Qatar University, Doha, Qatar
e-mail: Abayo@hamad.qa

I. Babarinsa · T. A. Jido · M. A. M. Shahata
Women's Wellness and Research Center, Hamad Medical Corporation, Doha, Qatar

S. Al Obaidly
Women's Wellness and Research Center, Hamad Medical Corporation, Doha, Qatar

Weill Cornell Medical College, Doha, Qatar

N. Shaikh et al. (eds.), *Updates in Intensive Care of OBGY Patients*,
https://doi.org/10.1007/978-981-99-9577-6_6

rhage. It has been demonstrated that routine delivery room drills, simulations, and quick multidisciplinary team involvement further improve care even when major bleeding happens suddenly. Proper application of all these should make maternal mortality purely due to hemorrhage a rare event.

Keywords Peripartum hemorrhage · Obstetrics hemorrhage · Postpartum hemorrhage · Placenta accrete spectrum · 4T · ROTEM · Hemorrhagic shock

1 Introduction

Peripartum hemorrhage is a global issue which is associated with both maternal and fetal morbidity and mortality. It is a major obstetric emergency complicating 1–10% of deliveries [1] and is a primary cause of death of about a quarter of all the estimated 287,000 women who die annually from complications of pregnancy and childbirth globally [2]. In the UK, tri-annual report of the inquiry on maternal mortality 2015–17, bleeding accounted for 8% of maternal deaths making it the sixth most common cause of maternal deaths during the period [3].

While peripartum hemorrhage (PeriPH) is still a major obstetrics problem and had been so since the advent of obstetrics practice, recent advances in practice and reports shows that most of these are preventable deaths. Therefore, women should not die for giving birth to life. With advances in pharmacology, anesthesia, blood transfusion/hematological support, and new surgical techniques, we now have the tools to prevent most, if not all, of these maternal deaths [4–7]. A ten-fold reduction in maternal deaths in the UK has been documented over a period of 60 years [8], this has been attributed to confidential case reviews, surveillance, and implementation of recommendations in care provision. Similar national initiatives have achieved commendable reduction in maternal mortality and morbidity in Japan [9]. Comparatively obstetrics bleeding accounted for a third of the 196,000 women who died from pregnancy-related complications in sub-Saharan Africa, where such resources and initiatives/good practices implementations are lacking [10]. Also, in Brazil Peru, Bolivia, and the Dominican Republic hemorrhage have been the leading cause of maternal death, thus the launch of a "Zero maternal death by hemorrhage initiative" by PAHO/WHO [11, 12].

Peripartum hemorrhage, however, remains a challenge and a huge burden even in well-resourced societies. In these societies, obstetric hemorrhage and its complications is one of the leading causes of maternal intensive care unit (ICU) admissions [13]. Countries like the USA also still have high maternal deaths because of hemorrhage due to inequalities in healthcare provision [14, 15].

The bleeding may be during the antenatal, intrapartum, or postpartum period. However, postpartum hemorrhage (PPH) is the main component of periPH and remains the leading cause of maternal morbidity and mortality worldwide.

Peripartum hemorrhage also has a huge negative impact on perinatal morbidity and mortality. This is due to premature delivery and intrauterine fetal compromise or death as a result of severe hemorrhage thereby making it a complex clinical issue to deal with.

To help in reducing/preventing these deaths and severe morbidity in mothers and their babies, it is essential to have proper definition, identification of etiology and risk factors and early structured interventions in the care of pregnant women.

2 Definitions and Classification

Peripartum hemorrhage is an all-encompassing term that refers to bleeding from 24+0 weeks of gestation up to 12 weeks after delivery. This includes bleeding in the antepartum, intrapartum, and the postpartum periods. It also includes all obstetric hemorrhage form 24 weeks of gestation as well as maternal bleeding in the third trimester, not related to the pregnancy, like splenic rupture due to trauma in the pregnant woman. This group of patients are uncommon, as such usually receive less focus in discussion of peripartum hemorrhage.

The diagnostic criteria and classifications depend on the period when the bleeding occurs in respect of the delivery of the baby. In antepartum hemorrhage (APH), the bleeding occurs, from 24 weeks of gestation, before the baby is delivered. Bleeding after delivery of the baby is PPH even occurring before the placenta is delivered. The term intrapartum bleeding is frequently used to refer to APH mostly and a times PPH when bleeding occurs before delivery of the placenta after the delivery of the baby. The most common bleeding in labor is show which represent the bloody mucoid discharge of the mucus plug. Any bleeding adjudged to be more than a show before the delivery of the baby is an APH while that occurring from the third stage of labor onward is postpartum hemorrhage if adjudged to be more than the physiologic loss that occurs with delivery of placenta. It is pertinent to note that in denoting the terms, APH represents any form of bleeding no matter how mild while the bleeding in PPH is based on a quantitative threshold.

The threshold for definition of PPH varies, traditionally this is defined as bleeding of 500 mL or more following vaginal delivery or 1000 mL or more associated with cesarean delivery [16]. The American College of Obstetrics and Gynecologists (ACOG) defined PPH as blood loss of 1000 mL or more irrespective of mode of delivery or any bleeding postpartum associated with signs and symptoms of hypovolemia and advised that blood loss of more than 500 mL after vaginal delivery is abnormal and warrant further investigation [17]. Belfort simply defined PPH as blood loss more than expected after delivery that is associated with signs and symptoms of hypovolemia.

The severity of hemorrhage may point to the etiology but more importantly guides management if severe morbidity and mortality is to be avoided. This is particularly so in antepartum hemorrhage where the definition represents any bleeding no matter how slight, and this is highlighted in the classification of severity of APH as shown in Table 1.

Table 1 Classification of bleeding in antepartum hemorrhage

Spotting	Staining, spot, or streak of blood noted on the underwear or sanitary pad
Minor hemorrhage	Blood loss of <50 mL and has settled
Major hemorrhage	A blood loss of between 50 and 1000 mL with no sign of maternal clinical shock or fetal compromise
Massive hemorrhage	A blood loss of >1000 mL and/or sign of maternal clinical shock or fetal compromise

Table 2 Advanced trauma life support classification

Class	Features
I	Loss of up to 15% blood volume; heart rate is minimally elevated or normal; no change in blood pressure, pulse pressure, or respiratory rate
II	Loss of 15–30% blood volume loss, tachycardia heart rate of 100–120 bpm, tachypnea of 20–24 breaths/min, decreased in pulse pressure (systolic blood pressure changes minimally if at all)
III	Loss of 30–40% blood volume, resulting in a significant drop in blood pressure and changes in mental status
IV	Loss of more than 40% blood volume, significant depression in blood pressure and mental status, hypotensive systolic blood pressure <90 mmHg and tachycardia >120 bpm

Assessment of severity of bleeding based on specified volumes is difficult in clinical practice and measurements in use are fraught with limitations. Methods include using graduated measurement containers like suction containers and V-drapes; visual assessment which gives rough estimates and subjective; gravimetry in which differences in weight of containment material are used and colorimetry [18]. Accuracy of measurement may be improved by combination of the above methods, where possible.

Estimation of blood loss in pregnant women with periPH must be done with caution as methods used have limitations, in some cases the main bleeding is concealed as in placental abruption, intra-abdominal bleeding and hematomas. Measured volumes must therefore be interpreted within the clinical context of the patient. Similarly, measured loss may be a false indicator of patient's condition in patients already compromised, as in anemia or underlying cardiac conditions, and should be carefully gauged against clinical findings to avoid severe morbidity and untoward outcomes.

The Advanced Trauma Life Support classification (Table 2) [19] is in common use and correlate volume estimates with clinical features of cardiovascular changes. This, however, is validated in trauma patients outside obstetrics. Pregnancy, as a compensated hemodynamic milieu may impact on the direct utility of this system. The California Maternal Quality Care Collaborative Staging System [20] is perhaps the most established staging system in obstetrics population.

Table 3 California Maternal Quality Care Collaborative Staging System

Stage 0	Every patient in labor/giving birth
Stage 1	Blood loss ≥500 mL vaginal birth or ≥1000 mL cesarean birth with continued bleeding or signs of concealed hemorrhage. Vital signs abnormal or trending (heart rate ≥110 bpm, blood pressure ≤85/45 mmHg, O_2 saturation <95%, shock index 0.9) or confusion
Stage 2	Continued bleeding or vital sign instability, and <1500 mL cumulative blood loss
Stage 3	Continued bleeding with cumulative blood loss >1500 mL or >2 units transfusion of packed red blood cells or abnormal vital signs or suspicion of disseminated intravascular coagulation

3 California Maternal Quality Care Collaborative Staging System

The California Maternal Quality Care Collaborative Group, obstetrics hemorrhage tool kit describes stages of severity of postpartum bleeding as in Table 3.

4 Risk Factors and Causes of Peripartum Hemorrhage

Some bleeding is almost an inevitable end of every pregnancy and all pregnant women are at risk of major hemorrhage. However, certain factors predispose patients to bleeding which if not timely and correctly managed may imperil the mother and/or fetus. While some of these factors are specific to certain forms of peripartum hemorrhage, a host of them are generic. In some instances, the bleeding is a consequence or complications of pregnancy-related interventions. Furthermore, the risk factors are dynamic and sometime changes during the antenatal and postnatal period.

Antepartum hemorrhage: placental abruption, a leading cause of APH, for example, is commonly associated with prolonged rupture of membranes, chorioamnionitis, hypertension, thrombophilia, previous placental abruption, and abnormal placentation. Smoking and substance misuse especially crack cocaine are recognized predispositions. Abruption may complicate procedures like external cephalic version [21, 22]. Other causes (Table 4) of APH, such as placenta previa, are strongly associated with previous uterine surgery, multiple pregnancy, and previous history.

The main causes of APH like placenta previa and placental abruption constitute risk for PPH, and some of the causes are both for APH and PPH (Table 4). PPH, in addition, is more common in grand multiparity, multiple pregnancy, previous uterine surgery, morbidly adherent placenta, induced labor, prolonged labor and precipitate labor, prolonged use of oxytocin, instrumental delivery and retained placenta. Patients with prepartum anemia and/or cardiac diseases may have limited

Table 4 Causes of peripartum hemorrhage

Antepartum	Postpartum
Placenta previa	Four Ts Tone Trauma Tissue Thrombin
Placental abruption	Uterine atony Uterine inversion
	Bleeding disorder
Placenta accreta, increta, and percreta	Retained placenta
Vasa previa	Genital tract trauma
Uterine rupture	Placenta accreta, increta, and percreta
Cervical varices	
Incidental: lower genital tract trauma, cervical inflammation/infection, polyps, carcinoma	
Splenic artery rupture	

tolerance to blood loss and may meet some diagnostic threshold for PPH even with smaller blood loss.

The etiopathogenesis of primary PPH is generally adapted in the frame 4Ts (Tone, Trauma, Tissue, and Thrombin). Most, over 70%, of primary PPH is associated with uterine atony or poor uterine contraction. The resulting bleeding can progress rapidly, and it is this category of PPH that account for most of the related maternal morbidity and mortality. Risk factors for uterine atony include multiple pregnancy, grand multiparity, chorioamnionitis, pelvic masses like fibroids, ovarian cyst, full bladder, and previous surgery. Others are labor-related factors like prolonged/obstructed labor and other labor dystocia [22].

Genital tract trauma involving the vagina, vulva, cervix, uterus, or the broad ligament area are the next common causes of primary PPH. This should be a specific consideration in patients with previous surgery (vaginal or uterine), precipitate labor, obstructed labor, following instrumental delivery, midline episiotomy, persistent occipito-posterior position and second-stage cesarean section. A ruptured uterus is also an important traumatic cause of PPH.

Tissue: Retained placenta and/or membrane or blood clots, morbidly adherent placenta, and improper management of the third stage of labor are the usually the risk factors associated with this cause.

Thrombin—in about 7% of cases, primary PPH is associated with coagulation disorders and/or bleeding diathesis. This may be hereditary as in Von Willebrand disease or more commonly a consequence of consumption coagulopathy seen in patients with severe abruption, preeclampsia/HELLP syndrome, thrombocytopenia, and chorioamnionitis.

Secondary PPH is commonly associated with retained products of conception and/or endometritis and rarely vascular abnormalities such as arteriovenous (AV) malformation.

5 Diagnosis/Recognition

Diagnosis of peripartum hemorrhage in the antenatal period is mainly based on bleeding from the genital tract. Rarely bleeding may be concealed. However, the severity of the bleeding needs to be recognized so appropriate management can be instituted. The classification and/or severity of bleeding are in Tables 1, 2, and 3.

In the postpartum period, some bleeding is expected and considered normal physiological part of delivery and puerperium. It is however vital to estimate the amount of blood loss, so abnormal bleeding can be recognized and treated early. Blood loss measurement should be complemented with assessment of the vital signs changes which may indicate severity of the blood loss and may be the first indicators of concealed bleeding or hematoma. Methods of measurement of blood loss include graduated containers like V-drapes/pocket/suction canister; visual assessment which is rough and subjective; gravimetry which uses weight containment materials and colorimetry. Combination of these methods, where possible, may improve accuracy of quantification of the blood loss.

Clinical recognition of severity of bleeding requires vigilance and high index of suspicion. All pregnant patients should be risk assessed for peripartum hemorrhage. Patients at high risk should have preventive measures prescribed and carried out at the appropriate stage. At presentation, it is essential to appraise clinical features in all patients, interventions should be targeted, focused, and timely as conditions may evolve rapidly.

A thorough history aimed at risk stratification and, where bleeding has started, determined the cause and extent of bleeding. Relevant records should be reviewed including antenatal care, ultrasound scans, and laboratory results. Once patient is stabilized, the gestational age and location of the placenta should be crosschecked as well as welfare of the fetus.

A detailed clinical examination to ascertain the general condition of the patient should be done. Abdominal examination eliciting distension and tenderness, or absence thereof is discerning. PeriPH associated with soft, non-tender abdomen in which fetal lie and presentation is easily palpated should raise the possibility of placenta previa in which case pelvic examination should be avoided. While a tense, tender rigid abdomen with/without FHR abnormality points to abruption of placenta.

The vital signs should specifically be watched in the clinical assessment of these patients. Heart rate >100 bpm should suggest non-physiological pregnancy changes and uncompensated loss and rates above 120 bpm indicate more severe blood loss.

Blood pressure, especially where baseline reading is known, is a good guide to the degree of blood loss. In all circumstances a systolic blood pressure of <100 mmHg needs to be scrutinized closely. Similarly, increased in respiratory rate may be indicative of severity of blood loss and should be complemented with the oxygen saturation SaO_2 low levels of which should promptly be corrected to avoid cerebral hypoxia commonly presenting as agitation, confusion, obfuscation, lethargy as features of major or severe blood loss.

Urinary output is a good clinical indicator of kidney perfusion and reliable measure of the extent of blood loss and/or volume replacement. Urine output of <30 mL/h suggest poor renal perfusion or inadequate volume replacement during resuscitation [23].

Changes in vital signs could be indicative of the degree of hemorrhagic shock. The Society of Obstetrics and Gynaecologists of Canada (SOGC) has provided a guide on interpreting the clinical picture in relation to the degree of shock.

6 Investigations

At the time of initial clinical assessment, urgent baseline laboratory investigations such as full blood count, blood group and hold/crossmatch, urea, electrolyte, creatinine, and lactate as well as coagulation profile, including fibrinogen level should be checked.

Fibrinogen level is an important predictor of major PPH and a more sensitive indicator of ongoing bleeding than activated partial thromboplastin time (APTT), prothrombin time (PT), and platelet count. Fibrinogen levels less than 2 g/L is predictive of major PPH and defines the need for transfusion of multiple units of blood and blood products, admission to the ICU and maternal death. Recently, the rotational thrombelastometry (ROTEM) test has been shown to be a faster and more specific test for coagulopathy in bleeding patients [24].

The Kleihauer-Betke test helps determine the amount of additional anti-D to be administered. Previous ultrasound reports should be reviewed where available. Targeted ultrasound scan to determine the gestational age, fetal viability as well as possible site and extent of bleeding should be performed as soon as the clinical situation allows.

7 Prevention/Potential Deterioration

Various attempts have been made with the hope of preventing obstetric hemorrhage. However, all the recommended measures do not necessarily prevent bleeding but can reduce the severity of blood loss and/or the consequences thereof. Correcting anemia in pregnancy, identification, and proper management of hemoglobinopathies, judicious use of oxytocic, active management of third stage of labor, proper management of retained placenta and control of bleeding, prompt suturing of episiotomies and vaginal tears reduce severity of hemorrhage and its consequences [25].

Perhaps, more importantly is patient and provider education aiming at early identification of patients at risk of obstetric hemorrhage so measures, outlined above, could be initiated to prevent the occurrence and mitigate the severity of bleeding where it ensued. All at risk patients should be advised to deliver in facilities with blood transfusion service.

In bleeding patients, quantitative assessment help identify patients early, allow earlier escalation within the multidisciplinary team hierarchy, streamline preventive and resuscitative efforts, and mitigate on the severity and sequalae of periPH [26, 27].

Prediction tools for peripartum hemorrhage have been developed to help prevent severe morbidity and mortality. In their recent guideline, the SOGC recommend assessment of all patients for PPH at the beginning of labor and regularly thereafter [28]. Peripartum hemorrhage is a rapidly evolving clinical situation where deterioration proceeds quickly in the absence of timely sequence of appropriate interventions that predict and mitigate severe morbidity, especially hypovolemic shock, which is the common pathway for all related morbidity and mortality.

All patients with obstetric hemorrhage should have a dynamic risk assessment as well as evaluation of cumulative blood loss whether it is during antenatal or postpartum period. Predictive measures in everyday practice like vital signs can be deceptive, especially in young healthy pregnant women. In the compensated state of shock, blood pressure and heart rate for instance are usually normal.

Algorithms such as Maternity Early Obstetrics Warning Signs (MEOWS) are widely deployed and validated internationally [29]. In Qatar, this is adapted as Qatar Early Warning Signs-QEWS, with additional hierarchy of responsibilities especially at senior clinician level to reflect the needs and peculiarities of our patient population, balanced against available resources, especially human resources.

Other algorithms are: Modified Early Warning Score (MEWS), Maternal Early Recognition Criteria (MERC), Maternal Early Warning trigger (MERT), and APACHE II score [30].

A recent advance has been the increased utilization of the Shock Index (SI)

$$\left\{ \mathrm{SI} = \frac{\text{Heart rate}}{\text{Systolic blood pressure}} \right\}$$

The Shock Index was proposed by Allgower et al. (1967) [31] as a quotient designed to improve detection of severe circulatory collapse in the setting of hypovolemic medical patients. It has since been validated in large retrospective studies to show that, compared to standard vital signs in isolation, it is more sensitive in the prediction of developing hypotension, the need for massive transfusion, and rates of post-intubation hypotension [32].

A 2014 systematic review of 351 publications on SI concluded that it is a readily available tool in predicting critical bleeding on arrival to hospital [33]. Its general validity in predicting PPH among 30,820 women following vaginal deliveries was reported by Ushida et al. (2021) [34]. Threshold of 0.9 is well established in critical care and trauma [35, 36], in obstetric population, Le Bas et al. (2014), found the normal SI to be 0.7–0.9 with values >1, as a useful adjunct in estimating blood loss in cases of massive PPH and a predictor for need of blood and blood products [37]. This threshold has been validated in an obstetrics population in Scandinavia [38]. It should be borne in mind that both heart rate and blood pressure are affected by common medications, such as anti-hypertensives, beta blockers, and inotropes, used in obstetric critical care. As such, consideration should be given in the interpretation of the SI where these are being used.

It has been reported that almost 90% of deaths due to PPH happen within the first 4 h of delivery. It is therefore essential to be vigilant during this period. Assessment of cumulative bleeding, vital signs and general condition of the patient should be closely monitored and interpreted within the frame of QEWS and SI as appropriate.

8 Management of Peripartum Hemorrhage

At the current stage of medical science and medical practice, we cannot prevent obstetrics hemorrhage. However, we must not allow women to die from obstetrics hemorrhage. This is because we have the knowhow and the tools to minimize severe morbidity and prevent death.

Obstetrics hemorrhage is one of those conditions that if not recognized and managed adequately in time can evolve from being a simple hemorrhage to a catastrophic situation of severe morbidity and even mortality. This fits well with the founder of Apple, Steve Jobs' dictum that "it was extremely difficult to make complex things simple, whereas it was easy to make simple things complex." Passage of time invariably increases the complexity of obstetrics hemorrhage where hypotension, shock, coagulopathy, and end-organ injury set in, in the absence of the correct and timely interventions [39, 40].

Successful management depends on early recognition, effective communication, accurate assessment, and timely application of coordinated, focused interventions through a multidisciplinary team [18, 28, 41, 42]. Once recognized it is important that patients and birthing partners are informed and immediate obstetrics, midwifery, anesthetic teams are alerted. Moderate to severe bleeding warrants involvement of blood transfusion services and senior members of the multidisciplinary team.

In managing periPH to achieve the desired goal, an initial general approach along with specific measures are essential and should comprise of:

1. Early resuscitation to avoid hypovolemic shock.
2. Management of bleeding and associated complications.
3. Identification and management of underlying cause(s) of the hemorrhage.

8.1 *Initial/General Approaches*

Women presenting with peripartum hemorrhage should have immediate assessment and coordinated management. The broad approach in management of peripartum hemorrhage is outline in Fig. 1. Focused history and clinical examination as well as investigations should be the first approach. This must be done simultaneously with prompt and early resuscitation to prevent and/or reverse hypovolemia.

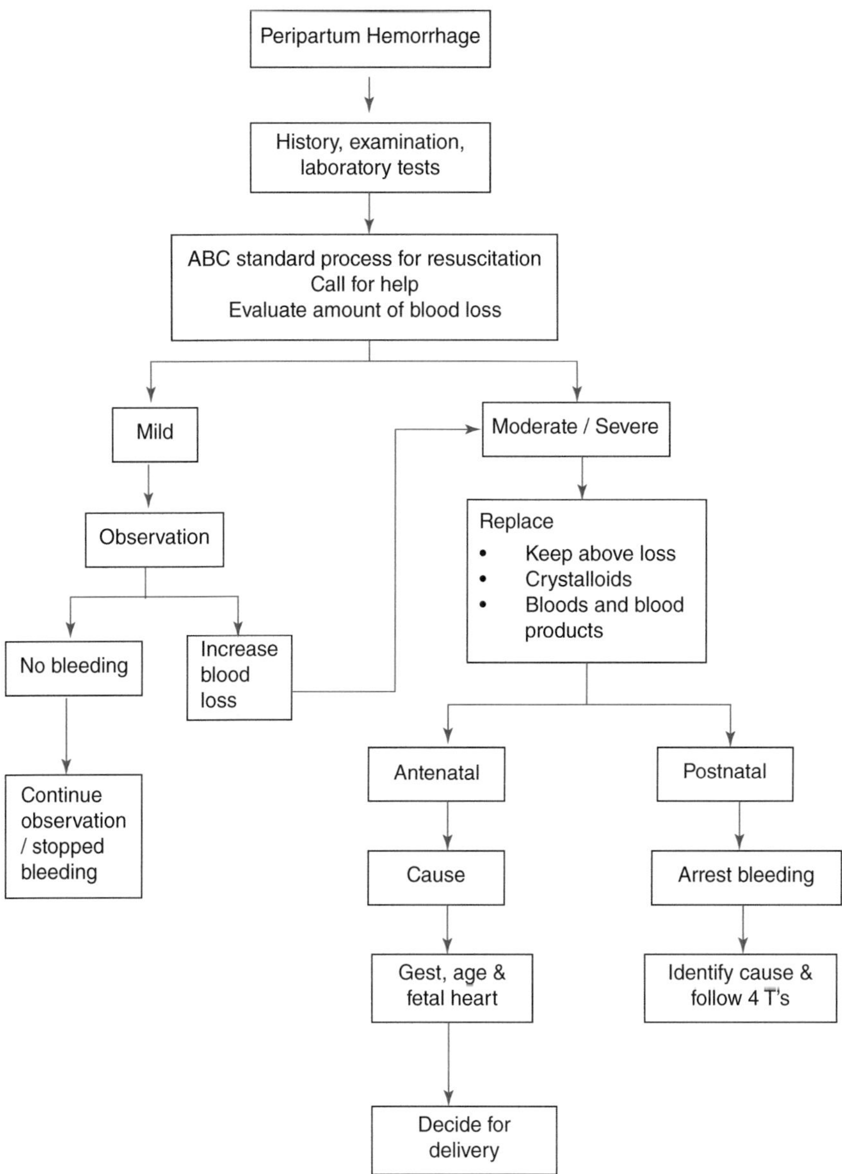

Fig. 1 Flow chart for management of peripartum hemorrhage

Minor PPH should be escalated, immediate intravenous access secured, group and hold, complete blood count, and coagulation screen including fibrinogen. They should be started on crystalloids. Monitoring should include pulse, blood pressure, respiratory rate, and oxygen saturation, initially every 15 min and if stable and bleeding stops hourly. Crossmatch 2 units of blood (PRBC) and give or increase rates of intravenous fluid to achieve normovolemia.

In major hemorrhage, immediate help should be summoned, and major hemorrhage declared. Theater should be notified and if not already arranged, an emergency team with clear roles and responsibilities should be constituted. Where possible consent for possible vaginal and/or abdominal exploration are obtained.

Resuscitation should proceed using ABC approach in standard manner. Patient is kept warm, placed in flat position with requisite tilt where appropriate, intravenous crystalloids commenced until blood is available. The rate and volume of bleeding is assessed continuously and recorded. High flow oxygen is administered at 15 L/m. A second wide bore IV cannula is inserted. In addition to the bloods above, Ca^{2+}, K^{+}, and lactate are checked. The vital signs are monitored every 5 min.

If required blood should not be delayed, including use of group O rhesus negative blood. Up to 3.5 L of crystalloids may be infused and the best available equipment may be required to facilitate rapid volume replacement. The anesthetist usually leads these aspects of resuscitation including administration of concentrated oxygen. Point-of-care tests, ABG, and ROTEM are increasingly becoming useful adjuncts in resuscitation [24].

Where bleeding continues or patient becomes unstable, massive PPH should be declared. Protocol for massive PPH should be activated, requiring blood bank hotline to be called, emergency team ascertained and if not already in theater the patient should be transferred as soon as is safe and practical. Additional help may be required, as such other obstetricians/gynecologic surgeons, anesthetists, and the intensive care unit should be notified.

Measures to control the bleeding are concurrently deployed by the obstetrics team. It is important to maintain clear communication with all members of the team. This may involve delivery in APH and bimanual compression and use of uterotonics or surgical interventions in PPH [41, 43, 44]. Finding the cause and arresting the hemorrhage is essential at this point. These patients should be monitored, closely having their heart rate, blood pressure, oxygen saturation, respiratory rates, urine output, and ECG continuously checked. Patients with major or massive hemorrhage would require high dependency care after the control of bleeding.

It is pertinent to note that there are no firm criteria for red blood cell transfusion and decision for this should be based on clinical and hematological indices jointly appraised by the senior members of the MDT. Other measures and surgical procedures required will depend on the cause of the bleeding and whether the abdomen is opened or not. These are highlighted under specific measures as outlined later in this chapter.

All units must have major obstetrics bleeding protocols in place. These includes a close liaison between clinical areas and hematology laboratory that will make products including O rhesus negative blood immediately available. Antibody positive patients with hemorrhage present a peculiar challenge and their management should be anticipatory, including making the right blood products available locally, before any potential bleeding episode. The absence of this should not delay lifesaving interventions. Special blood filters are not recommended in major periPH but where practical cell salvage may be considered.

Patients with ongoing bleeding who have received up to 4 units of packed RBC should be considered for fresh frozen plasma especially if hemostatic results are still awaited and where coagulopathy is suspected, and this should be earlier rather than later. A general approach of transfusing, in 1:1:1 ratio of PRBC: FFP: Platelets, corrects anemia, maintain perfusion, while maintaining hemostasis prior to outcome of coagulation panel, following which goal directed hemostatic management subsist. This is especially the case in situations like abruptio placenta, severe bleeding in Placenta Accrete Spectrum (PAS) disorder, amniotic fluid embolism, IUFD, and sepsis where coagulation may be normal at the beginning but deteriorates rapidly. Blood products order from the transfusion laboratory should be anticipatory to mitigate the impact of delay. In continuing bleeding, the principle is that replacement should aim not to lag behind the blood loss.

Where fibrinogen levels are <2 g/L, cryoprecipitate should be transfused. Similarly, the threshold for platelet transfusion in bleeding patients is $<75 \times 10^9$/L. Tranexamic acid should be given early as it is shown to reduce the severity of hemorrhage. The role of recombinant factor VII (rFVIIa) is limited to clinical trials [4, 41, 45].

In the event of massive transfusion, 4 units/h or 10 units in 24 h of PRBC administered, ionized Ca^{2+} and K^+ should be monitored and corrected.

Further management of peripartum hemorrhage depends on the cause and severity of the bleeding as well as whether it is occurring before the baby is delivered or after (antepartum or postpartum).

9 Antepartum Period

In the antepartum period, gestational age and condition of the baby are important considerations, as delivery of the baby may become inevitable; however, maternal consideration always supersede fetal consideration in making such decisions. In severe bleeding, the principle is to deliver the baby where:

(a) There is a significant risk to the life of the mother or fetus at any gestational age.
(b) At 34–36 weeks, there is an ongoing bleeding.
(c) At term (≥37 weeks), there has been a significant bleed, even if it has stopped, as subsequent bleeds are likely in these patients.

9.1 Placental Abruption

This is bleeding due to partial or complete separation of placenta after 24 weeks of gestation in a normally situated placenta. Risk factors include abdominal trauma, decompression of the uterus as in amniocentesis and vascular changes as in cocaine abuse, hypertensive disorders in pregnancy, smoking, uterine abnormalities, premature rupture of membranes, and multiple gestation. Previous placental abruption has a recurrence rate up to 20–30 times in subsequent pregnancies. This is especially common in antiphospholipid syndrome and congenital thrombophilia.

Between 0.4 and 1:100 [46, 47] pregnancies may be complicated by placental abruption. Three grades of placental abruption are described.

Mild (Grade I): Slight vaginal bleeding, uterine irritability with no signs of maternal shock or fetal compromise. This also includes asymptomatic patients with a retroplacental clot or infarct.

Intermediate (Grade II): Moderate vaginal bleeding, signs of uterine hypertonicity, maternal tachycardia although maternal blood pressure and fetal heart rate are normal.

Severe (Grade III): More severe vaginal bleeding with marked uterine tetany and changes in fetal heart rate. There may be persistent abdominal pain, maternal shock, and features of fetal compromise. This group comprises 15% of cases of placental abruption. In Grade IIIB, in addition there is coagulopathy.

The diagnosis of placental abruption is mainly clinical. Patients with placental abruption present with triad of vaginal bleeding, abdominal pain, and/or fetal heart abnormalities, depending upon the grade. The bleeding is usually associated with abdominal pain. The patient may notice the pain before or after the onset of bleeding. Clinical examination may reveal uterine tenderness and sometimes a woody hard uterus on palpation. The severity of bleeding or the whole episode of bleeding may be concealed in some cases. Such patient may present with only pain and the examination findings above. Fetal heart rate abnormality on cardiotocography (CTG) with typical sinusoidal pattern or bradycardia are common. In mild cases, the diagnosis may only be confirmed postpartum when retroplacental clot or infarct are seen. In some cases, ultrasound scan may reveal retroplacental clot and certainly confirm fetal viability otherwise its role is limited.

The major concern in placental abruption is of maternal and fetal compromise particularly in patients with placental abruption Grade III. It is a highly dynamic situation that can change from grade I to III rather quickly. Hemoglobin and coagulation profile are indicative of the severity of bleeding.

Immediate delivery of the baby by cesarean section is usually indicated in most cases of placental abruption. This is particularly applicable in patients with moderate to severe features.

In cases where there is intrauterine fetal death, vaginal delivery can be considered:

If there are no deteriorating in hemoglobin, coagulation profile or vital signs, the cervix is favorable, and there is no contra-indication to vaginal delivery. In the rare event of placental abruption in the second stage of labor, assisted vaginal delivery may be performed if it is deemed feasible and faster than a cesarean section. The mode of delivery in patients with coagulopathy must be carefully gauged against the risk of maternal hemorrhage and should be considered in consultation with anesthetic and hematology team.

In patients with milder condition (Grade I and II), a more measured and conservative approach may be considered, but continuous monitoring of the mother and fetus checking for features of deterioration is essential. In this situation, any signs of significant deterioration of mother and/or fetus should be an indication for immediate delivery.

Whether delivery is achieved vaginally or by cesarean section, continuous patient monitoring and re-evaluation is essential in the postpartum period, as this condition is associated with coagulopathy and is a risk for PPH. Immediate postpartum care should be High Dependency Unit (HDU) based.

9.2 Placenta Previa

In placenta previa, the placenta is wholly or partially located in the lower uterine segment. This complicates 4–5 per 1000 births and is commonly associated with previous uterine surgery, multiparity, assisted conception, multiple pregnancy, and previous placenta previa (with recurrence rate of 4–8% in subsequent pregnancies). Placenta previa is graded in relation to the placental lower edge location from the internal cervical os. With advances in imaging, current grading recommends three groups [18, 48, 49]:

Complete: The placenta partially or centrally covers the entire cervical os.

Incomplete: The placenta is in the lower uterine segment, the edge is within 2 cm of the internal cervical os, but not covering it.

Low-lying: The placenta is in the lower uterine segment, but the placental edge is between 2.0 cm and 3.5 cm from the internal cervical os.

This classification corresponds, to a certain degree, to the traditional classification of grades I–IV, placenta previa as: complete corresponds to grade III and IV; incomplete to grade I and II; and low lying to some cases in Grade I placenta previa and early low-lying placenta in the second trimester.

Ultrasonography is the mainstay of diagnosis of placenta previa. Clinical presentation with vaginal bleeding after 24 weeks that is typically painless and unprovoked. Initial bleeding is generally mild (warning bleed) the abdomen is usually soft and non-tender with fetal lie and presentations easily discerned. Fetal heart rate abnormalities are uncommon. In this clinical scenario, pelvic examination should be avoided until placental location is ascertained, so heavy bleeding is not provoked. In current practice, abnormal situation of the placenta if not heralded by an earlier bleed, as it is normally documented in earlier scan and requisite surveillance instituted mostly before the first bleed.

An expert group on ultrasound recommends placental position monitoring by ultrasound up to 32 weeks where the placenta covers or is within 2 cm of the internal os in mid-trimester anomaly scan. If at the 32-week examination, the placental edge is 2 cm or more from the internal os, the placenta position is reported as normal and no further ultrasound for placental position is indicated. If the placental edge covers or remains within 2 cm from the internal os, a further ultrasound scan should be performed at the 36th week [50]. If at the 36-week ultrasound follow-up, the placental edge is covering the internal os it is unlikely to migrate.

All patients with placenta previa covering the os should be delivered by cesarean section. However, if at the 36 weeks gestation ultrasound, the placenta is not covering the internal cervical os but is less than 2 cm from it, vaginal delivery may be considered, but keeping in mind that the risk of bleeding is increased. The risks and benefits of trial of labor or cesarean section should be discussed with these patients. The closer the edge of the placenta to the internal os the higher the risk of bleeding, furthermore associated conditions like vasa previa are common. Fetal head below the placental edge and anteriorly situated placentae are favorable features for vaginal delivery. A systematic review of 10 studies of patients with low-lying placenta undergoing trial of labor reported an emergency cesarean section rate of 45% and 10–14% in patient with placental edge to internal os of 0–10 and >10 mm, respectively [51].

Opinions vary on the timing of delivery in patients with stable placenta previa but is generally accepted that delivery should be after 36 weeks of gestation. Society for Maternal-Fetal Medicine and ACOG recommend delivery at 36 to 37+6 weeks of gestation [52, 53]. In the UK and in our practice, we deliver at 38–39 weeks. A recent retrospective study suggests 38+0 to 38+6 days as the optimal time for delivery, especially in uncomplicated cases [54].

In patients who have acute bleeding the timing of delivery remains the same as the principles outlined earlier in this chapter for termination of pregnancy in severe bleeding. Where the bleeding is not severe, with premature fetus, conservative management can be considered.

Whether conservative management is in hospital or at home remains a subject of debate. Observational data suggest that asymptomatic patients who had not experienced bleeding could be managed as outpatients until vaginal bleeding occurs or it is time for scheduled cesarean delivery. In deciding for outpatient management, risk factors such as short cervical length, rapid cervical shortening (>10 mm over 1–2-week period), the ability to get to the hospital promptly and home support should be considered [55].

Patients who have bleeding should be admitted to the hospital. If there is no significant bleeding and bleeding stopped for at least 24 h, they can be discharged and managed as outpatients. In our experience, most bleeds recur within 72 h, we therefore tend to observe select group of patients for this period before discharge. For patients who have had three or more bleeds during the pregnancy it is advisable that they stay in the hospital until delivery. A randomized trial of outpatient versus inpatient management of patients with placenta previa after an initial bleed that resolved, found no greater risk of morbidity in outpatient group than inpatients [56]. Another study found progressively increased risk of emergency cesarean section with more episodes of bleeding (OR 7.5, 14, and 27 for 1, 2, or 3 or more bleeds, respectively) [56, 57].

During the conservative management, it is important to optimize the hemoglobin and to keep blood ready in case of bleeding. A placenta previa bundle is recommended where specific details on who to be informed, anesthesia, preparation for delivery, and how to get blood ready is specified, particularly, when patients are admitted to the hospital.

At cesarean section oxytocin and other uterotonics should be administered as prophylaxis. Tranexamic acid should be given after delivery of the baby to help in controlling bleeding. Bleeding site injection of vasopressin, use of hemostatic, square sutures, ligation of uterine artery and uterine balloon tamponade, uterine compression sutures like B-Lynch are some of the measures that may be required. The need to use any of these depends on the bleeding. In rare situation, cesarean hysterectomy may become necessary as a last resort to stop bleeding. Patient with placenta previa must be closely monitored for PPH because of the increased risk of bleeding and possible coagulopathy.

In all cases of placenta previa effort must be made to exclude placenta accreta spectrum (PAS) because of their strong association. The presence of this is associated with more postpartum bleeding and sometime the need for hysterectomy.

9.3 Placenta Accreta Spectrum

PAS refers to morbidly adherent placenta (MAP) of various degrees of invasion of the myometrium (accreta, increta, and percreta). This mostly occurs in the lower uterine segment (Fig. 3a, b), but it can occur at other sites of placental insertions, away from lower segment [58, 59].

In further defining PAS, the FIGO Placenta Accreta Spectrum Disorder Diagnosis and Management Expert Consensus Panel came out with the following classification system that includes clinical and histologic criteria:

Grade 1: Abnormally adherent placenta; placenta adherent or accreta
Grade 2: Abnormally invasive placenta: increta
Grade 3: Abnormally invasive placenta: percreta

Subtype 3a: limited to uterine serosa
Subtype 3b: urinary bladder invasion
Subtype 3c: invasion of other pelvic tissue/organs

This spectrum of disease is thought to be because of uterine remodeling resulting in failure of normal decidualization and/or loss of normal decidua-myometrium layers and their replacement by scar tissue [60]. The risk factors associated with PAS are generally in situations where such uterine remodeling or scar formation has occurred such as a previous cesarean delivery and/or other uterine surgery. The most important risk factor for PAS is previous cesarean delivery, particularly when it is associated with a placenta previa in the index pregnancy. In a study of women with previous cesarean delivery and placenta previa [61], it was found that the frequency of PAS increased with the number of previous cesarean sections. PAS was reported in 11%, 40%, 61%, and 67% at the second, third, fourth, and fifth or more cesarean births, respectively. In the same study, in patients without placenta previa, it was found to be 0.2%, 0.1%, 0.8%, and 4.7% at the second, third, fourth or fifth and sixth or more cesarean births, respectively. Other surgical risk factors are previous myomectomy where the uterine cavity has been entered, hysteroscopic surgery, dilatation and curettage, endometrial ablation, resection of cornual ectopic pregnancy, manual removal of placenta. Non-surgical risk factors associated with PAS include pelvic irradiation, postpartum endometritis, multiparity, age greater than 35 years, multiple gestation, infertility, and/or Infertility procedures.

PAS without placenta previa is more likely to be associated with non-cesarean section risk factors outlined above. In a systematic review and meta-analysis [62], PAS without placenta previa was found to be less likely associated with prior cesarean birth.

The clinical presentation and diagnosis of PAS requires high index of suspicion taking into consideration the risk factors. This is particularly important when performing an early ultrasound scan.

In most cases the diagnosis of PAS would have been made earlier on ultrasound or MRI imaging. These patients may or may not present with painless vaginal bleeding, just as in placenta previa. Some of these patients are only diagnosed during surgery, particularly in healthcare settings where expertise and antenatal care is limited.

Ultrasound scan is the main diagnostic tool, but additional imaging may complement this in certain circumstances. Color Doppler for example is useful in confirming the diagnosis of PAS when combined with other ultrasound findings. MRI may be more useful in evaluation of a posterior PAS, assessment of depth of myometrial and parametrial or bladder involvement; and to evaluate the myometrium and placenta at the most lateral portions [63].

Laboratory investigations are limited in the diagnosis of PAS. Biomarkers such as maternal serum alpha fetoprotein (MSAFP) and pregnancy-associated plasma protein A (PAPP-A) have been suggested as associated findings with PAS but have not been found to be useful clinically [64, 65].

PAS is a serious condition which can result in more severe hemorrhage at delivery or postpartum and the management requires drilled, experienced multidisciplinary team. This is because the difficulty in controlling the associated hemorrhage, in view of neovascularization, and involvement of contiguous structures may result in severe maternal morbidity and sometimes mortality. Prematurity occasioned by early delivery increases perinatal morbidity and mortality.

Institutions need to have PAS Care Bundle for the management of these patients. These are set of standards aimed at improving the outcome of patients. These should normally be instituted before any antepartum bleeding occurs. An example of the care bundle and check list use in our institution is shown in Fig. 2a, b.

Once bleeding start, management is like that of major placenta previa. However, cesarean section is necessary in all cases of PAS, including cases with low-lying placenta and placentation away from the lower uterine segment. Unlike in placenta previa without morbid adherence, these patients should be delivered before term, even where bleeding has stopped or not occurred. In our practice, we deliver these patients at 34–36 weeks to forestall the eventuality of emergency bleeding and interventions when resources including personnel may not be optimal.

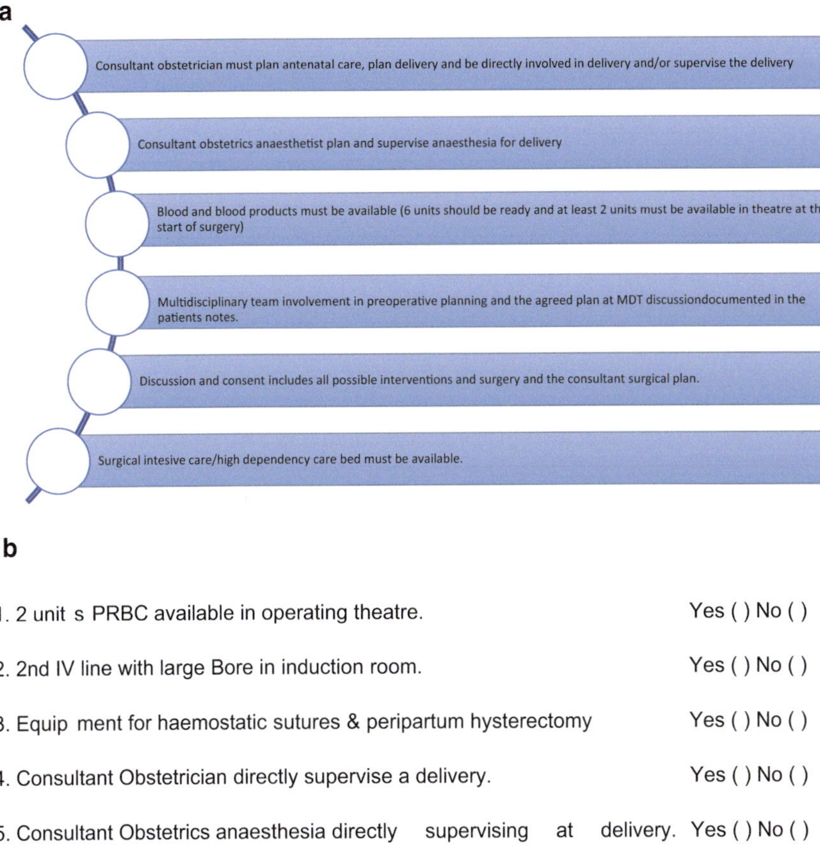

Fig. 2 (**a**) Care bundle for management of placenta accreta spectrum disorder: Women's Wellness and Research Center (WWRC). (**b**) Care bundle checklist and monitoring

At delivery, hysterectomy or conservative uterine sparing procedures may be performed. This is determined by depth of invasion, involvement of surrounding organs, depending on the severity/extent of invasion, availability of blood and blood products, reproductive wishes of the patient, sociocultural consideration, and most importantly expertise and experience of the multidisciplinary team. When deciding for hysterectomy, it is essential to understand that in many cases most of the bleeding is from placental invasion and neovascularization in areas outside the uterus such as the bladder, vaginal fornixes, parametrium, and broad ligament, which means hysterectomy may not always be the solution to the hemorrhage [63].

Conservative measures such as devascularizing sutures (uterine, ovarian, and internal iliac artery ligation), placental bed hemostatic sutures and uterine reconstruction may help in arresting the bleeding. Areas of invasion outside the uterus and neo-vascularization need to be treated separately to achieve full hemostasis, whether hysterectomy is to be performed or not. Where there is no bleeding, the placenta may be left in situ, to autolyze or to be removed later, but this carries a significant risk of secondary hemorrhage and severe infection.

Hysterectomy has been the traditional approach and widely practiced procedure. It could be technically difficult in some cases and may not be helpful in arresting bleeding from neovascularization and surrounding organ invasion. In cultures where high parity is the norm or there are beliefs against hysterectomy, it is not readily acceptable.

Many uterine sparing (conservative) measures are described and are deployed alone or in combination [63, 66–70].

- Manual removal of the placenta (extirpative technique) aimed to completely remove the placenta. This is, however, fraught with massive hemorrhage if not properly executed and most areas of bleeding controlled early.
- Leaving the placenta in situ. A transverse upper uterine incision is made away from the placenta to deliver the baby. The umbilical cord is ligated, the placenta is left undisturbed, and the uterus is closed. Patients are followed up with serial ultrasound scan (and occasionally, beta hCG), with the expectation that the placenta with decreasing vascular supply will eventually autolyze and/or be expelled. In this situation, the placenta is left alone, and patient followed up or done with additional procedures such as treatment using preventive devascularization (surgical/radiological).

Conservative surgical procedures: There are different types of these procedures performed in various centers, singly or in combination. Among these, FIGO guideline described the one-step conservative surgery, the triple-P procedure and the tamponade technique. In the one-step surgical technique where an upper segment hysterotomy is done to deliver the fetus, all invaded myometrial tissue and placenta is resected en-block, the myometrium is then reconstituted in two layers.

In the triple-P procedure, arterial balloon catheters are inserted preoperatively; no attempt is made to remove the entire placenta with large excision, no attempt to excise the myometrium with the PAS-disordered tissue, and no attempt to reconstitute the uterine defect.

In the tamponade technique, the cervix is inverted into the uterine cavity, and sutured to the wall of the lower uterine segment, to form a tamponade anteriorly or posteriorly depending on the area of involvement.

There are other conservative procedures performed in various parts of the world that are not captured by the FIGO group. In our institution, we use our own different method of uterine conservation. We aimed at uterine conservation in almost all cases owing to our peculiar sociocultural circumstances. Over the past 12 years, we have deployed the technique described below with considerable success in conserving the uterus, limiting maternal morbidity, no maternal or fetal mortality and good subsequent reproductive outcomes.

Our technique involves (some steps as given in Fig. 3a–c):

- Normal abdominal wall entry to access the lower uterine segment.
- Identification and ligation of abdominal wall and intra-abdominal wall adhesions and neovascularization with meticulous hemostasis.

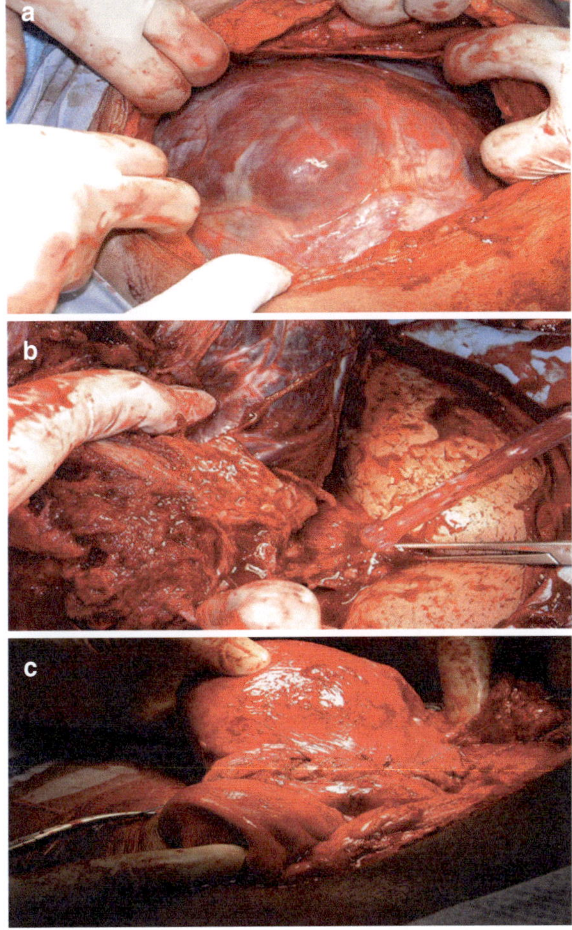

Fig. 3 (**a**) Placenta protruding through the lower uterine wall, with adherent bladder. (**b**) Placenta invading myometrium and its removal. (**c**) Reconstructed uterus. (© Dr. Arabo Ibrahim Bayo, 2024 All Rights Reserved)

- Dissecting the bladder off the lower uterine segment, while ligating vessels (including neovascularized vessels) between the uterus, bladder flap, and adjacent areas.
- Opening the uterus transversely, directly over the area of placental invasion/uterine defect and delivering the baby quickly through that.
- Immediately exteriorizing the uterus and manually compressing the uterine vessels by a firm hand grip posteriorly over the lower segment.
- Then removing most of the placental tissue.
- Then identifying and holding the edge of the internal cervical os with forceps.
- Placing hemostatic sutures at the angles of the uterine incisions and at the anterior portion of the lower flap of remaining lower segment onto the cervix.
- Then removing the remaining placental tissue.
- Attaching the remaining serosa and whatever myometrial tissue that remains to the identified upper cervix.

- Reconstructing the uterus using the serosa and myometrial remnant attached to the cervix taken along with the identified part of the internal cervical os and suturing these to upper myometrial/serosal flap.

Using this technique, in our institution, one of the authors has managed over 150 cases of PAS where only one patient proceeded to hysterectomy. This patient presented at 26th weeks gestation, with retroperitoneal hematoma that extended almost to the liver. The placenta had invaded retroperitoneally with MRI evidence of neovascularization from the ovarian vessels and aorta.

9.4 Uterine Rupture

Uterine rupture is the disruption of most or all layers of the pregnant uterus. It is complete where it involves the entire thickness of the uterine wall with the uterine cavity communicating with peritoneal cavity or "incomplete" where the uterine serosa remains intact. In the presence of a scar, the latter is described as a dehiscence. Overall incidence of rupture in the presence of prior cesarean scar is 3 per 1000 deliveries but more common among women undergoing trial of labor after cesarean birth [71].

The main risk factors are the presence of a uterine scar, previous uterine rupture, previous non-lower segment cesarean section, obstructed labor, injudicious use of oxytocics, myomectomy especially if endometrium was breached, grand multiparity, congenital uterine abnormalities, and maternal abdominal trauma [72, 73].

Uterine rupture usually occurs during labor but can occur before labor. It is difficult to predict thereby warranting vigilance in management especially of the at-risk patients. Presentation is acute or sudden onset of abdominal pain, vaginal bleeding, and abdominal tenderness on palpation. The fetal part may be easily palpable, cervical dilatation and station of the presenting part may regress and CTG abnormalities are common. Maternal cardiovascular instability, hematuria, and abnormal fetal heart (most commonly fetal bradycardia) are not uncommon. Other findings may include changes in uterine contraction pattern, including cessation.

Sometimes uterine rupture is diagnosed after vaginal delivery. Postpartum features include persistent vaginal bleeding, abdominal distension, maternal collapse, inability to maintain vital signs despite fluid resuscitation or persistent anemia despite blood transfusion.

Uterine rupture is a clinical diagnosis, but in stable patients where there is no maternal compromise or fetal heart rate changes, imaging may help to evaluate hemoperitoneum, disruption of the myometrium, fetal position outside the uterus and fetal viability [74, 75].

In some cases, uterine rupture may be difficult to distinguish from placental abruption, both present with acute abdominal pain, abnormal fatal heart rate, and vaginal bleeding. Also when acute abdominal pain occurs with normal or abnormal fetal heart in the absence of vaginal bleeding, traumatic rupture of abdominal viscus, hepatic rupture in pre-eclampsia and splenic artery rupture are differential diagnoses that require considering. Neuro-axial anesthesia is commonly associated with maternal hypotension and fetal heart abnormalities resulting from sympathetic blockade.

Once uterine rupture is suspected the management should be immediate and simultaneous; resuscitation and laparotomy by a multidisciplinary team comprising of Obstetricians, Anesthesiologists, Hematologists, Operating Theater staff, and Neonatologists. Arrangements should also be made for immediate blood products.

In most cases, the uterine defect needs to be repaired, and in rare situations hysterectomy becomes necessary. Evacuation of hemoperitoneum and repair of collateral organ damage such as bladder damage should then be undertaken. Postoperative management should include close monitoring, depending on hemodynamic stability of the patient [71].

9.5 *Vasa Previa*

Vasa previa is a rare complication where unprotected fetal blood vessels are coursing in the lower uterine segment over the cervical canal and are prone to injury at the time of amniotomy. Vasa previa occurs in multiple pregnancy, low lying placenta, velamentous insertion of the umbilical cord, bilobed placenta, and succenturiate lobe [76].

Patients usually present with mild to moderate vaginal bleeding associated with fetal heart rate abnormality, commonly sinusoidal pattern, or bradycardia. The amount of bleeding, usually mild, is disproportionate to the fetal heart rate abnormality because most of the blood loss is of fetal origin. The fetal blood vessels may rupture spontaneously in labor or more often inadvertently breached during amniotomy. The bleeding may sometimes be moderate when it consists of maternal blood. Rarely, a pulsating vessel may be palpated through the cervix or identified on scan; an important finding that obviates unintentional injury and fetal bleeding.

Diagnosis of vasa previa is clinical and requires high index of suspicion. Ultrasonography is confirmatory where there is no bleeding and color Dopplers are an important adjunct [77]. In the presence of bleeding, however, the expedience of management to save the baby supersedes confirmation of the diagnosis.

Immediate delivery by cesarean section and prompt resuscitation are the mainstay of management in these cases. The neonatal team should be informed of the diagnosis, so that arrangements can be made for red blood cell transfusion.

9.6 *Incidental Causes*

In many patients presenting with APH, the bleeding is because of non-placental causes including trauma, cervical ectopy, polyps, vulval or vaginal varices, and rarely cervical tumor and cervical varices.

The bleeding in this case is usually mild to moderate and the management is mainly resuscitation and suturing lacerations or removing polyps or hemostatic sutures applied to the vulval or vaginal varices [78].

10 Postpartum Hemorrhage

The definition, classification etiology, and risk factors for PPH are considered earlier in this chapter.

The etiology and management of PPH are closely linked to the type and severity of the bleeding. Hemorrhage within 24 h of delivery which by far is the most common and serious is primary PPH while bleeding, thereafter, up to 12 weeks postpartum is secondary PPH.

Morbidity and mortality in PPH are direct consequences of the amount of bleeding in all patients; therefore, successful management depends on accurate quantification, coordinated, focused, and timely interventions particularly replacement anchored on the background of effective communication in a multidisciplinary context. Multidisciplinary approach, control of bleeding, replacement of blood volume to foster adequate organs, tissue perfusion, and monitoring are the key elements of the management. These general measures are outlined in Table 5.

Assessment of bleeding, the central guide to management has been described earlier in this chapter.

PPH represent a sign of an underlying pathology which must be identified and managed. Resuscitation and assessment to identify the underlying cause should proceed *pari passu*. Effective communication and leadership help streamline the effort of the multidisciplinary team in resuscitation, control of the bleeding, and prevention of hypovolemic shock which is the common pathway to end-organ damage and mortality [41, 79].

Risk assessment of all patients in labor for PPH and identifying the at-risk patients (prediction) are essential. The SOGC in their recent guidance recommend risk assessment of all patients for PPH at the beginning of labor and regularly thereafter [28]. Preparation to prevent PPH can then be made for high-risk patients. This includes participation of personnel from different disciplines and specialties as would be highlighted. The degree of involvement depends on the severity of the PPH.

In minor PPH (blood loss 1000 mL or less), communication and general management of hemorrhage are described above. The situation is communicated to the senior midwifery, anesthetic, and obstetrics team. A wide bore 14G intravenous access is secured and specimen sent for complete blood count, liver function and renal function test, and coagulation screen including fibrinogen level. Four units of packed red cells are crossmatched. Resuscitation with warm IV crystalloid is commenced to maintain blood volume and tissue perfusion even if vital signs are stable. Women with minor PPH usually do not need blood product, except in those with anemia or other comorbidities. However, where blood transfusion is required, as in low hemoglobin, it should not be delayed.

Table 5 General measures in major and massive PPH

Major PPH	Massive PPH
• Initiate standard emergency resuscitation procedure of ABCs (airway, breathing, and circulation) • Assess rate and volume of bleeding • Monitor vital signs pulse, blood pressure, and pulse-oximetry continuously if possible or at 5–15 min interval • Administer oxygen by face mask on high flow oxygen 15 L/min and to keep $SpO_2 \geq 95\%$ • Establish two wide bore IV access—at least one 14 or 16G • Blood sample for full blood count, grouping and crossmatch, coagulation profile, full chemistry including fibrinogen level • Give IV warm crystalloids (Ringer's lactate) • Record cumulative total blood loss every 15 min until PPH is controlled • Keep the patient warm (temp >35 °C)	• As in major PPH above • Declare massive obstetric hemorrhage—ring Blood Bank hotline • Set up emergency team if it is not yet done • Move to theater if not already there • Call additional obstetrics/ gynecology surgeons as needed • Call additional anesthetist if needed • Notify Intensivist and Intensive Care Unit (ICU)

Control of hemorrhage involves emptying the bladder, bimanual compression of the uterus, and administration of medications. Oxytocin 10 IU, by intramuscular injection or by slow intravenous infusion of 5 IU. Ergometrine or its derivative methyl ergometrine (methergine) is a potent constrictor of smooth muscle and is effective in patients with PPH. Ergometrine should be avoided in hypertensive patients, Raynaud's phenomenon, and scleroderma. When bleeding is controlled, it is our practice to maintain uterine contraction with oxytocin infusion at rate of 10 IU/h (40 IU in 500 mL saline at 125 mL/h).

The use of tranexamic acid in PPH has recently gained traction, with a positive impact on overall blood loss [4, 80]. It is given at 1 g intravenously. Similarly, the efficacy of the synthetic prostaglandin misoprostol at a dose of 600–1000 mcg, sublingually or per rectum is well established. The main advantages of misoprostol and tranexamic acid are their low cost and stability which lend themselves to management of hemorrhage even in low resources settings.

In patients with major PPH (>1000 mL) and ongoing bleeding despite above measures, a second large bore peripheral canula should be secured and consideration given to arterial line and indwelling urethral catheter inserted. Intramuscular prostaglandin, carboprost is administered at a dose of 250 mcg and can be repeated after every 15 min. An anesthetic team should help with assessment and management of airway, breathing, and circulation [41].

In our practice, the management of patients with major PPH, who's bleeding persist after two doses of carboprost is to be transferred to the operating theater. Examination under anesthesia (EUA) to identify persistent uterine atony, genital tract trauma and/or retained products of conception is carried out in the theater. By this time, the result of the initial investigations including coagulation screen are available and a diagnosis is usually achieved. Subsequent definitive management depends on the diagnosis.

It is pertinent to note that resuscitation is a continuing process as the rate of hemorrhage is fast and the clinical situation evolve rapidly. Transfusion of blood must not be delayed and should be considered after 2.5–3 L of crystalloids bearing in mind there is no firm criteria for blood transfusion in a bleeding patient [81]. Fresh frozen plasma FFP is given at the rate of 12–15 mL/kg for every four units of blood transfused where hemostatic results are not available. But where PT and APTT are available and are >1.5 times more than 15 mL/kg of FFP will be required. The plasma fibrinogen should be maintained at >2 g/L in ongoing PPH. Low fibrinogen should be corrected with cryoprecipitate in liaison with the hematologist [82]. The threshold for platelet transfusion is in the region of 75×10^9/L. The preparation of these products takes time which requires early communication with the blood transfusion laboratory.

With ongoing bleeding, severe or massive PPH, examination of the patient under anesthesia helps establish the diagnosis. Uterine atony (tone) that is not responsive to uterotonics, and manual mechanical maneuvers is next managed by one or more compressions tamponade methods. Insertion of the Bakri balloon is a common and well-founded method. The Ebb's balloon has been used with similar outcome. Less commonly uterine packing with gauze is described. The technique of vacuum-induced tamponade has been recently introduced and is proving to be effective.

Where bleeding persists despite these measures, or where the abdomen is already opened, more invasive methods especially where bleeding ensued during cesarean section include the use of tamponade brace sutures. The B-lynch suture is the most common of these methods owing to its effectiveness and simplicity. Stepwise ligation of uterine and ovarian vessels can help in controlling bleeding. Internal iliac artery ligation is effective, but its safe application in the face of active bleeding operation field is limited and risk more bleeding especially in situation of coagulopathy. Also, the complexity of pelvic side wall dissection in this situation makes it a more common preserve of clinicians with requisite expertise and experience mostly with gynecology oncology support. Uterine artery embolization is now commonly used in the treatment of PPH where, preferably, in a bicameral theater with radiology facility available. Hysterectomy is a last resort measure to be considered where other methods failed but should be decided early.

Timely management (ligation and suturing) of trauma including early repair of episiotomy helps to stem bleeding. It is important to identify and repair, vulval and vaginal hematomas. Supralevator hematomas can be both diagnostic and therapeutic challenge owing to limited access in ligating the bleeding vessels. It extends upward into the broad ligament thus bleeding is concealed. Involvement of senior clinicians with experience in pelvic side wall surgery is pivotal to safe and effective management. The management of uterine rupture is considered earlier in this chapter. At EUA, the uterus should be evacuated of any retained products. The management of coagulopathy (thrombin) is outlined under resuscitation above.

Uterine inversion (IU): It is a rare but potentially difficult condition to diagnose. UI represent a subcategory of uterine atony in which there is focal atony of the uterine fundus and contraction of the lower uterine corpus resulting in inversion. Present with profound shock usually out of proportion with the bleeding. Diagnosis is clinical and requires a high index of suspicion. When recognize early, manual or hydrostatic replacement may be achieved. These may be aided by medications such as glyceryl trinitrate (GNT) and terbutaline that relax the smooth muscle in the lower segment constriction ring. Persistent cases may require surgery where the often-described Huntington and Haultain procedure may be carried out [83]. This involves gently pulling the round ligaments to reposition the uterine fundus. Where the lower constriction ring is too tight, this may be divided posteriorly by a vertical incision. This procedure is recently described using laparoscopic techniques.

11 Monitoring

Patients with major and massive PPH require close and intensive monitoring during the emergency management and the immediate period after the episode. Regular assessment for ongoing bleeding by assessment of lochia, uterine contraction is combined with vital signs monitoring and assessment. The pulse, blood pressure, temperature, ECG, oxygen saturation, and urine output monitored continuously during resuscitation and up to 24 h afterward. Hematological parameters including hemoglobin, platelets, white cell count, fibrinogen, and coagulation profile should be checked regularly. Biochemical markers of renal and liver function should be monitored. Where there is massive transfusion, ionized calcium and potassium should be measured. Arterial line and pulmonary wedge pressure monitoring helps in monitoring volume replacement and detection of volume overload. Strict input and output monitoring is the norm.

The immediate care after PPH is in high dependency or intensive care unit to monitor vital signs in cases of major or massive hemorrhage and/or where patient's condition is critical. For minor or moderate PPH where patient is stable, monitoring in delivery suite with half-hourly observations for 2 h before transferring to postnatal ward where uterine tone, blood loss, and vital signs are monitored, at least, 4 hourly thereafter.

Patient who are transferred to HDU/ICU should have blood loss closely monitored and recorded cumulatively. Vital signs should be monitored continuously. Hemoglobin should be checked 6 h after stabilization and repeated at least once within 24 h even if vital signs are stable, and there are no signs of external bleeding.

If vital signs are unstable or patient requires inotropes, more frequent assessment of hemoglobin and coagulation profile should be performed as needed. Bedside ultrasound should be performed if vital signs remain unstable and/or hemoglobin dropped without visible external bleeding. This will help to identify enlarging hematomas or intraperitoneal bleeding. Measure urine output hourly using graduated catheter bags.

In all cases of major or massive hemorrhage and where massive blood transfusion has occurred and/or there is continued concern about further bleeding, consider sequential compression devices and graduated elastic compression stockings to prevent venous thrombosis. Pharmacological thromboprophylaxis should be deferred until patient is stable without requiring inotropes and has no further bleeding or drop in hemoglobin.

Subsequent care is aimed at detecting adverse sequelae of PPH, such as acute lung injury, ARDS, respiratory failure, heart failure, and hepatic failure. Adequate monitoring and replacement are essential to prevent significant end-organ damage that will lead to multiple organ failure. Acute kidney injury (pre-renal) and acute MI are of particular concern in these patients.

Other complications that might occur include ischemic hepatitis, hepatic infarction, or hepatic failure and bowel sloughing due to splanchnic ischemia. Long-term sequelae like Sheehan's syndrome, degrees of neurological impairment because of cerebral ischemia are also seen in these patients.

12 Current Trends and Future Direction in the Management of PPH

12.1 Tranexamic Acid

Tranexamic acid delays clot breakdown by reducing plasmin activation by way of inhibiting the interaction between fibrin and plasminogen. The benefits of administering tranexamic acid within 180 min of delivery, once PPH is diagnosed clearly has different effects depending on whether this followed a vaginal or cesarean delivery [84, 85]. The epileptogenic risk of tranexamic acid is to be noted in women with complicated pregnancy-induced hypertension [86].

12.2 Identification of Factors in Event Recurrence

The apparent tendency for familial recurrence of PPH is a trend that warrants attention in the future, especially in closely-knit, ethnically homogeneous communities. Using data from the Medical Birth Registry of Norway, Statistics Norway and Central Population Registry of Norway, Linde et al. (2021) studied 1,002,687 mother-offspring, 84,164 father-off springs and 761,011 both-parents-offspring pairs. They found that PPH was more likely to be recurrent between full sisters (OR 1.47, 95% confidence interval 1.41–1.52) [87]. The risk appeared to be strongly influenced by the birthweight in the index pregnancy above a threshold of 4000 g. The odds ratio for PPH was also higher if the mother's sister or brother's partner had also previously experienced PPH. Although the specific etiology of PPH was not available from this study, the referred fetal weight suggests that the relative proportion of possible causes is unlikely to be at huge variance from the traditional dominance of about 70% of instances being attributable to atony.

12.3 *Translational Pharmacology*

With atony being the main cause of PPH, identification of factors that may impair uterotonic pharmacologic response is worth exploring. Syntocinon is among the first-line oxytocics administered to prevent and treat primary atonic PPH. However, even if stored optimally to ensure its efficacy, not all patients will respond appropriately. The implications of this were underscored by a recent small study by Erickson et al. (2022) [88, 89] who found that differences in the DNA sequence within one variant (r53576) of the oxytocin receptor may be associated with variable responses to exogenous oxytocin. The authors note that such a risk may only be important in women who had fewer risk factors for atonic PPH.

13 Conclusion

We know the effective and efficient approaches to managing peripartum hemorrhage. We have at our disposal, reliable uterotonics and many effective surgical procedures as well as therapeutic radiological tools to significantly contain hemorrhage in the obstetric patient. Regular delivery suite drills, prior simulations and prompt involvement of multidisciplinary teams have been shown to further optimize care even when massive bleeding occurs unexpectedly.

What appears needed now is to synchronize these pearls of practice across all practices, where pregnant mothers are cared for. Benchmarks and clinical protocols should complement regular audit to improve the confounding effect of human factors.

References

1. Borovac-Pinheiro A, Pacagnella RC, Cecatti JG, et al. Postpartum haemorrhage: new insights for definition and diagnosis. Am J Obstet Gynaecol. 2018;219(2):162–8.
2. WHO postpartum haemorrhage summit, Dubai, UAE, 7–10 Mar 2023.
3. Knight M. The findings of MBRRACE UK confidential enquiry into maternal deaths and morbidity. Obstet Gynaecol Reprod Med. 2019;29(1):21–3.
4. Cook L, Roberts I, WOMAN Trial Collaborators. Effect of early tranexamic acid administration on mortality, hysterectomy and other morbidities in women with postpartum haemorrhage (WOMAN): an international randomised double-blind placebo-controlled trial. Lancet. 2017;389(10084):2105–16.
5. Kellie FJ, Wandabwa JN, Mousa HA, Weeks AD. Mechanical and surgical interventions in treating primary postpartum haemorrhage. Cochrane Database Syst Rev. 2020;7(7):CD013663.
6. D'Alton ME, Rood KM, Smid MC, et al. Intrauterine vacuum-induced haemorrhage control device for rapid treatment of postpartum haemorrhage. Obstet Gynaecol. 2020;136(5):882–91.
7. Ring L, Landau R. Postpartum haemorrhage: anaesthesia management. Semin Perinatol. 2019;43(1):35–43.

8. Knight M, Nair M, Tuffnell D, Shakespeare J, Kenyon S, Kurinczuk JJ, on behalf of MBRRACE-UK. Saving lives, improving mothers care. UK confidential enquiries into maternal deaths and mortality 2015–2017. Oxford National Perinatal Epidemiology Unit, University of Oxford; 2017. p. 20–4.
9. Hasegawa J, Katsuragi S, Tanaka A, et al. Decline in maternal death due to obstetrics haemorrhage between 2010 and 2017 in Japan. Sci Rep. 2019;9(1):11026.
10. Sekpon AB. Drop in blood donations add to maternal health threats in Africa. Brazzaville: WHO Africa; 2021.
11. Zero maternal death by haemorrhage initiative. Guatemala: PAHO/WHO; 2021.
12. Osanan GC, Padilla H, Reis MI, Tavares AB. Strategy for zero maternal deaths by haemorrhage in Brazil: a multidisciplinary initiative to combat maternal morbimortality. Rev Bras Ginecol Obstet. 2018;40(3):103–5.
13. Padilla CR, Shamshirsaz A. Critical care in obstetrics. Best Pract Res Clin Anaesthesiol. 2022;36(1):209–25.
14. Vilda D, Wallace M, Dyer L, Harville E, Theall K. Income inequality and racial disparity in pregnancy related mortality in the US. SSM Popul Health. 2019;9:100477.
15. D'Alton ME, Bonanno CA, Berkowitz RL, et al. Putting the 'M' back in maternal-fetal medicine. Am J Obstet Gynaecol. 2013;208(6):442–8.
16. Kerr R, Eckert LO, Winikoff B, et al. Postpartum haemorrhage: case definition and guidelines for data collection, analysis and presentation of immunisation safety. Vaccine. 2016;34(49):6102–9.
17. Quantitative blood loss in obstetrics haemorrhage: ACOG practice guideline 794. Obstet Gynaecol. 2019;134(6):150–6.
18. Belfort MA. Overview of postpartum hemorrhage. In: Goffman D, Barss VA, editors. UpTodate. Wolters Kluwer; 2022. p. 1–58.
19. American College of Surgeons. Advance trauma life support (students manual). American College of Surgeons; 1997.
20. Lagrew D, McNulty J, Sakowski C, Cape V, McCormick E, Morton CH. Improving health care response to obstetrics hemorrhage, California Maternal Quality Care Collaborative Toolkit. CMQCC; 2022. www.cmqcc.org.
21. Li Y, Tian Y, Chen Y, Wu F. Analysis of 62 placental abruption cases: risk factors and clinical outcome. Taiwan J Obstet Gynaecol. 2019;58(2):223–6.
22. Sebghati M, Chandraharan E. An update on the risk factors for and management of obstetrics haemorrhage. Women's Health (Lond). 2017;13(2):34–40.
23. Bonnar J. Massive obstetric haemorrhage. Baillieres Best Pract Res Clin Obstet Gynaecol. 2000;14(1):1–18.
24. Seeble J, Lohr J, Kirchner M, Michaelis J, Merle U. Rotational thermoelectrometry (ROTEM) improves haemostasis assessment compared to conventional coagulation test in ACLF and non-ACLF patients. BMC Gastroenterol. 2020;20(1):271.
25. Giouleka S, Tsakiridis I, Kalogiannidis I, et al. Postpartum haemorrhage: a comprehensive review of guidelines. Obstet Gynaecol Surv. 2022;77(11):665–82.
26. Bell SF, Watkins A, John M, et al. Incidence of PPH defined by quantitative blood loss measurement: a national cohort. BMC Pregnancy Childbirth. 2020;20:271–6.
27. Shields LE, Wiesner S, Fulton J, et al. Comprehensive maternal haemorrhage protocols reduce the use of blood products and improve patient safety. Am J Obstet Gynaecol. 2015;212(3):272–80.
28. Robinson D, Bosso M, Chan C, Duckitt K, Lett R. Guideline no. 431: postpartum haemorrhage and haemorrhagic shock. J Obstet Gynaecol Can. 2022;44(12):1293–310.
29. Smith V, Kenny LC, Sandall J, Devine D, Noonan M. Physiological track-and-trigger/early warning systems for use in maternity care. Cochrane Database Syst Rev. 2021;9(9):CD013276.
30. Xu Y, Zhu S, Song H, et al. A new modified obstetrics early warning score for prognostication of severe maternal morbidity. BMC Pregnancy Childbirth. 2022;22(1):901–5.
31. Allgower M, Burri C. The shock index. Dtsch Med Wochenschr. 1967;92(43):1947–50.

32. Heffner A, Swords D, Nussbaum M, Kline J, Jones A. Predictors of complication of postintubation during emergency airway management. J Crit Care. 2012;27(6):587–93.
33. Olaussen A, Blackburn T, Mitra B, Fitzgerald M. Shock index for prediction of critical bleeding post-trauma: a systematic review. Emerg Med Australas. 2014;26(3):223–8.
34. Ushida T, et al. Shock index and postpartum haemorrhage in vaginal deliveries: a multicenter retrospective study. Shock. 2021;55:332.
35. Rady MY, Smithline HA, Blake H, Nowak R, Rivers E. A comparison of the shock index and conventional vital signs to identify acute, critical illness in the emergency department. Ann Emerg Med. 1994;24(4):685–90.
36. Mutchler M, Nienaber U, Munzberg M, et al. The shock index revisited—a fast guide to transfusion requirement? a retrospective analysis on 21,853 patients derived from the trauma register DGU. Crit Care. 2013;17(4):R172.
37. Le Bas A, Chandraharan E, Addei A, Arulkumaran S. Use of the obstetrics shock index as an adjunct in identifying significant blood loss in patients with massive obstetrics haemorrhage. Int J Gynaecol Obstet. 2014;124(3):253–5.
38. Nathan HL, et al. Shock index threshold to predict adverse outcomes in maternal haemorrhage and sepsis: a prospective cohort study. Acta Obstet Gynacol Scand. 2019;98(9):1178–86.
39. Karoshi M, Palacios-Jaraquemada J, Keith L. Managing the ten most common life-threatening scenarios associated with postpartum hemorrhage. Semanticscholar.org; 2012.
40. Green-top guideline no. 52. Prevention and management of postpartum haemorrhage. RCOG; 2016. p. 1–44.
41. Gallos ID, Williams HM, Price MJ, et al. Uterotonic agents for prevention and treatment of postpartum haemorrhage: a network meta-analysis. Cochrane Database Syst Rev. 2018;4(4):CD011689.
42. Dahlke JD, Mendez-Figueroa H, Maggio L, et al. Prevention and management of postpartum haemorrhage: a comparison of 4 national guidelines. Am J Obstet Gynaecol. 2015;213(1):76.
43. Hofmeyr GJ, Abdel-Aleem H, Abdel-Aleem M. uterine massage for preventing postpartum haemorrhage. Cochrane Database Syst Rev. 2013;(7):CD006431.
44. Papadopoulou A, Man R, Athanasopoulos N, et al. Uterotonics agents for preventing postpartum haemorrhage: a network meta-analysis. Cochrane Database Syst Rev Update. 2018;12(12):CD011689.
45. McLintock C. Prevention and treatment of postpartum haemorrhage: focus on haematological aspects of management. Haematol Am Soc Haematol Educ Program. 2020;1:542–6.
46. Tikkanen M, Riihimaki O, Gissler M, et al. Decreasing incidence of placental abruption in Finland during 1980-2005. Octa Obstet Gynaecol Scand. 2012;91(9):1046–52.
47. Qui Y, Wu L, Xiao Y, Zhang X. Clinical analysis, and classification of placental abruption. J Matern Fetal Neonatal Med. 2021;34(18):2952–6.
48. Jain V, Bos H, Bujold E. Guideline no. 402: diagnosis and management of placenta praevia. J Obstet Gynaecol Can. 2020;42(7):906–17.
49. Oppenheimer LW, Farine D. A new classification of placenta previa: measuring progress in obstetrics. Am J Obstet Gynaecol. 2009;201(3):227–9.
50. Reddy UM, Abuhamad AZ, Lenine D, et al. Fetal imaging: executive summary of a joint Eunice Kennedy Shriver National Institute for Child Health and Human Development, Society for Maternal-Fetal Medicine, American Institute of Ultrasound in Medicine, ACOG, American College of Radiology, Society for Paediatrics Radiology, and Society of Radiologists in Ultrasound Fetal Imaging workshop. J Ultrasound Med. 2014;33(5):745–57.
51. Lockwood CJ, Russo-Stieglitz K. Placenta previa: management. In: Berghella V, Barss VA, editors. UpToDate. Wolters Kluwer; 2022. p. 1–20.
52. Society for Maternal-Fetal Medicine, Gyamfi-Bennerman C. SMFM consult series no. 44: management of bleeding in the late preterm period. Am J Obstet Gynaecol. 2018;138:e35.
53. ACOG Committee on Obstetrics practice, Society of Maternal-Fetal Medicine. Medically indicated late preterm and early preterm deliveries: ACOG committee opinion no. 831. Obstet Gynaecol. 2021;138:e35.

54. Schwartz A, Chen D, Shinar S, Agrawal S, Yogev Y. Timing of cesarean delivery in women with uncomplicated placenta previa. J Matern Fetal Neonatal Med. 2022;35:10559.
55. Love CD, Fernando KJ, Sargent L, Hughes RG. Major placenta previa should not preclude outpatient management. Eur J Obstet Gynaecol Reprod Biol. 2004;117(10):24–9.
56. Wing DA, Paul RH, Millar LK. Management of the symptomatic placenta previa: a randomised controlled trial of inpatient versus outpatient expectant management. Am J Obstet Gynaecol. 1996;175(4):806–11.
57. Ruiter L, Eschbach SJ, Burgers M, et al. Predictors for emergency cesarean delivery in women with placenta previa. Am J Perinatol. 2016;33:1407.
58. Jauniaux E, Ayres-de-Campos D, Roos JL, et al. FIGO classification for the clinical diagnosis of placenta accreta spectrum disorder. Inter. J Obstet Gynaecol. 2019;146(1):20–4.
59. Ishibashi H, Miyamoto M, Iwahashi H, et al. Criteria for placenta accreta spectrum in the international federation obstetrics and gynaecology classification and topographic invasion area are associated with massive haemorrhage in patients with placenta previa. Octa Obstet Gynaecol Scand. 2021;100(6):1019–25.
60. Cahil AG, Beigi R, Heine RP, Silver RM, Wax JR. Placenta accreta spectrum. Am J Obstet Gynaecol. 2018;219(6):B2–B16.
61. Silver RM, Landon MB, Rouse DJ, et al. Maternal morbidity associated with multiple repeat caesarean deliveries. Obstet Gynaecol. 2006;107:1226.
62. Hessami K, Salmanian B, Einerso BD, et al. Clinical correlates of placenta accreta spectrum disorder depending on the presence or absence of placenta previa: a systemic review and metanalysis. Obstet Gynaecol. 2022;14(4):599–606.
63. Jauniaux E, Alfirevic Z, Bhide AG, et al. Placenta previa and placenta accreta: diagnosis and management: Greentop guideline no. 27a. BJOG. 2019;126(1):e1–e48.
64. Bartels HC, Postle JD, Downey P, Brennan DJ. Placenta accreta spectrum: a review of pathology, molecular biology, and biomarkers. Dis Markers. 2018;2018:1507674.
65. Zhang T, Wang S. Potential serum biomarkers in prenatal diagnosis of placenta accreta spectrum. Front Med. 2022;9:860186.
66. Sentilhes L, Kayem G, Chandraharan E, et al. FIGO consensus guidelines on placenta accreta spectrum disorders: conservative management. Int J Gynecol Obstet. 2018;140:291–8.
67. Sentihes L, Kayem G, Silver RM. Conservative management of placenta accreta spectrum. Clin Obstet Gynaecol. 2018;61(4):783–94.
68. ACOG, Society for Maternal-Fetal Medicine. Obstetrics care consensus no. 7: placenta accreta spectrum. Obstet Gynaecol. 2018;132(6):e259–75.
69. Durukan H, Durukan OB, Yazici FG. Placenta accreta spectrum disorder: a comparison between fertility sparing techniques and hysterectomy. J Obstet Gynaecol. 2021;41(3):353–9.
70. Shmakov RG, Vinitskly AA, Chuprinin VD, et al. Alternative approaches to surgical haemostasis in patients with morbidly adherent placenta undergoing fertility-sparing surgery. J Matern Fetal Neonatal Med. 2019;32(12):2042–8.
71. Landon MB, Frey H. Uterine rupture a life-threatening pregnancy complication. In: Berghella V, Barss VA, editors. UpToDate. Wolters Kluwer; 2022. p. 1–21.
72. Vachon-Marceau C, Demers S, Goyet M, et al. Labour dystocias and the risk of uterine rupture in women with prior caesarean. Am J Perinatal. 2016;33:577.
73. Hasselman S, Lampa E, Wikman A, et al. Time matters—a Swedish cohort study of labour duration and risk of uterine rupture. Acta Obstet Gynecol Scand. 2021;100:1902.
74. Kamaya A, Ro K, Benedetti NJ, et al. Imaging and diagnosis of postpartum complications: sonography and other imaging modalities. Ultrasound Q. 2009;25:151.
75. Hunter TJ, Maouris P, Dickinson JE. Prenatal detection and conservative management of partial fundal uterine dehiscence. Fetal Diagn Ther. 2009;25:123.
76. Pavalagantharajah S, Villani SA, D'Souza R. Vasa previa and associated risks factors: a systematic review and meta-analysis. Am J Obstet Gynecol MFM. 2020;2(3):100117.
77. Ruiter L, Kok N, Limpens J, et al. Systematic review of accuracy of ultrasound in the diagnosis of vasa previa. Ultrasound Obstet Gynecol. 2015;45(5):16–22.

78. Young JS, White LM. Vaginal bleeding in late pregnancy. Emerg Med Clin North Am. 2019;37(2):251–64.
79. Escobar MF, Nassar AH, Theron G, et al. FIGO recommendations on the management of postpartum hemorrhage. Int J Gynecol Obstet. 2022;157(Suppl 1):3–50.
80. Kumaraswami S, Butwick A. Latest advances in postpartum hemorrhage management. Best Pract Res Clin Anaesthesiol. 2022;36(1):123–34.
81. Diaz V, Abalos E, Caroli G. Methods for blood loss estimation after vaginal birth. Cochrane Database Syst Rev Metan. 2018;9:CD010980.
82. Wikkelso A, Wetterslev J, Moller AM, Afshari A. Thromboelastography (TEG) or Rotational thromboelastometry (ROTEM) to monitor hemostatic treatment in bleeding patients: a systematic review with meta-analysis and trial sequential analysis. Anaesthesist. 2017;72:519.
83. Coad SL, Dahlgren LS, Hutcheon JA. Risks and consequences of puerperal uterine inversion in United States, 2004 through 2013. Am J Obstet Gynaecol. 2017;217(3):377e1–6.
84. Sentiles L, Senat MV, Le Lous M, et al. Tranexamic acid for prevention of blood loss after Cesarean section. N Engl J Med. 2021;384(17):1623–34.
85. Sentiles L, Meriot B, Madar H, et al. Postpartum hemorrhage: prevention and treatment. Expert Rev Hematol. 2016;9(11):1043–61.
86. Idialisoa R, Jouffroy R, Philippe P, et al. Beware of using tranexamic acid in parturients with eclampsia. Anaesth Crit Care Pain Med. 2016;35(3):231–2.
87. Linde LE, Ebbing C, Moster D, et al. Recurrence of postpartum haemorrhage in relatives: a population-based cohort study. Acta Obstet Gynaecol Scand. 2021;100(12):2278–84.
88. Erickson EN, Myatt L, Danoff JS, et al. Oxytocin receptor DNA methylation is associated with exogenous oxytocin needs during parturition and postpartum hemorrhage. Commun Med. 2023;3(11):113.
89. Erickson EN, Krol KM, Perkeybile AM, Connely JJ, Myatt L. Oxytocin receptor single nucleotide polymorphism predicts atony-related postpartum hemorrhage. BMC Pregnancy Childbirth. 2022;22:884.

Trauma in Pregnancy-Requiring Intensive Care

Abdulgafoor Tharayil, Gustav Frans Strandvik, Sujith M. Prabhakaran, Ahmed Obeidat, Adnan A. Saadeddin, Aboobacker K. A. Thode, and Nissar Shaikh

Abstract Trauma to the parturient is uniquely challenging because of the physiological changes that could happen during pregnancy, as well as the fact that two lives, rather than one, are in danger. Trauma during pregnancy ranges in severity; it can be as minor as a simple bump, or as severe as a gunshot. Even minor trauma during pregnancy may result in fetal loss. The commonest causes of trauma during pregnancy are domestic abuse and road traffic accidents. Appropriate assessment and timely management of pregnant trauma patients are crucial to avoid maternal and fetal complications. The approach to pregnant trauma patients is similar to non-pregnant trauma patients, which includes the primary survey, secondary survey, and use of adjunct diagnostic tests. Assessment of the fetus and fetal monitoring is essential in any pregnant patient with trauma.

This chapter offers an overview of trauma management during pregnancy, including the initial management as per Advanced Trauma Life Support (ATLS) protocols and the management in the intensive care unit.

A. Tharayil (✉) · S. M. Prabhakaran · A. Obeidat · N. Shaikh
Surgical Intensive Care Unit, Department of Anesthesia, Hamad General Hospital, Hamad Medical Corporation, Doha, Qatar
e-mail: atharayil@hamad.qa

G. F. Strandvik
Trauma Intensive Care Unit, Department of Surgery, Hamad General Hospital, Hamad Medical Corporation, Doha, Qatar

A. A. Saadeddin · A. K. A. Thode
Department of Anesthesia, Hamad Medical Corporation, Doha, Qatar

N. Shaikh et al. (eds.), *Updates in Intensive Care of OBGY Patients*,
https://doi.org/10.1007/978-981-99-9577-6_7

Keywords Pregnancy · Trauma · Fetal monitoring · Physiological changes · Parturient · Maternal medicine · Placenta previa · Abruptio-placenta · Uterine rupture

1 Introduction

Pregnancy or conception state is a unique physiological and psychological condition. It is the greatest gift of life but carries a lot of emotional and physiological stress to the parturient mother, which progresses day by day till the time of delivery. During these 40+ weeks of highly demanding period, a conceived mother will try to adapt all her physiology and emotional state to safeguard her pregnancy towards a healthy delivery. But unfortunately, we cannot predict a smooth natural course always, and sometimes unexpected events happen during this period. One of these is trauma to the parturient.

Over the ages, trauma in pregnancy has raised so many concerns. This can occur in different magnitudes, from an accidental minor bump to the abdomen while walking past a table, to a penetrating gunshot to the gravid uterus which can lead to both maternal and fetal mortality or significant injuries. While hemorrhagic shock or direct head trauma can be a major cause of death in the mother, maternal death in most cases leads to fetal mortality or pregnancy loss.

The main challenge in the management of a parturient trauma victim is the physiological and anatomical changes that may affect the timing of diagnosis and initiation of the management.

Different authors have described many mechanisms of injury and established various guidelines of how to deal with them, from diagnosis to admission criteria and levels of monitoring both the mother and the fetus, based on the nature and the distribution of such traumas in different communities, and the availability of healthcare resources in those communities.

In this chapter, we will try to highlight in detail what changes we expect in a pregnant woman throughout her gestational period, the impact of different types of trauma in relation to the gestational age in trimesters, and what guidelines are proposed to approach such patients, or what modification is implemented to the already existing trauma management guidelines and recommendations in comparison to a non-conceiving woman.

2 Epidemiology

The incidence of trauma in pregnant women in North America is reported to be 6–8% [1], other regions of the world have reported similar percentages; the differences are in the etiology of this trauma which most probably will be linked to the overall trauma causes in the particular population.

Expected complications to the mother include uterine rupture, maternal hemorrhage, premature rupture of membranes, or contractions which might be challenging to distinguish from benign contractions. Expected complications to the products of conception include fetal hemorrhage, placental abruption, intrauterine fetal demise, and preterm birth [2].

Some regions of the world have reported motor vehicle accidents as the leading cause of trauma in pregnancy, but some systematic reviews have identified domestic violence as a leading cause of trauma in pregnancy [3]. We believe that the reported number of traumas in pregnancy does not reflect the actual incidence for many reasons. Many trauma victims may not be identified as pregnant, especially in their first trimester of pregnancy, many domestic violence injuries are unreported worldwide, and some underestimated minor traumas that may lead to slowly progressing complications in any organ, may be detected either during gestation or after delivery.

Seat belt bruising has been described as one of the causes of injury, but it is counterbalanced by the fact that the use of the seatbelt is helpful in lowering the severity of abdominal injury and fewer hospital stay days [4].

Psychological trauma has been given more attention in the past years including post-traumatic stress disorder, traumatic sexual abuse, or previous traumatic birth.

Despite the mild inconsistencies in reported numbers by different authors and researchers, we can agree on and identify the main reasons for trauma worldwide, as follows:

1. Motor vehicle collisions and other road traffic-related events
2. Domestic violence
3. Falls either from a standing position or from heights
4. Thermal injuries which may include burns, heat stroke, or electrical injuries
5. Homicides including both blunt and penetrating wounds
6. Psychological trauma.

Each type of trauma can include various categories and subcategories, which mirror the epidemiology of trauma in non-pregnant women; what matters most are the classifications crucial in initiating the management, which prompt certain steps to enable early prediction of possible complications, and measures to avoid or mitigate them.

3 Physiologic Changes During Pregnancy

Pregnancy imposes certain anatomic and physiological changes to the conceived body. A wide spectrum of physiologic and anatomic changes is expected to occur to accommodate the growing fetus and to prepare the mother for delivery and postpartum provision. Such changes are well tolerated in most pregnancies and generally reversible, but in some pregnancies, such physiologic adaption may be challenging and carries certain risks.

3.1 Respiratory System

The first significant change at early conception is the increasing level of progesterone, which by its stimulatory effects in both respiratory rate and tidal volume, results in respiratory alkalosis that is compensated by the decreased absorption of sodium bicarbonate in the kidneys. This is to meet the increasing metabolic demand of oxygen during pregnancy.

Respiratory changes can be summarized as follows:

- Increased oxygen demand and consumption (20%).
- Increased PO_2 of 10 mmHg secondary to increased minute ventilation and cardiac output [5].
- Decreased PCO_2 of 10 mmHg also secondary to increased minute ventilation [5].
- Cephalad displacement of the diaphragm with growing gravid uterus size.
- This will affect the volumes of the lung in terms of low Functional Residual Capacity (FRC) (20% decrease) and increasing Tidal Volume (TV) (10–15%) [5].
- Airway edema results from estrogen-induced fluid retention during pregnancy and vascular engorgement, which can be exacerbated by pregnancy-induced hypertension, fluid overload, the head-down position, presence of oxytocin infusion (antidiuretic effect), prolonged Valsalva efforts during delivery, and β-adrenergic tocolytic therapy [6]. Such edema may increase the airway resistance by 6 cm H_2O.
- Less affinity of maternal hemoglobin to oxygen. This is a very important physiological adaptation to increase oxygen delivery to the fetus. So, any changes in the mother's serum pH can affect the fetal oxygen exchange significantly [7].

3.1.1 Special Considerations

- Relative changes in the upper airway anatomy might lead to a more difficult airway.
- Bleeding can occur relatively easier with minimal instrumentation to the upper airway.
- Difficult instrumentation of the esophagus, either by a nasogastric tube or scope.
- Any drop in the blood PO_2 of less than 60 mmHg can lead to significant fetal hypoxia and acidosis [7].
- Trauma to the chest can lead to abdominal injuries.
- Dilutional anemia and dilutional hypoalbuminemia, which make the lungs more prone to edema.

3.2 Cardiovascular System

Most of these changes start to be noticed by the end of the first trimester and are prominent in the third trimester, apart from cardiac output which normalizes around 24 weeks in the post-partum period. Other cardiovascular changes almost normalize at 6 weeks of the puerperium period [8]. Changes in cardiovascular system in pregnancy are depicted in Figs. 1, 2, 3, and 4. Figure 5 summarizes the changes.

Cardiovascular changes can be summarized in the following key points:

- Systemic vascular resistance (SVR) decreases (mechanism not fully understood yet) 35–40% by mid-second trimester which leads to a decreased after-load and mild hypotension [9].
- Cardiac output increases gradually up to 50% at 32 weeks gestational age (hypervolemic high cardiac output state).
- Increased demand is met by increased cardiac output.
- Heart rate slightly increases 15–20 beats per minute by term (ranges 82–91 Beats per minute by term [10].
- Blood volume expansion leads to an increased preload.
- Engorged pelvic vasculature, with stiff placental vessels and absent autoregulation.
- Aortocaval compression, which should be considered after 20 weeks gestation. Supine position leads to inferior vena cava occlusion by 80% and aortic occlusion by 30%, which is partially compensated by collateral circulation later.
- Physiological left axis deviation with heart displacement upward and to the left that should be considered during cardiac massage if CPR commenced.

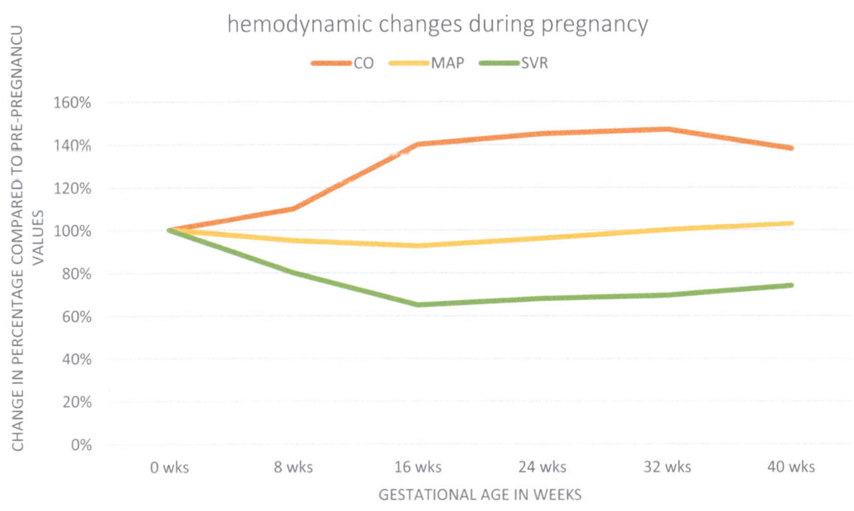

Fig. 1 Data from: Cardiac output and related haemodynamics during pregnancy: a series of meta-analyses
Meah VL, Cockcroft JR, Backx K, Shave R, Stöhr EJ, Heart. 2016;102(7):518. Epub 2016 Jan 21

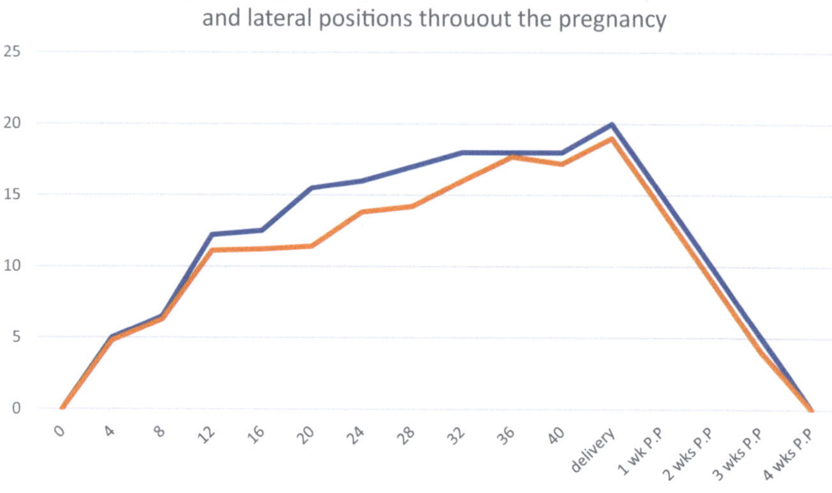

Fig. 2 Data from: Cardiac output and related haemodynamics during pregnancy: a series of meta-analyses. *WKS* weeks, *P.P* post partum
Meah VL, Cockcroft JR, Backx K, Shave R, Stöhr EJ, Heart. 2016;102(7):518. Epub 2016 Jan 21

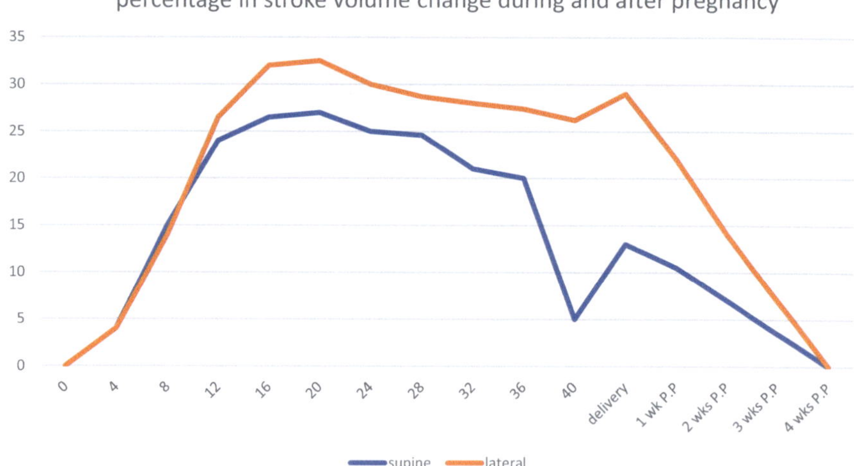

Fig. 3 Data from: Cardiac output and related haemodynamics during pregnancy: a series of meta-analyses. *WKS* weeks, *P.P* post partum
Meah VL, Cockcroft JR, Backx K, Shave R, Stöhr EJ, Heart. 2016;102(7):518. Epub 2016 Jan 21

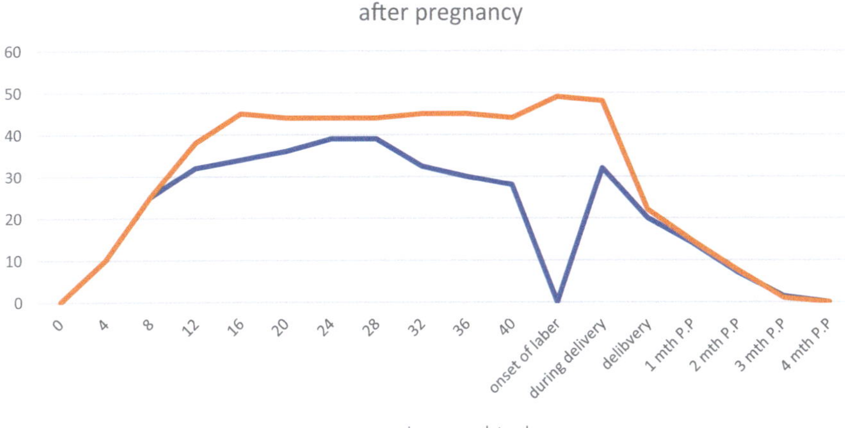

Fig. 4 Data from: Cardiac output and related haemodynamics during pregnancy: a series of meta-analyses. *Mth* months, *P.P* post-partum
Meah VL, Cockcroft JR, Backx K, Shave R, Stöhr EJ, Heart. 2016;102(7):518. Epub 2016 Jan 21

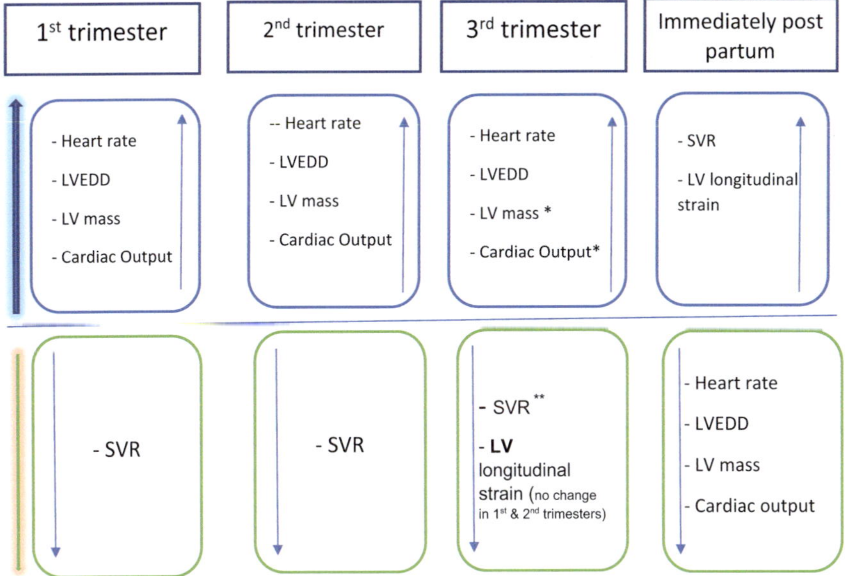

Fig. 5 Data from: Ashrafi R, Curtis SL. Heart disease in pregnancy. Cardiol Ther. 2017 Dec;6(2):157–173. doi: 10.1007/s40119-017-0096-4. Epub 2017 Jul 5

3.2.1 Special Considerations

- It might be challenging to assess hemorrhagic shock state with the pre-existing physiological state of relative tachycardia and hypotension in the parturient. However, a heart above 115 beats/min mandates an evaluation.
- Benign palpitations are more common during pregnancy, but the approach of such complaint does not differ from a non-pregnant woman.
- Uteroplacental circulation is dependent on the cardiac output, and fetal distress can occur at a relatively small drop in blood supply.
- Pelvic trauma can carry a higher than usual risk of bleeding, so even minor traumas must be evaluated thoroughly and carefully.
- A 30-degree left lateral decubitus position is a crucial step in positioning a lying pregnant woman.

3.3 Hematology and Coagulation

- High metabolic demand increases serum Erythropoietin levels which leads to red blood cells expansion by 30% (250–450 mL), at the same time if the conceived mother is not on iron supplementation during pregnancy the red cells expansion will reach a maximum of 15% only [11].
- The plasma expands by 50%, which leads to dilutional anemia of around 15–20% of non-pregnant women (Fig. 6).

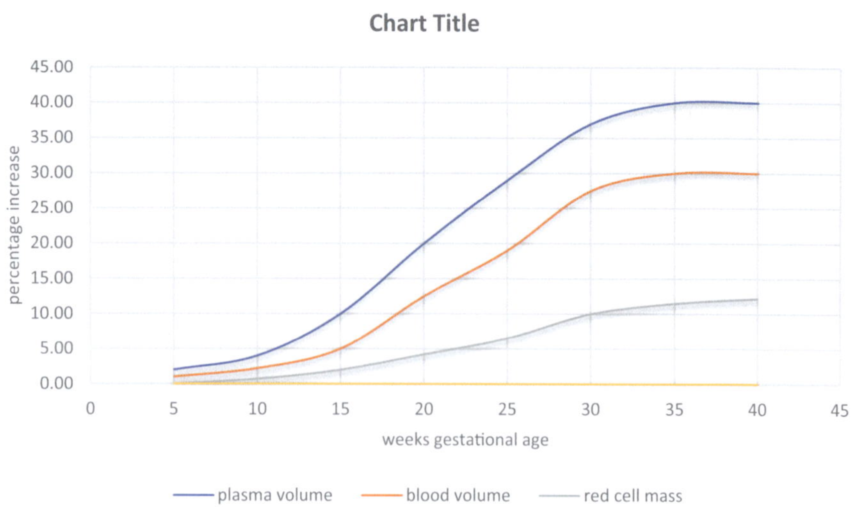

Fig. 6 Data From: Lund CJ, Donovan JC. Blood volume during pregnancy. Significance of plasma and red cell volumes. Am J Obstet Gynecol 1967; 98:394

- Overall blood volume increases from 70 mL per kgBW to 100 mL per kgBW by term.
- Hypercoagulability with a relatively higher risk of thrombus formation.
- Enlarged spleen.

3.4 *Gastrointestinal System*

Pregnancy affects the gastrointestinal tract mainly by two factors: first is the progesterone levels and its effects on motility (intrinsic factor), and second is compression by the gravid uterus and displacing effect on the abdominal contents (mechanical effect), while secretion and absorption might be unaffected.

Most of these changes return to the non-pregnant state upon delivery or shortly after that.

Key Changes:

- Swollen gingiva and edematous oral mucosa.
- Sialorrhea or excessive salivation (mechanism not fully understood).
- Relaxed esophageal sphincter.
- Decreased motility with preserved gastric emptying and delayed emptying of both small and large bowel, especially in diabetic mothers.
- Inhibition of the adaptive responses of the sphincter.
- Lower gastric PH (low level of evidence).
- Nausea and vomiting in more than 50% of pregnancies, and less frequently the aggressive form of hyperemesis gravidarum.
- Upward displacement liver of about 4 cm at term and is rarely palpable in the abdomen.
- Upward displacement of the bowels by the gravid uterus protects the bowel from injuries in the lower abdomen.
- Serum alkaline phosphatase increases, alanine aminotransferase and aspartate aminotransferase slightly decrease, and bilirubin remains unchanged or slightly decreases.
- Displaced appendix.

3.5 *Kidneys and Renal Tract*

Gestational changes of the kidneys and renal tract are profound during pregnancy to accommodate the expansion in blood volume, changes in the hemodynamic system and increased metabolic demand.

- Increased plasma blood flow of around 80% by 12 weeks driven by many factors which leads to an increased renal blood flow, which will result in an increased glomerular filtration rate of 40–50% by the second trimester [12].

- Creatinine levels drops at early pregnancy and normalizes towards the gestation term, which means a normal creatinine could indicate a deteriorating Glomerular Filtration Rate (GFR) [13].
- Slight drop in osmolality and sodium levels is expected.
- Increased excretion of proteins and glucose in urine compared to a non-pregnant woman.
- Renal excretion of sodium bicarbonate increases simultaneously to accommodate the state of respiratory alkalosis during gestation.
- Serum bicarbonate decreases to 22 mmol/L; pH remains in high-normal range [14].
- Ureters are more elongated, less motile, and less contractile as a result of increased progesterone levels.
- The urinary bladder is slightly distended in early pregnancy and compressed to a smaller than normal size by the third trimester with a congested hyperemic mucosa [15].

4 Management of the Pregnant Trauma Victim

The challenge in managing a pregnant trauma victim is dealing with two lives simultaneously. Early optimization of the mother plays an important role for survival of both the mother and fetus. Even though there are various physiological changes in pregnancy, the initial management remains similar to that of non-pregnant trauma victims.

The assessment is divided into primary survey and secondary survey as per the Advanced Trauma Life Support (ATLS) Course protocols. First is the primary survey and resuscitation of the mother, then assessment of the fetus followed by secondary survey of the mother [16, 17].

4.1 Prehospital Care

The prehospital care of the pregnant trauma patient is the same as that of a non-pregnant patient. It includes rapid assessment, performance of necessary first aid treatments to stabilize the patient, and then transfer to the appropriate medical facility. During the initial assessment period, the history should also include the obstetric history if possible. An estimation of the last menstrual period and thus the gestational age will be very helpful in deciding on the appropriate hospital facility and for the treating physician to arrange specific expert clinicians at the destination. Regardless of the trauma severity, any pregnancy >20 weeks shall be transferred to a trauma center according to the Centers for Disease Control and Prevention update on the "Guidelines for Field Triage of Injured Patients" [18].

Any patient in the later stages of pregnancy should be transported in the left lateral decubitus position to prevent the development of supine hypotension syndrome

[19]. Place the mother on oxygen supplementation and secure wide-bore intravenous access while transferring.

4.2 Primary Survey with Simultaneous Resuscitation

During the primary survey follow ATLS principles. This includes the ABCDEF approach: airway, breathing, circulation, disability, and exposure/environmental control. For the pregnant patient, "D" also stands for "displacement" of the uterus. Manual displacement of the uterus can help to improve maternal hemodynamics. "F" refers to fetus. This indicates that the fetus is enclosed in the primary survey but only after the initial assessment and stabilization of the mother [20]. Management of a pregnant trauma patient requires a multidisciplinary approach including emergency physicians, trauma surgeons, anesthesiologists, obstetricians, and pediatricians.

4.2.1 Airway and Breathing

The first step is to assess airway patency. Protect the cervical spine prior to airway manipulation. Anticipate difficulty in securing a patent airway, and possibly difficult intubation in a pregnant patient.

This is due to mucosal edema caused by increased capillary engorgement, which leads to increased risk of bleeding during airway manipulation and further difficulty in laryngoscopy [21]. The physiological changes that occur during pregnancy in the respiratory system such as decreased functional residual capacity (FRC) and less oxygen reserve and increased oxygen requirements, exacerbate hypoxia risk. The fetus is extremely sensitive to maternal hypoxia. The possibility for faster desaturation and hypoxia mandates oxygen supplementation for all pregnant women involved in trauma. Maintain saturation >95% and it is safer if an early elective planned intubation is considered than an emergency intubation.

Pregnant patients are at increased risk for aspiration of gastric contents because of delayed gastric emptying and decreased lower esophageal sphincter tone [22]. If chest tube insertion is required, avoid the usual intercostal space. As the diaphragm is pushed up by the gravid uterus, there are chances of chest tube entering abdominal cavity if inserted in the usual anatomical space. Ideally, a chest tube should be placed one to two intercostal spaces higher than in normal patients [23]. Consider ultrasound-guided chest tube insertion as it may be safer and prevent complications.

4.2.2 Circulation

The third step of the primary survey is the evaluation of the circulatory status. Signs and symptoms of shock and identifying active sites of bleeding should be the initial focus. The common cause for shock in any trauma victim is hemorrhage, but other causes such as direct cardiac injury, cardiac tamponade, or tension pneumothorax may also lead to reduce cardiac output and shock. In pregnant patients, the possibility of "supine hypotension syndrome" should be considered and addressed immediately. Cardiac output can be reduced by 30% in pregnant patients after mid-pregnancy because of compression of the vena cava by gravid uterus. If maternal spinal injury is not a concern, place the back board at a slight leftward tilt (15°) or place a wedge under the right hip.

Hemorrhagic shock classification is the same as that of any adult patient, but a few points to be considered. Due to the increase in intravascular volume status in pregnancy, the clinical signs of hypovolemia will be present later after significant blood loss. In cases of maternal hypotension, vasopressors should be avoided unless the patient is unresponsive to replenishment of intravascular volume by fluid administration [24]. Bicarbonate should be used with caution; avoid rapid correction of maternal acidosis because it may reduce compensatory hyperventilation [25]. Management of hemorrhagic shock is like any other trauma patients. Initiate judicious administration of IV crystalloids until blood products are available. To avoid alloimmunization in Rh (−) females, uncross matched type O Rh (−) blood can be administered until type-specific blood is available [26]. Hypothermia should be avoided as it worsens bleeding. The "triad of death in trauma" includes hypothermia, coagulopathy, and acidosis [27].

4.2.3 Disability

After airway breathing and circulation is stabilized, a rapid neurological examination should be performed. Glasgow coma score, pupillary size and reaction, and lateralizing signs should be assessed. However, seizures in a pregnant patient should be evaluated carefully. In pregnancy, seizures could be due to head injury or eclampsia. Eclamptic fits are associated with hypertension, proteinuria, and peripheral edema. Head computed tomography (CT) scan, if necessary, should be done in all patients. The indications for CT scan remain the same as in non-pregnant patients.

Measures to identify and manage raised intracranial pressure should be done as in non-pregnant patients. Hypertonic saline or mannitol and acute hyperventilation can be safely instituted in cases of acute rises in ICP. Prophylactic anticonvulsant therapy with levetiracetam or phenytoin should be administered to prevent seizures as seizures may have deleterious effect on both mother and fetus.

Radiation exposure of the fetus of less than 5–10 rad causes no significant increase in risk of congenital malformations, intrauterine growth retardation, or miscarriage [27]. Radiation dose from the CT scan of the head is approx. 0.05 rad. While doing a head CT scan, the abdomen of the mother should be shielded with a lead apron.

4.2.4 Exposure

Like any other trauma patient, expose and screen for any other life-threatening injuries. While examining the abdomen inspect for distension and palpate for guarding and rigidity to assess for intraabdominal hemorrhage, perforation of viscus, and uterine rupture. In uterine examination, fundal height, shape, uterine tone, and tenderness should be evaluated. Uterine contractions occur in almost 40% of cases of trauma but in 90% cases resolve with time with no adverse fetal effects [28].

Routine tocolytics are not indicated in trauma patients as most of the contractions stop spontaneously and those contractions that are not self-limited are often pathological in origin and are contraindication to tocolytic therapy. The decision to use them should be made by the obstetrician. Placental abruption occurs in 5–50% of cases [29]. The signs of placental abruption are vaginal bleeding, uterine tenderness, uterine irritability, and tetany. Abruption near term can be managed by urgent vaginal delivery or cesarean section depending on the mothers' vitals, in early abruption, continuous and vigilant monitoring is required and consider urgent delivery if irritability increases [30].

Uterine rupture is rare. It is seen in only 0.6% of all trauma patients. Uterine rupture is suggested by abdominal fetal lie [oblique or transverse] or palpation of fetal parts along with guarding and rigidity. Once uterine rupture is identified consider urgent laparotomy to control bleeding and resuscitation of patients. Trauma can lead to two-fold increased risk of preterm delivery [31]. Placental abruption, traumatic injury to uterus directly, or premature rupture of membranes can initiate preterm labor. Early neonatology consultation and injection of steroid if the fetus is viable should be considered.

4.2.5 Fetus

Fetal heart sounds should be auscultated for fetal assessment. Before 10 weeks of gestation, they can be auscultated with Doppler ultrasound. After 20–24 weeks of gestation, continuous fetal monitoring with tocodynamometer should be done. The normal fetal heart rate is 120–160 beats/min; fetal bradycardia, tachycardia, repetitive decelerations, and the absence of beat-to-beat variability are signs of impending maternal or fetal decompensation which should prompt immediate consultation with an obstetrician.

According to ATLS principles [17], patients with no risk factors for fetal loss should be monitored continuously for 6 h. If there are risk factors for fetal loss or placental abruption, monitoring should be continued for 24 h. Risk factors include maternal heart rate >110, an injury severity score (ISS) >9, evidence of placental abruption, fetal heart rate >160 or <120, ejection during accident, motorcycle or pedestrian collisions [17]. Indications to perform any radiographic studies should be done like any other non-pregnant trauma patients; the benefits certainly outweigh potential risk to the fetus. Figure 7 illustrates an example protocol to guide the primary survey of a pregnant trauma victim.

Victorian State Trauma System
Obstetric Trauma
TRAUMA
VICTORIA
Make early contact with ARV for advice from the major trauma services and to initiate retrieval.
• Fetal survival depends on effective maternal resuscitation.
• Maternal position – 1 or 2 handed manual uterine displacement or left tilt 15-30°
• Maternal hypovolaemia will significantly impact on fetal outcomes.
Early Activation
• Gather vital information
• Activate Trauma Team
• Designate roles
• Set up to receive patient
• Ensure safety using PPE
Primary Survey
AIRWAY / C-SPINE
• Protect Airway
• Be prepared for difficult intubation
• Maintain full spinal precautions if indicated
BREATHING
• Identify and treat any life threats
• Assess RR, work of breathing, SpO_2 & symmetry
• Oxygen therapy to maintain SpO_2 94% - 98%
• $ETCO_2$ monitoring if ventilated
• Intercostal Catheter should be inserted 1-2 rib spaces higher
CIRCULATION
• Position patient with manual left uterine displacement or tilt if > 20 weeks gestation
• Insert x 2 large bore IV cannulas & commence fluid resuscitation if required
• Assess HR/BP/Cap refill
• Identify and control source of haemorrhage
DISABILITY
• Assess level of consciousness
• Check pupils
• Check BSL
EXPOSURE / ENVIRONMENT
• Fully expose patient
• Prevent heat loss
• Log roll
ADJUNCTS
• Ultrasound / CTG monitoring
• X rays: Chest, Pelvis
• Take blood: Hb, Group & X-Match, coagulation studies
• 12 lead ECG
• Consider IDC
• Orogastric tube if intubated
Does patient meet potential Major Trauma criteria for Inter-hospital transfer?
N
Y
• Monitor closely
• Perform secondary survey
• Observe in facility for at least 2 hours
• Provide required care, discharge and follow up as necessary
Notify ARV to conduct case assessment
Patient meets potential major trauma criteria?
N
Y
• Perform complete trauma evaluation including secondary survey
• Obtain an early and accurate obstetric history
• Assess fetal well being
• Perform cervical exam if qualified obstetric staff available
• Take advice from MTS via ARV coordinators
• Make early contact if any deterioration in patient's condition occurs
• Prepare patient for retrieval and definitive care
• Optimise oxygenation
• Continue fluid resuscitation
• Continuously monitor patient
• Assess fetal well-being
• Commence secondary survey if time allows
• Ensure clear, accurate & concise documentation
• Seek advice from MTS via ARV
• Communicate any new clinical developments or significant deterioration
• Support family and friends
PERIMORTEM CAESAREAN SECTION is indicated where the mother is in cardiac arrest with a fetus of > 20 weeks gestation. In these cases, caesarean section is performed to help restore circulating volume to the mother and fetal survival is not the primary indication. Rarely, where complications of trauma indicate that maternal survival is unlikely and the fetus is > 24 weeks gestation, a caesarean section may be performed to rescue the fetus.
Key points
Maternal Resuscitation
• Fetal survival is improved by optimizing maternal resuscitation and avoidance of hypovolaemia. Haemorrhage control may be impossible without emergent surgical intervention.
Fluid resuscitation
• Initiate if hypovolaemia is suspected to maintain both maternal and fetoplacental perfusion. Note that a pregnant patient may not display signs of haemorrhage until as much as 30% of her blood volume is lost.
• Crystalloid fluids: Initial treatment with Normal Saline is recommended up to 20 - 30 mL/kg.
• Blood products: if minimal response to fluids, administration of Rhesus negative packed red blood cells should be given.
Maternal oxygenation
• Maternal hypoxia is associated with poor fetal outcomes. Maintain oxygenation >94%. Apply supplemental oxygen as required.
Patient positioning
• Patients greater than 20 weeks gestation should be deliberately positioned to protect blood flow and venous return. This can be achieved by using 1 or 2 handed manual left uterine displacement or with a left sided tilt of 15 - 30° to facilitate blood flow and venous return.
Manual displacement with 1 or 2 hands or left lateral tilt 15 - 30°
30°
Obstetric Trauma Considerations
Pregnancy Related Complications
• Placental abruption.
• Premature labour.
• Uterine rupture.
• Feto-maternal haemorrhage.
Obstetric assessment is important to identify signs of labour, fetal well-being, perineal injury and concealed or contained haemorrhage.
Cervical examination should only be performed by qualified obstetric staff.
Fetal well-being: CTG monitoring is important to institute where possible to assess fetal status. If not available, auscultate fetal heart sounds and / or ask the mother when she last felt fetal movement.

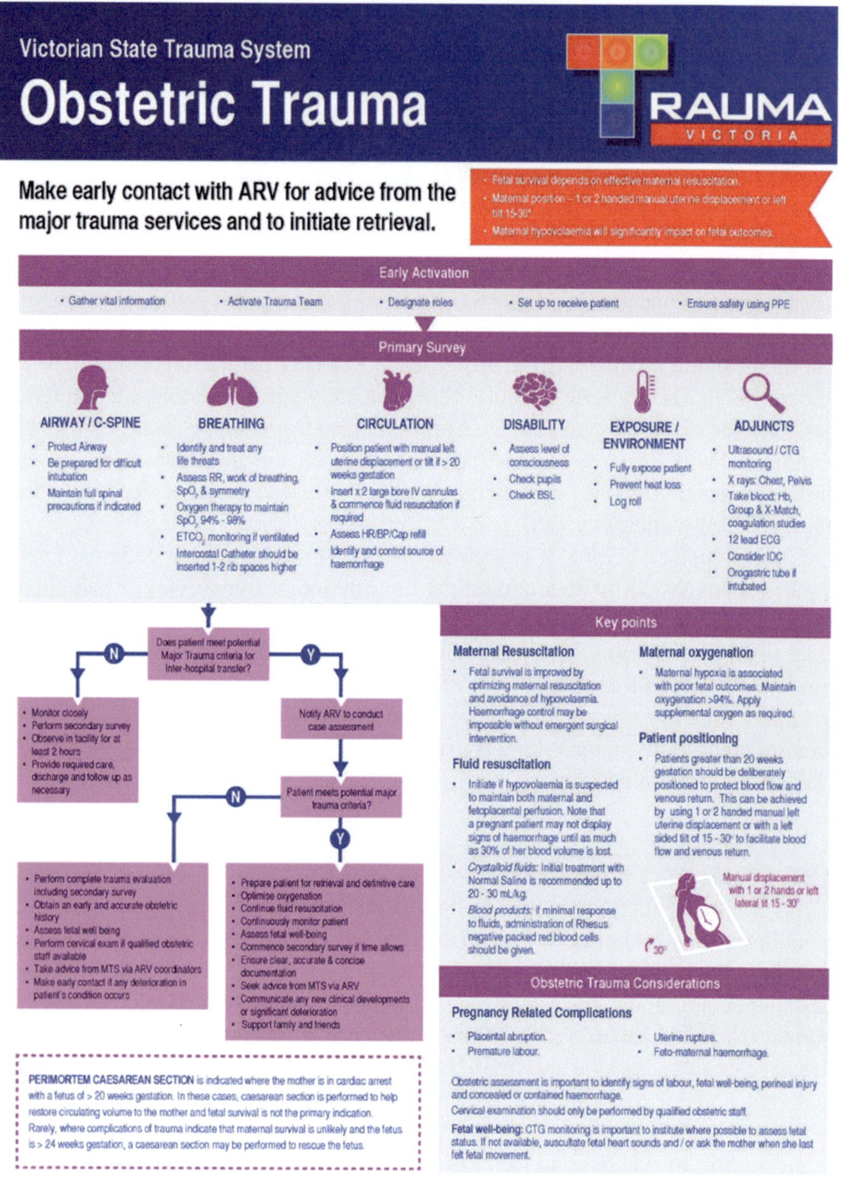

Fig. 7 With permission from: Victoria State trauma system obstetric trauma pathway

4.3 Secondary Survey

There is no difference in the secondary assessment of pregnant and non-pregnant patients. The secondary survey is started only after primary survey and life-threatening injury management have been completed. It comprises history, and a complete, detailed evaluation of the patient.

History—A brief history is taken which is the same as in non-pregnant patients. The mnemonic AMPLE is used [17]:

- A—History of allergies
- M—Medication
- P—History of past illness
- L—Last meal taken
- E—Events leading to injury

Apart from this history, one should also gain the past obstetric history and history of the current pregnancy. Any leakage of fluid, vaginal bleeding, abdominal pain, and contractions should be enquired about. Secondary survey includes examination of head, maxillofacial structures, cervical spine and neck, chest, abdomen, and pelvis with extra care to assess for uterine contractions and fetal examination. Examination for injuries should also include the perineum and vagina.

There is no difference between pregnant and non-pregnant patients in terms of initial assessment and management of trauma, indication for CT scan, focused assessment with sonography for trauma (FAST) or diagnostic peritoneal lavage (DPL). Diagnostic peritoneal lavage (DPL) has largely been replaced by FAST although when FAST is ambiguous, DPL may have a role. If DPL is performed, place the catheter above the umbilicus using an open technique. The presence of amniotic fluid in the vagina, evidenced by a fluid pH of above 4.5, suggests ruptured chorioamniotic membranes.

Vaginal bleeding in the third trimester may indicate disruption of the placenta and impending death of the fetus; a vaginal examination is imperative although repeated vaginal examinations are best avoided. The decision for emergency cesarean section is made in consultation with an obstetrician [17]. Various feto-maternal complications should be kept in mind. These include disseminated intravascular coagulation due to placental abruption and uterine rupture, amniotic fluid embolism, preterm labor and delivery, and uterine rupture requiring emergency cesarean section.

4.3.1 Isoimmunization of the Mother in Rh-Negative Woman

Feto-maternal bleeding has been reported in 2.6–30% of pregnant trauma patients [32]. As small as 0.01 mL of Rh-positive blood can sensitize 70% of Rh-negative women, thus mandating Rh immunoglobulin therapy. All Rh-negative pregnant trauma patients should receive Rh immunoglobulin therapy (single dose of 300 mg) within 72 h of injury; exceptions are when the injury is far away from the uterus such as isolated to the extremities or head [26].

Table 1 Estimated fetal radiation exposure [35]

Radiological exam	Estimated fetal radiation exposure (rad)
Thoracic spine radiograph	<0.001
Chest (posteroanterior/lateral)	0.001
CT head	<0.01
Hip radiograph	0.13
Pelvis radiograph	0.17
Abdominal radiograph	0.24
Lumbar spine radiograph	0.34
CT abdomen/pelvis	1–2

4.4 Adjuncts to the Secondary Survey

Any diagnostic tests mandated by the clinical presentation may be performed during the secondary survey to identify injuries. CT scan, X rays, angiography, bronchoscopy, esophagoscopy, contrast urography, and other diagnostic procedures may all be performed.

In 2004, the American College of Obstetricians and Gynecologists supported the use of the 5 rad cut-offs. Stochastic carcinogenic effects of radiation, by definition, are random and have no threshold value. According to the American College of Radiology, there is a 0.4% increase in the cumulative lifetime incidence of cancer when a fetus is exposed to 10 mGy (1 rad) [33, 34]. Table 1 summarizes the estimated fetal radiation exposure with each radiological investigation.

4.4.1 Perimortem Cesarean Section

This is initiated after CPR has commenced. The data in support of perimortem cesarean section are limited. The two main indications for postmortem cesarean section are: [7, 36].

1. To salvage the mother—if cardiopulmonary resuscitation has not been effective; should be performed within 4 min of maternal cardiac arrest. The rationale behind this is the improved efficacy of maternal chest compression and resuscitation as aortocaval compression is alleviated after delivery. It should be done only in pregnancies more than 23–24 weeks when the uterus is large enough to cause aortocaval compression [16].
2. To salvage the fetus—if survival of the mother is not possible, a multidisciplinary decision must be made to salvage the fetus. Fetal compromise may have started well before mothers' hemodynamic instability, and the fetus may have suffered prolonged hypoxia, so this decision should not be made lightly.

4.5 *Intensive Care Management*

A pregnant trauma victim may be admitted to an intensive care unit for the monitoring of mother and fetus as indicated by the severity and type of injury. As trauma impacts the lives of two human beings, meticulous follow-up is paramount in the care of a parturient trauma victim. Sometimes fetal monitoring may reveal signals about maternal deterioration due to direct trauma to the uterus, placental abruption, and uterine rupture.

Common indications for Intensive Care Unit admission:

1. **Signs of abruptio-placenta:**

   Incidence varies from 7.4 to 66% of cases of severe trauma to the abdomen [37, 38]. Significant direct abdominal trauma, abdominal or uterine tenderness, or vaginal bleeding are suggestive of an abruptio-placenta and should be monitored.

   Maternal monitoring: Excessive uterine activity is one of the cardinal signs of placental abruption. More than four contractions per hour may be indicative of abruption and more than eight contractions per hour in the first 4 h following trauma is consistent with the diagnosis of placental abruption [40]. Eighty percent occur within 6 h of monitoring but presentation may be delayed for up to 48 h or longer.

   Along with important maternal findings, associated non-reassuring cardiotocographic findings may occur on fetal monitoring. Fetal distress is predictive of abruptio-placenta in 60% of all cases [41]; this may not happen until 30% of the placenta is separated from the uterus, and 50% or more uteroplacental separation is consistently associated with fetal fatality [7].

   Sonographic and laboratory abnormalities are not consistently present with abruption but support the diagnosis. CT and MRI, though not routinely used to diagnose placental abruption, will give a definite indication about abruption if done as a part of routine screening for trauma.

2. **Signs of uterine rupture:**

   Uterine rupture can happen due to sharp or blunt trauma to the abdomen. This should be suspected in cases of assault and in individuals with pelvic fractures, direct perineal trauma, or penetrating injury to the pelvis. It usually happens towards term and in patients with a previous uterine scar. The injury may range from a small tear up to complete avulsion of the uterus. Urinary bladder injury may be coexisting.

   Patients may present with hypovolemic shock, vaginal bleeding, abdominal tenderness, features of peritonitis, and abnormal fetal CTG or fetal death. As these features are not specific for uterine rupture and may mimic abruption, solid organ injuries, and pelvic fractures, the diagnosis will often be confirmed at laparotomy. These patients should be admitted to the intensive care unit and stabilized perioperatively.

3. **Non-obstetric Indications:** Examples include patients with moderate and severe head injuries, thoracic and solid organ injuries in the abdomen, and life-threatening pelvic injuries. Admission to the ICU may be required for monitoring, perioperative stabilization and optimization, or for conservative management as decided by the trauma team.
4. **Trauma-related pulmonary embolism (venous thromboembolism or amniotic fluid)**: Although rare these may be life-threatening conditions [39]. The mechanism of amniotic fluid embolism is believed to be a sudden increase in amniotic fluid pressure at impact in the presence of vascular wounds [40]. Patients present with sudden respiratory distress with hypoxia, severe hypotension, circulatory shock, seizures, coma, and cardiac arrest. Half of these cases will present with Disseminated Intravascular Coagulation (DIC) if they survive [40]. Echocardiography may show right heart strain or failure and increased pulmonary artery pressure [41]. These patients must be admitted to the Intensive Care Unit for cardiopulmonary support including extracorporeal techniques in some cases [41, 42]. Decisions about thrombolysis in venous thromboembolism should be made promptly in conjunction with decisions about fetal delivery. In addition to the obstetrician, thoracic surgeons and interventional radiologists should be immediately involved in decision-making and management.
5. **Other obstetric complications**: Premature contractions, premature rupture of membranes, and preterm labor are expected in patients admitted with trauma to the intensive care unit. The risk of preterm delivery is two times higher in pregnant trauma patients [7]. This happens commonly after premature rupture of the membranes (PROM). PROM can also result in umbilical cord prolapse, compression of the cord causing fetal distress, infection, pulmonary hypoplasia, and orthopedic deformities of the fetus [7, 43]. A fibronectin test or cervical length assessment may be used to assess the risk for preterm labor in cases of regular uterine contractions [7].

4.6 *Fetal Monitoring in Intensive Care Unit*

Assessment for the viability of the fetus should be done immediately after trauma and periodically throughout the ICU stay. If the fetus is viable, fetal monitoring should be commenced immediately.

Feto-maternal hemorrhage (FMH): This is expected in case of major trauma to the parturient. It happens due to transplacental passage of fetal blood into the maternal circulation. Apart from isoimmunization of the Rh−ve mother, FMH may also result in fetal exsanguination, anemia, distress, or demise [20]. Other complications of FMH are neonatal neurological damage and hemolytic anemia of the newborn [43]. The Kleihauer-Betke (KB) test quantifies the presence of fetal cells in the maternal circulation. Though used traditionally to test isoimmunization of the Rh-ve mother, the usefulness of this test to assess the degree of FMH in Rh+ve mother is not well validated. Flow cytometry using fetal middle cerebral artery flow velocity also has been suggested to estimate fetal anemia and the possibility of FMH [43]. In rare cases, intrauterine blood transfusion may be required to salvage the fetus [1].

Fetal monitoring helps in the following aspects [7]:

- Uteroplacental compromise or placental abruption resulting in impending hypoxemic fetal injury or death can be detected early by fetal monitoring.
- Trauma-related complications of pregnancy including placental abruption, preterm delivery, and spontaneous rupture of the membranes, can be detected early by fetal monitoring.
- Feto-maternal hemorrhage and resultant anemia can be diagnosed by advanced fetal monitoring methods.
- Fetal injuries can be detected by ultrasound-guided fetal monitoring.
- Decreased placental perfusion caused by maternal hypovolemia can be identified by fetal monitoring.

Although a fetus more than 23 weeks of gestation is considered viable, it may be difficult to get details of gestational age from the history. Fundus examination helps to estimate the gestational age. Ultrasound estimation of the fetus is an alternative solution in these cases.

Fetal heart rate monitoring: Electronic Fetal Monitoring (EFM) is highly recommended in any maternal trauma, the duration of which is decided by the severity of injury and further progress of events. It helps in not only assessing fetal well-being but also in the early detection of maternal obstetric complications as described above. In major maternal injuries, the incidence of fetal loss is up to 61% and in minor injuries up to 27% [44]. However, EFM has low sensitivity (62%) and specificity (49%) in predicting adverse obstetric outcomes. The combined use of physical examination and normal EFM tracing has a good negative predictive value. Alarming signs of fetal compromise include decelerations, bradycardia, tachycardia, and loss of variability. Many patients will respond to supplemental oxygen, IV fluids, and left lateral decubitus position; a small proportion of cases (2.4–7.2%) may end up in emergency cesarean section to salvage the fetus. Emergency cesarean section in a trauma victim is a significant predictor of maternal death [45].

The duration of fetal monitoring is controversial. A 4-h minimum is generally accepted, but it may be required for up to 24 h. The Society of Obstetricians and Gynecologists of Canada (SOGC) recommends extended monitoring if any of the following high-risk features are present [7]:

- Uterine tenderness
- Significant abdominal pain
- Vaginal bleeding
- Contraction frequency of more than once per 10 min during a monitoring period of 4 h
- Rupture of the membranes
- Atypical or abnormal fetal heart rate pattern (fetal tachycardia, bradycardia, or decelerations)

– High-risk mechanism of injury (motorcycle, pedestrian, high-speed collision), or serum fibrinogen <200 mg/dL

Monitoring for 4 h is sufficient to rule out major trauma-related complications in low-risk patients without the above-mentioned risk factors.

Direct Fetal Injury: As the fetus is protected by the uterus, maternal soft tissues and amniotic fluid, direct fetal injury is uncommon in minor trauma, and usually results from high-impact trauma. It occurs in less than 1% of maternal trauma cases [46], seems more prevalent in pelvic trauma, and often involves the fetal skull and brain.

4.7 ICU Care Issues

It is important to remember the physiological changes of pregnancy, and that these may continue for some time post-delivery. The intensive care team thus need to remain alert to changes in volume management, nutritional tolerance, and coagulation status. This is relevant even if the trauma incident has resulted in fetal delivery.

Dedicated nursing staff familiar with obstetric management should be co-opted to assist with care; post-delivery lactation management is important, as is psychological support for a critically injured woman who may have lost her child, or been separated from her infant due to emergent delivery.

5 Outcome of Pregnancy in Trauma

Trauma is a leading cause of morbidity and mortality in the parturient. The severity of injury is directly related to maternal death [47]. Pregnant trauma victims may have a 1.6-fold higher rate of mortality compared to non-pregnant trauma victims; and are more likely to be dead on arrival or die during their hospital course [48].

Unless complicated by maternal hypotension or pelvic injury, trauma-related pregnancy loss is uncommon in the first trimester [49]. Among patients who sustain life-threatening trauma, fetal loss can reach 40–50% [49].

In a population-based retrospective cohort, 25% of patients admitted in the third trimester had normal delivery during the hospital course and others in subsequent admissions [50]. Those who delivered remotely from their trauma event had more complications such as abruption, preterm birth, and low birth weight; it is hypothesized that this may be due to subclinical chronic abruption [49].

In another retrospective cohort, 83% of patients discharged following trauma had a sustained risk of risk of adverse pregnancy outcomes when compared to pregnant non-trauma cases. Interestingly, the Injury Severity score (ISS) was a poor predictor of adverse outcomes [50].

6 Summary

A pregnant trauma victim is admitted to the intensive care unit for monitoring and management of the mother and fetus. A proper understanding of the differences in physiology and anatomy helps us to focus our attention and to tailor the management accordingly. Fetal monitoring is an important tool to identify maternal complications early and to take appropriate measures to safeguard the mother and maintaining the normal physiology of the mother is the best approach to salvage the fetus.

A coordinated approach involving trauma surgeons, anesthesiologists, neonatologists, intensivists, midwives, and nurses results in the best outcome for the mother and fetus.

References

1. Huls CK, Detlefs C. Trauma in pregnancy. Semin Perinatol. 2018;42(1):13–20. https://doi.org/10.1053/j.semperi.2017.11.004.
2. World Health Organization. Global burden of disease. Geneva: World Health Organization; 2007. Available: www.who.int/healthinfo/global_burden_disease/en/ (accessed 23.03.17)
3. Mendez-Figueroa H, Dahlke JD, Vrees RA, Rouse DJ. Trauma in pregnancy: an updated systematic review. Am J Obstet Gynecol. 2013;209(1):1–10. https://doi.org/10.1016/j.ajog.2013.01.021.
4. Schellenberg M, Ruiz NS, Cheng V, Heindel P, Roedel EQ, Clark DH, Inaba K, Demetriades D. The impact of seat belt use in pregnancy on injuries and outcomes after motor vehicle collisions. J Surg Res. 2020;254:96–101. https://doi.org/10.1016/j.jss.2020.04.012.
5. Cugell DW, Frank NR, Gaensler EA, Badger TL. Pulmonary function in pregnancy. I. Serial observations in normal women. Am Rev Tuberc. 1953;67(5):568–97. https://doi.org/10.1164/art.1953.67.5.568.
6. Munnur U, Suresh MS. Airway problems in pregnancy. Crit Care Clin. 2004;20(4):617–42. https://doi.org/10.1016/j.ccc.2004.05.011.
7. Jain V, Chari R, Maslovitz S, Farine D, Maternal Fetal Medicine Committee, Bujold E, Gagnon R, Basso M, Bos H, Brown R, Cooper S, Gouin K, McLeod NL, Menticoglou S, Mundle W, Pylypjuk C, Roggensack A, Sanderson F. Guidelines for the management of a pregnant trauma patient. J Obstet Gynaecol Can. 2015;37(6):553–74. https://doi.org/10.1016/s1701-2163(15)30232-2.
8. Robson SC, Dunlop W, Moore M, Hunter S. Combined Doppler and echocardiographic measurement of cardiac output: theory and application in pregnancy. Br J Obstet Gynaecol. 1987;94(11):1014–27. https://doi.org/10.1111/j.1471-0528.1987.tb02285.x.
9. Meah VL, Cockcroft JR, Backx K, Shave R, Stöhr EJ. Cardiac output and related haemodynamics during pregnancy: a series of meta-analyses. Heart. 2016;102(7):518–26. https://doi.org/10.1136/heartjnl-2015-308476.
10. Green LJ, Mackillop LH, Salvi D, Pullon R, Loerup L, Tarassenko L, Mossop J, Edwards C, Gerry S, Birks J, Gauntlett R, Harding K, Chappell LC, Watkinson PJ. Gestation-specific vital sign reference ranges in pregnancy. Obstet Gynecol. 2020;135(3):653–64. https://doi.org/10.1097/AOG.0000000000003721.

11. Metcalfe J, Ueland K. Maternal cardiovascular adjustments to pregnancy. Prog Cardiovasc Dis. 1974;16(4):363–74. https://doi.org/10.1016/0033-0620(74)90028-0.
12. Maynard SE, Thadhani R. Pregnancy and the kidney. J Am Soc Nephrol. 2009 Jan;20(1):14–22. https://doi.org/10.1681/ASN.2008050493.
13. Hladunewich MA, Myers BD, Derby GC, Blouch KL, Druzin ML, Deen WM, Naimark DM, Lafayette RA. Course of preeclamptic glomerular injury after delivery. Am J Physiol Renal Physiol. 2008;294(3):F614–20. https://doi.org/10.1152/ajprenal.00470.2007.
14. Anon. Maternal physiology. In: Cunningham F, Leveno KJ, Bloom SL, Dashe JS, Hoffman BL, Casey BM, Spong CY, editors. Williams obstetrics. 25th ed. McGraw Hill; 2018. Accessed December 15, 2022. https://accessmedicine.mhmedical.com/content.aspx?bookid=1918§ionid=144754618.
15. Nel JT, Diedericks A, Joubert G, Arndt K. A prospective clinical and urodynamic study of bladder function during and after pregnancy. Int Urogynecol J Pelvic Floor Dysfunct. 2001;12(1):21–6. https://doi.org/10.1007/s001920170089.
16. Aggarwal R, Soni KD, Trikha A. Initial management of a pregnant woman with trauma. J Obstet Anaesth Crit Care. 2018;8(2):66–72.
17. American College of Surgeons. Trauma in pregnancy and intimate partner violence. In: Advanced trauma life support student course manual. 10th ed. Chicago, Ill: American College of Surgeons; 2018. p. 228–39.
18. Sasser SM, Hunt RC, Faul M, Sugerman D, Pearson WS, Dulski T, Wald MM, Jurkovich GJ, Newgard CD, Lerner EB, Centers for Disease Control and Prevention (CDC). Guidelines for field triage of injured patients: recommendations of the National Expert Panel on Field Triage, 2011. MMWR Recomm Rep. 2012;61(RR-1):1–20.
19. Humphries A, Mirjalili SA, Tarr GP, et al. Hemodynamic changes in women with symptoms of supine hypotensive syndrome. Acta Obstet Gynecol Scand. 2019;1:371.
20. Pearce C, Martin SR. Trauma and considerations unique to pregnancy. Obstet Gynecol Clin N Am. 2016;43:791–808.
21. Biro P. Difficult intubation in pregnancy. Curr Opin Anaesthesiol. 2011;24:249–54.
22. Heidemaun BH, McClure JH. Changes in maternal physiology during pregnancy. CEACCP. 2003;3:65–8.
23. Mendez-Figueroa H, Dahlke JD, Vrees RA, Rouse DJ. Trauma in pregnancy: an updated systematic review. Am J Obstet Gynecol. 2013;209:10.
24. Sperry JL, Minei JP, Frankel HL, West MA, Harbrecht BG, Moore EE, et al. Early use of vasopressors after injury: caution before constriction. J Trauma. 2008;64:9–14.
25. Atta E, Gardner M. Cardiopulmonary resuscitation in pregnancy. Obstet Gynecol Clin N Am. 2007;34:585–97.
26. Fung Kee Fung K, Eason E, Crane J, Armson A, De La Ronde S, Farine D, et al. Prevention of Rh alloimmunization. J Obstet Gynaecol Can. 2003;25(765):73.
27. Holcomb JB, Jenkins D, Rhee P, et al. Damage control resuscitation: directly addressing the early coagulopathy of trauma. J Trauma. 2007;62:307–10.
28. Connolly AM, Katz VL, Bash KL, McMahon MJ, Hansen WF. Trauma and pregnancy. Am J Perinatol. 1997;14:331–6.
29. Goodwin TM, Breen MT. Pregnancy outcome and fetomaternal hemorrhage after non-catastrophic trauma. Am J Obstet Gynecol. 1990;162:665–71.
30. Oyelese Y, Ananth CV. Placental abruption. Obstet Gynecol. 2006;108:1005–16.
31. Guth AA, Pachter L. Domestic violence and the trauma surgeon. Am J Surg. 2000;179:134–40.
32. Chames MC, Pearlman MD. Trauma during pregnancy: outcomes and clinical management. Clin Obstet Gynecol. 2008;51(2):398–408.
33. Committee ACOG. on Obstetric Practice. ACOG Committee Opinion. Number 299, September 2004 (replaces No. 158, September 1995). Guidelines for diagnostic imaging during pregnancy. Obstet Gynecol. 2004;104(3):647–51. https://doi.org/10.1097/00006250-200409000-00053.

34. American College of Radiology. ACR–SPR practice parameter for imaging pregnant or potentially pregnant adolescents and women with ionizing radiation. https://www.acr.org/-/media/ACR/Files/Practice-Parameters/pregnant-pts.pdf.
35. Cohn DC, Ramaswamy B, Blum K. Malignancy and pregnancy. In: Greene MF, Creasy RK, Resnik R, et al., editors. Creasy and Resnik's maternal-fetal medicine principles and practice. 6th ed. Philadelphia: Saunders Elsevier; 2009. p. 889.
36. Katz VL. Perimortem cesarean delivery: its role in maternal mortality. Semin Perinatol. 2012;36(68):72.
37. Schiff MA, Holt VL. Pregnancy outcomes following hospitalization for motor vehicle crashes in Washington State from 1989 to 2001. Am J Epidemiol. 2005;161(6):503–10. https://doi.org/10.1093/aje/kwi078. Erratum in: Am J Epidemiol. 2005 Jul 15;162(2):197
38. Esposito TJ. Trauma during pregnancy. Emerg Med Clin North Am. 1994;12(1):167–99.
39. Einav S, Sela HY, Weiniger CF. Management and outcomes of trauma during pregnancy. Anesthesiol Clin. 2013;31:141–56. https://bit.ly/3kV0h65
40. Rossignol M. Trauma and pregnancy: what anesthesiologist should know. Anaesth Crit Care Pain Med. 2016;35:S27–34. https://bit.ly/34bbEkg
41. Lucia A, Dantoni SE. Trauma management of the pregnant patient. Crit Care Clin. 2016;32:109–17. https://bit.ly/314wxeY
42. Oxford CM, Ludmir J. Trauma in pregnancy. Clin Obstet Gynecol. 2009;52:611–29. https://bit.ly/349aCFr
43. Petrone P, Marini CP. Trauma in pregnant patients. Curr Probl Surg. 2015;52:330–51.
44. Rothenberger D, Quattlebaum FW, Perry JF Jr, Zabel J, Fischer RP. Blunt maternal trauma: a review of 103 cases. J Trauma. 1978;18:173–9.
45. Morris JA Jr, Rosenbower TJ, Jurkovich GJ, Hoyt DB, Harviel JD, Knudson MM, et al. Infant survival after cesarean section for trauma. Ann Surg. 1996;223:481–91.
46. Van Hook JW. Trauma in pregnancy. Clin Obstet Gynecol. 2002;45:414–24.
47. Drost TF, Rosemurgy AS, Sherman HF, et al. Major trauma in pregnant women: maternal/fetal outcome. J Trauma. 1990;30:574.
48. Deshpande NA, Kucirka LM, Smith RN, Oxford CM. Pregnant trauma victims experience nearly 2-fold higher mortality compared to their nonpregnant counterparts. Am J Obstet Gynecol. 2017;217(5):590.e1–9. https://doi.org/10.1016/j.ajog.2017.08.004.
49. ACOG. Obstetric aspects of trauma management. ACOG Educ Bullet. 1998;251:1.
50. El-Kady D, Gilbert WM, Anderson J, et al. Trauma during pregnancy: an analysis of maternal and fetal outcomes in a large population. Am J Obstet Gynecol. 2004;190:1661.

Eclampsia: An Update

Firdos Ummunnisa, Umm E Amara, Umme Nashrah, M. M. Nainthramveetil, Naseera Aboobacker, Zeba Alami, and Nissar Shaikh

Abstract Eclampsia is an acute and urgent clinical condition during pregnancy. Frequently, it is a convulsive manifestation of preeclampsia. Fortunately, eclampsia is decreasing in developed countries but is still a major obstetric issue in the developing countries. The exact pathophysiology of eclampsia is not completely understood. The risk factors for eclampsia ranges from being primigravida to multifetal gestation. Eclampsia occurs after 20 weeks of gestation, with proteinuria, hypertension, and seizure activity, but is also increasingly detected without hypertension. The main management of eclampsia patients includes prevention of maternal hypoxia and injury, reducing the raised blood pressure, prevention of reoccurrence of seizure activity, and prompt delivery of the fetus. Eclampsia can cause multiorgan dysfunction and a majority of patients will have posterior reversible encephalopathy syndrome (PRES), preterm delivery. Overall eclampsia increases the fetomaternal mortality risk.

Keywords Anticonvulsant · Antihypertensive · Eclampsia · Hypertensive disorder of pregnancy · Preeclampsia · Pregnancy · Posterior reversible encephalopathy syndrome · Preterm · Seizures

F. Ummunnisa (✉)
Dr. Halima Al Tamimi, Obstetrics and Gynaecology Centre, Doha, Qatar

U. E Amara
Apollo Institute of Medical Sciences and Research, Hyderabad, Telangana, India

U. Nashrah
Deccan College of Medical Sciences, Hyderabad, Telangana, India

M. M. Nainthramveetil · N. Shaikh
Surgical Intensive Care: Hamad Medical Corporation, Doha, Qatar

N. Aboobacker · Z. Alami
OBGY Department, Al Khor Hospital/Hamad Medical Corporation, Doha, Qatar

N. Shaikh et al. (eds.), *Updates in Intensive Care of OBGY Patients*,
https://doi.org/10.1007/978-981-99-9577-6_8

1 Introduction

It is estimated that worldwide 10% of pregnancies are complicated by hypertensive disorders.

Eclampsia and preeclampsia occur in around 50% of these patients. Although these hypertensive disorders of pregnancy have been recognized for decades, there is a lack of understanding in many aspects of the disease [1]. Eclampsia is a convulsive manifestation of preeclampsia and one of the most serious acute complications of pregnancy. Eclampsia has higher morbidity and mortality for the mother and fetus. In spite of recent developments in diagnosis and management, these hypertensive disorders remain a common cause of maternal and fetal morbidity and mortality in developing countries.

Eclampsia commonly occurs in the third trimester of pregnancy, and 80% of eclampsia seizures occurs intrapartum or within the first 48 h following delivery. Rarely eclampsia is reported before 20 weeks gestation or up to 23 days postpartum. In the literature, various studies explored various techniques and biomarker predictors of patients at risk of eclampsia, apart from early diagnosis of preeclampsia, no other reliable test or symptom can predict the development of eclampsia. Eclampsia is reported to be responsible for around 1,00,000/annum mortality worldwide [2] and every 3 min a woman dies because of preeclampsia or eclampsia in the world. These hypertensive disorders are preventable and incidences are decreasing in particularly developed countries, still number of cases reported are classified as unpreventable [3].

2 Epidemiology

In last half century, the rate of eclampsia decreased in developed countries, with a stability of 1.5–10 cases per 10,000 deliveries [4]. Whereas the developing countries, rate of eclampsia reported to be higher in the ranges from 50 to 151 per 10,000 deliveries. These higher incidences and complication rates in developing countries are due to lack of disease awareness, absence of regular antenatal care, and delay in referral of seriously ill eclampsia cases [5].

3 Definitions

Eclampsia is defined as new-onset generalized tonic-colonic convulsions or unexplained coma during pregnancy or postpartum in cases with signs or symptoms of preeclampsia. Eclampsia occurs after the 20th week of gestation, intrapartum or in the postpartum period [5].

4 Pathogenesis

The exact pathophysiology of eclampsia is not well understood. There are two theories based on the role of hypertension with changes in cerebral blood flow and autoregulation causing hypertensive encephalopathy and the disruption of blood–brain barrier (BBB). The autoregulation of cerebral circulation is important to maintain a continuous blood flow in the brain with variation in the blood pressure. The elevated blood pressure causes cerebral vasoconstriction, when the blood pressure is lower it in turn, leads to cerebral vasodilation. According to the first theory, hypertension episode leads to the breakdown of the cerebral autoregulation, causing increased perfusion, endothelial dysfunction, cytotoxic and/or vasogenic edema causing seizures. The second theory states that hypertension with normal cerebral autoregulation causes cerebral vasoconstriction hence hypoperfusion, ischemia, endothelial malfunction, leading to cytotoxic and/or vasogenic edema [6]. The more recent experimental study did not show any variation in cerebral blood flow or autoregulation changes in pregnant and non-pregnant animal models [7].

The more recent literature showed that the vascular endothelial growth factor (VEGF) and placental growth factor (PlGF) will increase the permeability of BBB [8]. The blood–brain barrier (BBB) is rearranged due to increased levels of oxidized low-density lipoprotein (oxLDL) in preeclampsia patients [9]. Increased oxidative stress in placental circulation in preeclampsia patients leads to oxidative conversion of LDL into oxLDL; this oxLDL initiates multiple pathways in endothelial as well as in vascular smooth muscle, by binding to oxLDL receptor (LOX1); subsequently, oxLDL binding to LOX-1 produces complex stimulating cascades causing induction of the inflammatory interleukins, thus increasing the production of superoxide in cerebral endothelial cells causing vascular dysfunction [10]. The superoxide decreases the nitric oxide concentration by binding and forms peroxynitrite which has a deleterious effects on endothelial function, increased BBB permeability and causing vasogenic brain edema [11, 12].

The BBB dysfunction is described as an important etiology in seizure activity in preeclampsia patients [13]. The increased BBB permeability allows leakage of serum constituents into the brain causing microglial activation. Microglial activation decreases seizure threshold by secreting pro-inflammatory cytokines [13].

5 Risk Factors

Risk factors for preeclampsia, eclampsia, or gestational hypertension are the same. These risk factors are described in Table 1.

Magnesium sulfate prophylaxis protocols use in severe hypertension and preeclampsia can prevent the progress to eclampsia, the occurrence of seizures severe preeclampsia patients is 0.6% in those receiving magnesium sulfate compared to those patients not receiving magnesium sulfate is 2.0% [15].

Table 1 Risk factors [14]

Risk factors
Nulliparous
Black and Hispanic race
Preterm delivery at <32 weeks of gestation
Multifetal gestation
Advanced maternal age
No prenatal care

Table 2 Differential diagnosis for eclampsia

Differential diagnosis
Known case of seizure disorder
Traumatic/atraumatic brain injury and lesions
Amniotic fluid embolism
Thrombotic thrombocytopenic purpura
Drug or substance overdose or withdrawal
Systemic lupus erythematosus
Liver or renal failure
Hypoglycemia
Hyponatremia
Hyperosmolar osmotic state

6 Presentation and Diagnosis

Eclampsia is clear if a pregnant patient presents with hypertension, proteinuria, and convulsions, during or after 20 weeks of gestation. Hypertension considered essential in the diagnosis of eclampsia; it is absent in around 25% of the patients and it is also reported that the severe hypertension is frequent in patients developing antepartum eclampsia compared to postpartum eclampsia [11]. Several clinical symptoms are indicative of eclampsia, such as persistent occipital or frontal headaches, epigastric or right upper quadrant pain, blurred vision, photophobia, and altered level of consciousness in 59–75% of the patients; one of these symptoms is present before the occurrence of the seizure [11]. Differential diagnosis for eclampsia is described in Table 2.

7 Management

The main management of an eclampsia patient is to control the seizures, blood pressure and stabilization, and immediate delivery of the fetus. The eclampsia patients at term should be managed in a level 2 or 3 hospital with adequate intensive care therapy unit (ITU). Initial management of a convulsing pregnant patient is A (airway securing), B (breathing support), C (circulatory support and stabilization), D (assess disability and manage), and E (exposer and rolled onto their left side).

Following issues should be addressed immediately:

1. Maternal hypoxia and trauma prevention.
2. Hypertension treatment.
3. Seizure control and prevention.
4. Recurrent seizures prevention.
5. Immediate delivery of the fetus.

Eclampsia patients with status epilepticus, focal neurological signs, and/or seizure recurrence are highly suggestive of intracranial lesion/stroke. These patients should be managed by multidisciplinary team, including OBGY, anesthetist, intensivist, and neurologist. Further imaging studies and other blood investigations should be requested.

7.1 *Maintenance Oxygenation and Protection from Injuries*

The patient is placed in a lateral position, 8–10 L/min oxygen supplementation through a nasal cannula or nonrebreather face mask during the convulsion [13]. Insertion of oral airway and raising of padded bedrails will protect from injuries.

7.2 *Hypertension Treatment and Stabilization*

Antihypertensive therapy (Table 3) is essential to control the blood pressure as well as prevention of the stroke; stroke causes death in 15–20% of eclampsia patients; stroke risk correlates with severity of hypertension and maternal age [16]. The

Table 3 Guidelines for the treatment of severe hypertension with different medications

Labetalol	Hydralazine	Nifedipine
20 mg	5–10 mg	10 mg
Systolic blood pressure (SBP $\geq$ 160) or Diastolic blood pressure (DBP $\geq$ 110 mmHg) – 40 mg of labetalol bolus		
Still SBP $\geq$ 160 or DBP $\geq$ 110 mmHg – 80 mg	If SBP $\geq$ 160 or DBP $\geq$ 110 mmHg – 10 mg	If SBP $\geq$ 160 or DBP $\geq$ 110 mmHg – 20 mg
If SBP $\geq$ 160 or DBP $\geq$ 110 mmHg – 10 mg Hydralazine	Monitor blood pressure	
Check blood pressure If SBP $\geq$ 160 or DBP $\geq$ 110 mmHg – 40 mg Labetalol	Monitor blood pressure	SBP $\geq$ 160 or DBP $\geq$ 110 mmHg – 20 mg
If still SBP $\geq$ 160 or DBP $\geq$ 110 mmHg – 20 Labetalol, inform to physician		

Fishel Bartal. Eclampsia in the twenty-first century. Am J Obstet Gynecol 2022 cerebral vessels in patients with chronic hypertension may tolerate higher systolic pressures without any complications, whereas patients with known normal blood pressures may benefit therapeutic interventions earlier when initially blood pressure high. It is common practice to start antihypertensive therapy if sustained diastolic pressures equal or more than 110 mmHg or/and systolic blood pressures equal or more than 160 mmHg.

Intravenous hydralazine and labetalol bolus and infusion is considered as a first-line therapy. Labetalol should be avoided in patients with asthma, heart disease, or congestive heart failure. Oral nifedipine 10–20 mg is alternative, if labetalol and/or hydralazine contraindicated or ineffective in controlled blood pressure. Use of intravenous infusions of nicardipine and clevidipine in pregnancy has limited data. Sodium nitroprusside is used in extremes of hypertensive emergencies due to concerns of cyanide, thiocyanate toxicity, and the risk of raising the intracranial pressure. It is optimal to treat hypertensive emergencies in eclampsia patients in a monitored area, and with intravenous infusion. Fishel Bartal described the initial treatment with various antihypertensive (Table 3).

7.3 Anticonvulsant Medication (Fig. 1)

7.3.1 Persistent Seizure Activity

Two intravenous (IV) cannula should be placed as early as possible. The tonic-colonic phase of an eclampsia seizure usually resolves within 2 min, at which time magnesium sulfate should be started to prevent recurrent seizures (see "Magnesium sulfate prophylaxis" below).

If the patient is actively seizing for >5 min: Administer lorazepam 4 mg intravenous bolus; may need to repeat at 3–5 min if the seizure continues. If IV access has not been established, midazolam 10 mg intramuscularly is usually effective.

7.3.2 Prevention of Recurrent Seizures

Magnesium Sulfate Prophylaxis

Magnesium sulfate is the anticonvulsant of choice as it potentially prevents the reoccurrence of the convulsions along with control of initial seizure activity. Around 10% of eclampsia patients will have repeated convulsions if managed expectantly [1]. Literature suggest that in eclampsia the magnesium sulfate is more safer, pharmacological, and cost-effective compared to the phenytoin, diazepam, and lytic cocktail in prevention and control of recurrent seizures [17].

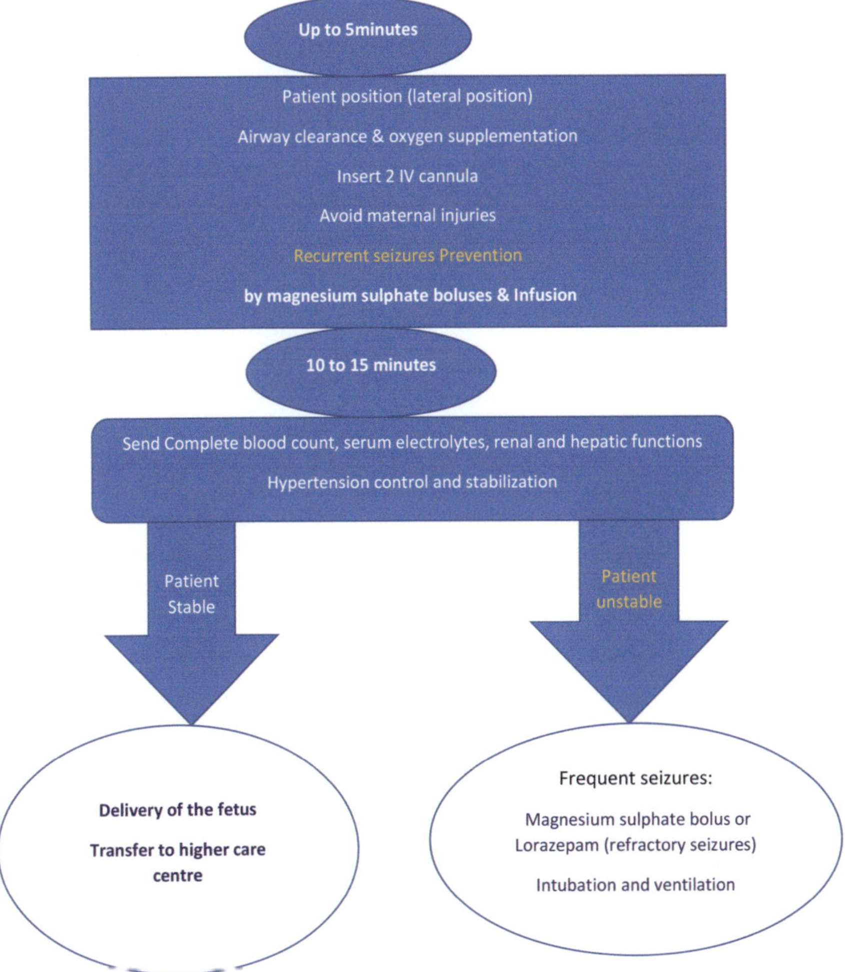

Fig. 1 Algorithm for eclampsia seizure management

7.4 *Dosing and Toxicity*

7.4.1 Loading Dose

A loading dose of magnesium sulfate—6 g intravenous over 15–20 min is recommended [18]. Other alternative dose and route of magnesium sulfate that can be administered is 5 g intramuscularly (IM) into each buttock with total 10 g. In this IM administration, the onset of action will be delayed and it is painful; mixing the magnesium sulfate with lidocaine 2% will decrease the pain. The loading doses can be administered safely in patients with renal impairment.

7.4.2 Maintenance Dose

Infusion of magnesium sulfate with 2 g/h started and continued for 24 h after the last seizure if the renal function is normal. The maintenance dose of 1–2 g/h is frequently used. Otherwise if infusion is not possible, magnesium sulfate 5 g should be given intramuscularly per 4 h; a lower dose maintenance regimen 2.5 g intramuscularly every 4 h found to be effective and cost-effective in resource-limited areas [19].

The maintenance phase is given and continued with monitoring clinically for the presence of deep tendon reflex, conscious level, urine output, with renal functions to avoid the hypermagnesemia or toxicity, following serum magnesium levels is not needed if patients pass adequate urine and there is no abnormality with the kidney functions. In cases with renal impairment or chronic kidney diseases, the maintenance dosing can be lowered after discussion with the clinical pharmacist or nephrologist, and magnesium levels should be monitored. It is advised to hold the magnesium sulfate infusion if the serum creatinine is >133 mmol/L or urine output decreases to <20 ml/h and checks the serum magnesium level after 6 h. In patients with mild increase in serum creatinine is 88–133 μmol/L and passing adequate urine output, the magnesium sulfate infusion should be reduced to 1 g/h with rechecking the magnesium level in 6 h. As reported, about 10% of the eclampsia patient's recurrent seizures after receiving magnesium sulfate [20]. In these patients, second bolus 2 g of magnesium sulfate should be given IV slowly over 5 min [20].

7.4.3 Therapeutic Magnesium Level

There is no threshold magnesium concentration in prevention of convulsion is described, serum magnesium levels of 1.9–3.5 mmol/L (4.8–8.4 mg/dL) is recommended, and serum magnesium levels should be monitored, as recurrent seizures may raise concerns of toxicity [20]. The dose adjustment should be done as per the clinical situation of the patients.

7.5 Magnesium Sulfate Toxicity and Side Effects

The most fearsome adverse effects of magnesium sulfate are respiratory depression and cardiac arrest that occur due to its toxicity. Hence, it is essential to monitor the serum magnesium levels in the management of these patients.

- Loss of deep tendon reflexes occurs at a serum magnesium level of 7 mEq/L (9 mg/dL).
- Respiratory depression occurs at 10 mEq/L (12 mg/dL).
- Cardiac arrest occurs at 25 mEq/L (30 mg/dL).

The eclampsia patients with impending respiratory depression or arrest may require intubation and ventilation and elevated serum magnesium should be corrected with IV calcium gluconate over 3 min. Serum magnesium levels should be monitored 4–6 h in eclampsia patients with renal impairments in patients with magnesium toxicity, the magnesium sulfate infusion should be stopped, and serum magnesium levels should be monitored every 2 h. Once the serum level is reduced to 7 mEq/L (<8.4 mg/dL), infusion should be resumed at a lower rate [21].

The use of calcium channel blockers along with the magnesium sulfate can cause hypotension. Magnesium sulfate is contraindicated in cases of myasthenia gravis as it can cause myasthenic crisis [21].

7.6 *Recurrent Seizures Management*

In patients with recurrent seizures on magnesium treatment, a serum magnesium level should be obtained. Administer a 4 g of magnesium sulfate bolus and 3 g/h maintenance infusion to patients with recurrent seizures and normal renal function with clinical and serum magnesium level monitoring [21].

When more than two recurrences occur after the above measures, discontinue magnesium sulfate, administering fosphenytoin or phenytoin infusion, along with cardiac monitoring and vital signs monitoring, and book urgent consultation with the neurology service.

8 Fetal Resuscitation

In eclampsia patients, fetal bradycardia for several minutes is a frequent finding during and after convulsions; it does not dictate an emergency cesarean delivery of the fetus. If the fetal heart rate tracing does not improve within 10–15 min in spite of maternal and fetal resuscitation, the possibility of an abruption of placenta is suspected and it indicates emergency delivery of the fetus [21]. The resuscitation of mother, control of seizure activity, hypertension, and maintaining oxygen will help the fetus recover from the effects of maternal eclampsia crisis such as hypoxia, hypercarbia, and uterine malperfusion [21].

9 Timing and Route of Fetus Delivery

The definitive therapeutic approach for eclampsia is immediate delivery of the fetus; still one can try induction and a trial of labor [22]. Once an eclampsia patient is stabilized, the factors which decide the mode of delivery will be whether the patient is already in labor or not, gestational age, condition of the cervix, and condition and position of the fetus. Patients with gestational age of 32–34 or earlier gestational age with a favorable Bishop score can have induction of labor; pharmacological agents can be used for cervical ripening and improving the Bishop score. Longer induction periods should be avoided and the treating team should have a clear plan for the delivery fetus.

10 Anesthesia

Labor analgesia will provide pain-free delivery; the presence of coagulopathy or severe thrombocytopenia is contraindication for regional anesthesia. From the recent literature it is reported that patients with a platelet count less than 100,000/mL and received a neuraxial anesthesia and analgesia, the risk of epidural hematoma is less than 0.2% [22].

In eclampsia patients due to airway edema, the general anesthesia will increase the risk of pulmonary aspiration and failed endotracheal. These patients with airway edema may be difficult to intubate; hence, the difficult intubation trolley including fibrotic bronchoscopes and tracheostomy set should be available immediately [22].

11 Postpartum Care

The eclampsia patients should be admitted to high dependency unit (HDU) or Intensive care unit (ICU) in the postpartum period for close monitoring of vital signs, input, output, and symptoms for 48–72 h. The patients with impaired renal function will have increased risk of pulmonary edema; hence, judicious fluid administration is essential [22].

11.1 Magnesium Sulfate Therapy Duration

In eclampsia patients, the seizures will resolve in postpartum period, within hours to days, occurrence of polyuria, with greater urine output of more than 4 L/day is the indicator of resolution of preeclampsia/eclampsia. Magnesium sulfate therapy should be continued for 24 h after delivery, and 24 h from the last seizure activity. During the magnesium sulfate therapy, decisions for maternal oral intake, physical activity, and care of the newborn should be on a case-by-case basis [22].

11.2 Treatment of Hypertension in Postpartum

In eclampsia patients, it is most important to control the blood pressure to prevent the occurrence of stroke. Patient's antihypertensive medications before the delivery or in antepartum period are frequently continued in postpartum period; it is essential that these drugs should be compatible with breastfeeding. The blood pressure target will be the same as in the antepartum period. Eclampsia patients with persistent hypertension may need to transfer to oral antihypertensive medications. If the patient was normotensive in the antepartum period, oral antihypertensive medications should be continued for 3 weeks and then can be stopped with continuous follow-up and monitoring of blood pressure [22, 23].

11.3 Neurological Follow-up

Eclampsia patients with neurological manifestation of, persistent neurologic deficits, prolonged loss of consciousness, onset of seizures more than 48 h in postpartum, seizures before 20 weeks of gestation, or with seizures on magnesium sulfate therapy should consult the neurologist in the postpartum period.

12 Complications

12.1 Maternal

Eclampsia slightly increases the risk of maternal death in developed countries, whereas the maternal mortality remained higher (7%) in developing countries [24]. A recent study from 29 countries concluded that the risk of death in eclampsia patients increased compared to those without eclampsia. In one of the Middle Eastern countries, the maternal morality remained zero for more than a decade [4].

Around 70% of eclampsia patients develop one or other complications such as hepatocellular damage, renal impairment, systemic coagulopathy, persistent hypertension, and neurologic complications, which resolve quickly following the delivery of fetus. The posterior reversible encephalopathy syndrome (PRES) is a frequent central nervous system complication in eclampsia patients [25]. Around 97% of eclampsia patients complicate into PRES, frequent risk factors including, eclampsia on presentation, recurrent seizures, postpartum eclampsia, cesarean delivery and labetalol use were associated with increased risk of PRES [26]. PRES is the leading cause of mortality and morbidity in patients with eclampsia [24, 26].

12.2 Fetal and Neonatal

In eclampsia, pregnancies with placental abruption, intrauterine asphyxia, preterm birth are the frequent causes of perinatal mortality. It is reported that the fetal death rates in eclampsia patients compared to pregnancies with no eclampsia were 10.8 and 4.1/1000 total births, respectively. The neonatal death rates were 7.5 and

2.2/1000 live births, respectively [25]. Literature from the developing countries of Africa mention that the overall rate of stillbirth or neonatal mortality in eclampsia patients ranges from 41/1000 to 231 per 1000 in Malawi and Uganda [25]. Eclampsia patients had a five- to sevenfold increased risk of preterm birth, 73% will have respiratory distress syndrome, and 21% of newborns will be small for gestational age [25].

13 Eclampsia Prevention

In patients with multifetal pregnancy, hypertension, diabetes, chronic renal disease, and autoimmune disease, use of low-dose aspirin ranging from 60 to 150 mg/day has been reported to reduce preeclampsia by up to 15% [25]. Hence, aspirin should also be administered if there is more than one of the risk factors, history of preeclampsia, low birth weight, previous adverse pregnancy outcome, 10-year or more pregnancy interval, primigravida, obesity, African American race, lower socioeconomic status, age of ≥35 years, and personal history factors. Measures to prevent the development of eclampsia can be by regular antenatal care of gestational hypertension, preeclampsia patients, and use of antihypertensive medications for blood pressure control, prompt delivery of fetus and use of magnesium sulfate in patients with preeclampsia with severe features [27].

In 40% of eclampsia patients, convulsions occur without prior symptoms; in 60%, seizure is the first sign of eclampsia [26]. In patients with preeclampsia, magnesium sulfate therapy prevents occurrence seizures, magnesium sulfate reported to be superior to diazepam, nimodipine, phenytoin for the prevention of eclampsia preeclampsia patients and hence considered the treatment of choice for the prevention of a seizure [27]. Magnesium sulfate also prevent the recurrence of seizures compared to the diazepam, phenytoin [27].

14 Conclusion

Eclampsia is a clinical diagnosis of occurrence of new-onset tonic-colonic convulsions, and the absence of other metabolic or neurological etiology for seizures, in hypertensive disorder of pregnancy patients. Although eclampsia is increasingly reported in patients with hypertension, eclampsia patients can present with focal or multifocal, repeated seizures or coma. Majority of eclampsia seizures occur during labor or intrapartum period, or within the first 48 h of delivery. Maternal oxygenation, prevention of injury, control of blood pressure and seizure activity, and delivery of the fetus is the therapy for eclampsia. These patients should be managed in HDU or ICU by multidisciplinary team. The maternal complications of eclampsia include hepatocellular damage, renal impairment, systemic coagulopathy, persistent hypertension, and PRES. PRES is the complication responsible for major maternal morbidity and mortality although many developed countries have achieved zero mortality. The frequent perinatal complication of eclampsia includes intrauterine asphyxia, preterm birth, and intrauterine growth retardation. Eclampsia increases perinatal mortality. The use of magnesium sulfate in severe preeclampsia and aspirin in high-risk pregnant patients decreases the risk of the eclampsia.

References

1. Altman D, Carroli G, Duley L, et al. Do women with pre-eclampsia, and their babies, benefit from magnesium sulphate? The Magpie Trial: a randomised placebo-controlled trial. Lancet. 2002;359:1877–90.
2. Fujita Y, Nakanishi TO, Sugitani M, Kato K. Placental elasticity as a new non-invasive predictive marker of pre-eclampsia. Ultrasound Med Biol. 2019;45(1):93–7.
3. Ghulmiyyah L, Sibai B. Maternal mortality from preeclampsia/eclampsia. Semin Perinatol. 2012;36:56–9.
4. Sharara HA, Shaikh N, Ummunnisa F, Aboobacker N, Tamimi HA. Changes in trends and outcomes of eclampsia: a success story from Qatar. Qatar Med J. 2019;2019(1):10.
5. Fong A, Chau CT, Pan D, Ogunyemi DA. Clinical morbidities, trends, and demographics of eclampsia: a population-based study. Am J Obstet Gynecol. 2013;209(3):229-e1.
6. Marra A, Vargas M, Striano P, Del Guercio L, Buonanno P, Servillo G. Posterior reversible encephalopathy syndrome: the endothelial hypotheses. Med Hypotheses. 2014;82(5):619–22.
7. Amburgey OA, Chapman AC, May V, Bernstein IM, Cipolla MJ. Plasma from preeclamptic women increases blood-brain barrier permeability: role of vascular endothelial growth factor signaling. Hypertension. 2010;56:1003–8.
8. Schreurs MP, Houston EM, May V, Cipolla MJ. The adaptation of the blood-brain barrier to vascular endothelial growth factor and placental growth factor during pregnancy. FASEB J. 2012;26:355–62.
9. Arifin R, Kyi WM, Che Yaakob CA, Yaacob NM. Increased circulating oxidised low-density lipoprotein and antibodies to oxidized low-density lipoprotein in preeclampsia. J Obstet Gynaecol. 2017;37:580–4.
10. Itabe H. Oxidative modification of LDL: its pathological role in atherosclerosis. Clin Rev Allergy Immunol. 2009;37:4–11.
11. Johnson AC, Tremble SM, Chan SL, et al. Magnesium sulfate treatment reverses seizure susceptibility and decreases neuroinflammation in a rat model of severe preeclampsia. PLoS One. 2014;9:e113670.
12. Sibai BM. Magnesium sulfate prophylaxis in preeclampsia: lessons learned from recent trials. Am J Obstet Gynecol. 2004;190:1520–6.
13. Cooray SD, Edmonds SM, Tong S, Samarasekera SP, Whitehead CL. Characterization of symptoms immediately preceding eclampsia. Obstet Gynecol. 2011;118:995–9.
14. Shah AK, Rajamani K, Whitty JE. Eclampsia: a neurological perspective. J Neurol Sci. 2008;271:158–67.
15. Demir BC, Ozerkan K, Ozbek SE, et al. Comparison of magnesium sulfate and mannitol in treatment of eclamptic women with posterior reversible encephalopathy syndrome. Arch Gynecol Obstet. 2012;286:287.
16. Eclampsia Trial Collaborative Group. Which anticonvulsant for women with eclampsia? Evidence from the Collaborative Eclampsia Trial. Lancet. 1995;345:1455.
17. Ambia AM, Wells CE, Yule CS, et al. Fetal heart rate tracings associated with eclamptic seizures. Am J Obstet Gynecol. 2022;227(622):e1.
18. Anon. Gestational hypertension and preeclampsia: ACOG Practice Bulletin Summary, Number 222. Obstet Gynecol. 2020;135:1492.

19. Tukur J, Umar NI, Khan N, Musa D. Comparison of emergency caesarean section to misoprostol induction for the delivery of antepartum eclamptic patients: a pilot study. Niger J Med. 2007;16:364.
20. Lee LO, Bateman BT, Kheterpal S, et al. Risk of epidural hematoma after neuraxial techniques in thrombocytopenic parturients: a report from the Multicenter Perioperative Outcomes Group. Anesthesiology. 2017;126:1053–63.
21. Vousden N, Lawley E, Seed PT, Gidiri MF, Goudar S, et al. Incidence of eclampsia and related complications across 10 low- and middle-resource geographical regions: secondary analysis of a cluster randomised controlled trial. PLoS Med. 2019;16:e1002775.
22. Sibai BM, Caritis SN, Thom E, et al. Prevention of preeclampsia with low-dose aspirin in healthy, nulliparous pregnant women. The National Institute of Child Health and Human Development Network of Maternal-Fetal Medicine Units. N Engl J Med. 1993;329:1213–8.
23. Meher S, Duley L, Hunter K, Askie L. Antiplatelet therapy before or after 16 weeks' gestation for preventing preeclampsia: an individual participant data meta-analysis. Am J Obstet Gynecol. 2017;216:121–8.
24. Roberge S, Nicolaides K, Demers S, Hyett J, Chaillet N, Bujold E. The role of aspirin dose on the prevention of preeclampsia and fetal growth restriction: systematic review and meta-analysis. Am J Obstet Gynecol. 2017;216:110–20.
25. Duley L, Henderson-Smart D. Magnesium sulphate versus phenytoin for eclampsia the Cochrane library issue 3. Oxford Publishers; 2003.
26. Shaikh N, Nawaz S, Ummunisa F, Shahzad A, Hussain J, Ahmad K, Almohannadi HS, Sharara HA. Eclampsia and posterior reversible encephalopathy syndrome (PRES): a retrospective review of risk factors and outcomes. Qatar Med J. 2021;2021(1):4.
27. Lewington S, Clarke R, Qizilbash N, et al. Age-specific relevance of usual blood pressure to vascular mortality: a meta-analysis of individual data for one million adults in 61 prospective studies. Lancet. 2002;360:1903.

Intensive Care Therapy Requirement in the Management of the Gynecological and Obstetric Patients

Firdos Ummunnisa, Umm E Amara, Umme Nashrah, M. A. Rahman, Shafee Shaikh, Wael Khalaf, and Nissar Shaikh

Abstract The advances in medical and surgical care, combined with improved access to healthcare, have greatly reduced maternal and neonatal morbidity and mortality rates. However, the rise in the rate of lower section cesarean section, maternal age with comorbidities, and assisted reproduction have increased maternal mortality rate (MMR), resulting in high-risk pregnancies. Critically ill pregnant patients requiring intensive care support should be classified based on their conditions, including those with hypertensive disorders, peripartum cardiomyopathies, comorbidities exacerbated during pregnancy, and those with a higher risk of complications during pregnancy. The initial management of these patients should follow the ABCDE approach, similar to non-pregnant patients. The use of regional anesthesia and analgesia techniques has significantly decreased anesthesia-related issues and ICU admissions. However, obstetric hemorrhage remains the leading cause of ICU utilization. Sepsis is responsible for 15% of maternal deaths worldwide. The most common cause of septic shock in obstetric patients is pyelonephritis, chorioamnionitis, and endometritis. Hypertensive disorders of pregnancy contribute to around 10% of all maternal deaths worldwide, while amniotic fluid embolism has a maternal mortality rate as high as 40%. Management of these conditions is mainly supportive, with the use of lipid emulsion therapy as a lipid sink to protect the myocardium from local anesthetic toxicity. It is crucial to prioritize the initial management of these patients, as it lays the foundation for their overall treatment and recovery. Understanding the risks and management of these conditions is critical for improving maternal health outcomes.

F. Ummunnisa
Dr Halima Al Tamimi OBGY Clinic, Doha, Qatar

U. E Amara (✉)
Apollo Institute of Medical Sciences and Research, Hyderabad, Telangana, India

U. Nashrah
Deccan College of Medical Sciences, Hyderabad, Telangana, India

M. A. Rahman · S. Shaikh · W. Khalaf · N. Shaikh
Surgical Intensive Care, Hamad Medical Corporation, Doha, Qatar

N. Shaikh et al. (eds.), *Updates in Intensive Care of OBGY Patients*,
https://doi.org/10.1007/978-981-99-9577-6_9

Keywords Critical care · Gynecological · Hypertensive disorders of pregnancy · Intensive care therapy · Local anesthesia toxicity · Maternal · Maternal sepsis · Morbidity · Mortality · Neonatal · Obstetrical · Peripartum hemorrhage

1 Introduction

The advances in science, particularly medical and surgical care in combination with improved access and availability of healthcare system has improved maternal and neonatal morbidity and mortality [1]. There are increasing comorbidities in gynecological patients, perioperative ventilation, and hemorrhage which require post-surgical monitoring and intervention thus needing intensive care support. Although the obstetric patients are younger and majority of them complete the pregnancy cycle without any complication, fewer of these patients require intensive care therapy due to hemorrhage, hypertensive or septic complication.

The anatomical and physiological changes during pregnancy, with potential side effects of medication on fetus, make intensive care management of the obstetric patients unique and challenging. When these patients are admitted to general intensive care units, relative lack of knowledge, orientation, management of these unique medical emergencies makes situation tough and confusing; hence, it is suggested nowadays with different level (e.g., ICU, HDU, IMCU) for better understanding management and outcome of these patients [2].

2 Epidemiology

The maternal mortality rate (MMR) is defined as a significant indicator of maternal and child healthcare. MMR increased from 12/10,000 to 28/10,000 from 1990 to 2013, mainly due to increased rate of lower section cesarean section (LSCS) maternal age with comorbidities and in combination with assisted reproduction which results in high-risk pregnancies along with advanced age pregnant patients with comorbidities [3].

Due to poor living conditions lack of health services and insufficient follow-up care services, increases the MMR 15 times more in developing countries compared to developed ones [4].

In the late 2000, WHO (World health Organization) proposed near missed, severe maternal morbidity (SMM) and severe associated maternal mortality (SAMM), indication of the level of healthcare, required for critically ill patients [5]. The reported incidence of OBGY patients requiring intensive care therapy for gynecological patients is 2.3/1000 women undergoing gynecological procedures and 9/1000 deliveries in obstetric patients with lowest ICU requirements in developed countries. The majority of OBGYN (obstetric and gynecological) patients requiring intensive care therapy is in the postoperative and post-partum period (>90%); the obstetric patients ICU stay is shorter ranging from 1 to 2 days [6].

After review of maternal deaths in the UK, interestingly 50% of maternal death can be prevented with early recognition and intensive care intervention [7].

3 Anatomical and Physiological Changes During Pregnancy

During pregnancy, a variety of anatomical as well as physiological changes occur, and it is essential to know all these changes to optimally manage the critically ill pregnant patients requiring intensive care support.

Details of these changes are given in Table 1.

3.1 *Indication for Intensive Care Therapy*

The frequent gynecological indications are described in Table 2 [8].

The indications mentioned in Table 2 gynecological patients requiring intensive care are due to post-surgical hemorrhage and infections along with comorbidities.

Table 1 Showing anatomical and physiological changes during pregnancy

Anatomical changes:	1. Vena cava syndrome 2. Enlarged uterus 3. Elevated diaphragm 4. Delayed gastric emptying 5. Edema of upper airway 6. Breast engorgement
Physiological changes:	1. Cardiovascular increase in stroke volume and heart rate; up to 50% increase in blood volume 2. Blood: Anemia of pregnancy; up to 50% increase in plasma volume 3. Coagulation: increase in procoagulant, thrombin and fibrinogen and decrease anticoagulation 4. Respiratory: decrease in residual functional capacity 5. Renal: increase in creatinine clearance up to 160 ml/min

Table 2 Indication for intensive care therapy

Gynecological indications:	1. Postoperative hemorrhage (43%) 2. Infection (39%) 3. Cardiovascular disease (30%) 4. Procedure-related complication (9%) 5. Pulmonary embolism (4%) 6. Ovarian hyperstimulation syndrome (4%)

4 Assessment

The obstetric patients requiring intensive care therapy are categorized according to condition ranging from hypertensive disorders to peripartum cardiomyopathies as seen in Table 3. Other group is patients with comorbidities exaggerated during pregnancy which ranges from autoimmune diseases to asthma. Third group of patients are patients with pregnancy and increased risk of complications such as urinary tract infection to the thromboembolism and last group of pregnant patients requiring intensive care therapy are those where pregnancy and disease occur coincidentally, for example, road traffic accidents to appendicitis.

Scoring systems in pregnancy as per the available literature, lesser number, and percentage of the obstetric patients critically ill are admitted to intensive care therapy although significant number of pregnant patients suffer with severe complications.

The intensive care units are specialized units with higher quality of care and should not be neglected if needed. As most of the obstetric and gynecological complications, patients require a noninvasive monitoring and supportive care only; these patients can be managed in specialized units or level 1 of intensive care, headed by OBGY senior leader; these units are commonly called IMCU (Intermediate Medical

Table 3 Obstetric indications for the intensive care admission [9]

Preexisting disease worsened during pregnancy	1. Myasthenia gravis 2. Autoimmune thyroiditis 3. Pulmonary hypertension 4. Cardiomyopathies 5. Congenital heart diseases 6. Asthma 7. Epilepsy 8. Diabetes mellitus
High-risk conditions during pregnancy	1. Infections (urinary tract infections and pneumonias) 2. Thromboembolic disease (deep venous thromboembolism and pulmonary embolism)
Coincidental during pregnancy	1. Road traffic accidents 2. Appendicitis 3. Cholecystitis 4. Rupture of cerebral aneurysm
Pure obstetrical	1. Peripartum hemorrhage 2. Ectopic pregnancy 3. Eclampsia 4. Pre-eclampsia 5. Microangiopathies of pregnancy 6. Chorioamnionitis 7. Amniotic fluid embolism 8. Acute fatty liver of pregnancy 9. Peripartum cardiomyopathy 10. Anaphylactic shock

Care Unit). OBGY leader should be ultimate decision-makers, but sure need of anesthesiologist and internal medicine specialists in combination they should design the diagnostic and management algorithm. These team also dictate which patient should be upgraded to HDU and ICU (high dependency intensive care units), respectively.

The predominant models and scoring system are essential to determine the requirement for the admission of acutely ill gynecological and obstetric patients to the intensive care therapy units. The established scores such as acute physiology and chronic health evaluation (APACHE II), sequential organ failure assessment (SOFA), simplified acute physiology score (SAPS) score and abstract trick early warning score OEWS (obstetric early warning system) are frequently used for assessing intensive care therapy these scores used in abstract trick and gynecological parameters are compatible to nano BG vial parameters of the same age [10].

There are no benefits of using specific sepsis-related obstetrical scores for predicting sepsis pathology [11].

Level 1 and level 2 refer to patients requiring invasive monitoring of single organ dysfunction. Level 3 refers to the patients requiring invasive monitoring, invasive ventilation, or requiring care of two to three organ dysfunctions or failure [12].

As far as the severity scores are concerned, the APACHE score is cumbersome to calculate, and physiological changes in pregnancy can lead to a high calculated score thus overestimation of mortality. SOFA score considers six vital organ dysfunctions to failure; each vital organ has four maximum points, thus easy to calculate and assess.

The OEWS (obstetric early warning system) seems to be accurate in estimation out of critically ill obstetric patients (Table 4): it also which level of care patients is required.

Table 4 Shows QEWS (obstetric early warning system)

Score	3	2	1	0	1	2	3
Temperature		<35 ºc	35-35.9 ºc	36-37.4 ºc	37.5-37.9 ºc	38.0-38.9 ºc	≥39 ºc
Systolic BP	≤70	71-79	80-89	90-139	140-149	150-159	≥160
Diastolic BP			≤49	50-89	90-99	100-109	≥110
Pulse		<40	40-49	50-99	100-109	110-129	≥130
Respiratory Rate	≤10			11-20	21-24	25-29	≥30
Oxygen Saturations	≤94%			≥95%			
AVPU				Alert	Responds to Voice	Responds to Pain	Unconscious
Urine output mLs/hr	<10	<30		Not Measured			

5 ICU (Intensive Care Unit) Management of Gynecological and Obstetric (OBGY) Patients

All these patients should be managed by multidisciplinary team consisting of intensivist, OBGY, neonatologist, clinical pharmacist, and paramedical staff. Management of this obstetric patient is given in the following subheadings.

5.1 General Care

Overall maternal hemodynamic optimization with fetal wellbeing must be the aim of general care of these patients. Fetal monitoring should be every 4–6 h and as required, and pregnant patients admitted to the ICU for 24 h should be prepared for LSCS (Lower Section Cesarean Section).

5.2 Initial Management

It should be similar to non-pregnant patients, and we should follow ABCDE approach (airway, breathing, circulation, disabilities, and exposure).

The monitoring of these patients should be the same as non-pregnant patients. Noninvasive ventilation in patients had higher risk of aspiration, can be used with precautions, and there should be low threshold for intubation and invasive ventilation. Airway edema can cause difficulties in securing the airway the difficult intubation kit should be stand by and standard ventilation with adaption to the changes of pregnancy should be considered. For those patients having resistance hypoxemia, ECMO (Extracorporeal Membrane Oxygenation) should be considered [13].

Most of the sedatives and opioid analgesia can be used safely in the post-partum period, whereas in the prepartum period they can cross placenta with variability. Involved clinical pharmacist, neonatologist to give the input.

Intensive care therapy physicians should be aware of group of contraindicated medications in the prepartum and immediately post-partum period. Penicillin, Cephalosporin, macrolides, and acyclovir are Group A medications that can be safely used, whereas aminoglycosides and quinolones are category C medications. Fluconazole is contraindicated. Enteral nutrition with antacid prophylaxis is a choice in parturient patients. Increase caloric requirement by 2.5 times, adding zinc, folate, and vitamin B12 in the first trimester.

Thromboprophylaxis should be considered early, during labor or late pregnancy unfractionated heparin is better choice due to easy reversibility with protamine sulfate.

5.3 *Specific Condition*

Anesthesia-related issues and ICU admission from difficult intubation to sleep apnea are much decrease after increased in use of regional anesthesia and analgesia techniques [14, 15].

5.3.1 Obstetrical Peripartum Hemorrhage

Obstetric hemorrhage remained the foremost cause of intensive care therapy utilization. It caused 10–30% of maternal mortality from high-income to low-income countries. Obstetric hemorrhage occurs due to placentation abnormalities, uterine atony, or surgical or genital tract injuries. Use of uterotonic medications, uterine artery embolization or ligation, and even peripartum hysterectomy may not be able to control post-partum hemorrhage (PPH).

Vasoelastic hemostatic assay (ROTEM, TEG) gives real-time information about coagulation status, whereas the traditional parameters (PT, aPTT, INR) are time consuming. In PPH, hypofibrinogenemia is a greater risk and causes severe PPH. For each decrease in 1 g/L of fibrinogen, there is 2.6-fold increase in severe PPH [16]. The earlier fibrinogen administration possible with thromboelastography, the FIBTEM result is available in 10 min indicating the fibrin polymerization which serves as early indicator for earlier intervention as fibrin polymerization decline more rapidly than fibrinogen [17]. The use of tranexamic acid and factor VII also help in prevention of peripartum hysterectomies [18].

5.3.2 Sepsis

Sepsis is responsible for 15% of overall maternal death in the world. Puerperal sepsis and urosepsis are common causes of sepsis in developed countries, whereas in developing countries, malaria, HIV, community acquired pneumonia are frequent causes of sepsis. Commonly septic shock in obstetric patients is due to pyelonephritis, chorioamnionitis, and endometritis [19].

Sepsis can be diagnosed earlier by raised inflammatory markers (WBC, CRP, and PCT), white blood cell count, C-reactive protein, and procalcitonin, respectively. Management should be guided by the recent surviving sepsis campaign guidelines.

5.3.3 Hypertensive Disorders of Pregnancy

Hypertensive disorders of pregnancy cause around 10% of total world maternal death [20]. Eclampsia and pre-eclampsia are rising all over the world, particularly in the developed countries [21]. Early diagnosis graded decrease in blood pressure, management as per hospital guidelines, and prevention of complications are essential for better outcome.

5.3.4 Amniotic Fluid Embolism

Amniotic fluid embolism has as high as 40% maternal mortality. Still re diagnosis of exclusion, sudden cardiovascular collapse and coagulopathy. Management of amniotic fluid embolism is supportive. Cardiac disorders causes 10–15%, maternal mortality it includes congenital heart diseases, peripartum cardiomyopathy, myocardial infarction and pulmonary hypertension should be detected and managed peripartum cardiomyopathy can be fatal should be treated as obstetrical emergency with monitoring and anti-cardiac failure medication [22].

5.3.5 Local Anesthetic Toxicity

Pregnancy increases the risk for local anesthetic toxicity due to changes of pregnancy causes epidural venous distention, increased cardiac output and decreased plasma protein binding increases the absorption availability of free fraction of local anesthetic. Increased neuronal susceptibility and hormonal effect on myocardium decreases the seizure threshold and increases susceptibility for arrhythmia [23]. The management is supportive and use of lipid emulsion therapy lead to the protection of myocardium from local anesthetic toxicity.

6 Conclusion

Despite the significant progress made in medical and surgical care and improved healthcare accessibility, the maternal mortality rate has increased due to factors such as the rise in lower section cesarean section, maternal age with comorbidities, and assisted reproduction. The proper classification and management of critically ill pregnant patients based on their specific conditions are crucial. The initial management of these patients should follow the ABCDE approach, and the use of regional anesthesia and analgesia techniques has notably reduced anesthesia-related issues and ICU admissions. However, obstetric hemorrhage, sepsis, hypertensive disorders of pregnancy, and amniotic fluid embolism remain significant concerns. Understanding the risks and management of these conditions is vital to improving maternal health outcomes. It is essential to prioritize the initial management of critically ill pregnant patients, which lays the foundation for their overall treatment and recovery. This highlights the significance of providing specialized and comprehensive care to this vulnerable patient population.

References

1. Minville V, Vidal F, Loutrel O, Castel A, Jacques L, Vayssière C, Parant O, Guerby P, Asehnoune K. Identifying predictive factors for admitting patients with severe pre-eclampsia to intensive care unit. J Matern Fetal Neonatal Med. 2022;35(16):3175–81.
2. Baird SM, Martin S. Framework for critical care in obstetrics. J Perinat Neonatal Nurs. 2018;32(3):232–40.
3. Zieleskiewicz L, Chantry A, Duclos G, Bourgoin A, Mignon A, Deneux-Tharaux C, Leone M. Intensive care and pregnancy: epidemiology and general principles of management of obstetrics ICU patients during pregnancy. Anaesth Crit Care Pain Med. 2016;35(Suppl. 1):S51–7.
4. Hogan MC, Foreman KJ, Naghavi M, Ahn SY, Wang M, Makela SM, Lopez AD, Lozano R, Murray CJ. Maternal mortality for 181 countries, 1980–2008: a systematic analysis of progress towards Millennium Development Goal 5. Lancet. 2010;375(9726):1609–23.
5. Gaffney A. Critical care in pregnancy—is it different? Semin Perinatol. 2014;38(6):329–40.
6. Anon. ACOG Practice Bulletin No: 211. Critical care in pregnancy. Obstet Gynecol. 2019;133(5):e303–19.
7. Cantwell R, Clutton-Brock T, Cooper G, Dawson A, Drife J, Garrod D, Harper A, Hulbert D, Lucas S, McClure J, Millward-Sadler H, Neilson J, Nelson-Piercy C, Norman J, O'Herlihy C, Oates M, Shakespeare J, de Swiet M, Williamson C, Beale V, Knight M, Lennox C, Miller A, Parmar D, Rogers J, Springett A. Saving mothers' lives: reviewing maternal deaths to make motherhood safer: 2006–2008. The eighth report of the confidential enquiries into maternal deaths in the United Kingdom. BJOG. 2011;118(Suppl. 1):1–203.
8. Heinonen S, Tyrväinen E, Penttinen J, Saarikoski S, Ruokonen E. Need for critical care in gynaecology: a population-based analysis. Crit Care. 2002;6(4):371–5.
9. Koukoubanis K, Prodromidou A, Stamatakis E, Valsamidis D, Thomakos N. Role of critical care units in the management of obstetric patients (Review). Biomed Rep. 2021;15(1):58.
10. el-Solh AA, Grant BJ. A comparison of severity of illness scoring systems for critically ill obstetric patients. Chest. 1996;110:1299.
11. Aarvold AB, Ryan HM, Magee LA, von Dadelszen P, Fjell C, Walley KR. Multiple organ dysfunction score is superior to the obstetric-specific sepsis in obstetrics score in predicting mortality in septic obstetric patients. Crit Care Med. 2017;45(1):e49–57.
12. Edwards Z, Lucas DN, Gauntlett R. Is training in obstetric critical care adequate? An international comparison. Int J Obstet Anesth. 2019;37:96–105.
13. Nair P, Davies AR, Beca J, Bellomo R, Ellwood D, Forrest P, Jackson A, Pye R, Seppelt I, Sullivan E, Webb S. Extracorporeal membrane oxygenation for severe ARDS in pregnant and postpartum women during the 2009 H1N1 pandemic. Intensive Care Med. 2011;37(4):648–54.
14. Shaikh N, Imran MA, Zubair M, Ehfeda M, Ummunnisa F. Scoline apnoea and pregnancy: SICU experiences. Qatar Med J. 2019;2019(2):69.
15. Khawaga S, Ei SN, Shaikh N, Mustafa G, Kettern MA, Hafiz A. Critical care of gynecological and obstetric patients: a decade of surgical intensive care experience. Qatar Med J. 2010;2:22–4.
16. Butwick AJ, Goodnough LT. Transfusion and coagulation management in major obstetric hemorrhage. Curr Opin Anaesthesiol. 2015;28(3):275–84.
17. de Lange NM, Lancé MD, de Groot R, Beckers EA, Henskens YM, Scheepers HC. Obstetric hemorrhage and coagulation: an update. Thromboelastography, thromboelastometry, and conventional coagulation tests in the diagnosis and prediction of postpartum hemorrhage. Obstet Gynecol Surv. 2012;67(7):426–35.
18. James AH, McLintock C, Lockhart E. Postpartum hemorrhage: when uterotonics and sutures fail. Am J Hematol. 2012;87(Suppl. 1):S16–22.
19. van Dillen J, Zwart J, Schutte J, van Roosmalen J. Maternal sepsis: epidemiology, etiology and outcome. Curr Opin Infect Dis. 2010;23(3):249–54.

20. Chappell LC, Cluver CA, Kingdom J, Tong S. Pre-eclampsia. Lancet. 2021;398(10297):341–54.
21. Sharara HA, Shaikh N, Ummunnisa F, Aboobacker N, Tamimi HA. Changes in trends and outcomes of eclampsia: a success story from Qatar. Qatar Med J. 2019;2019(1):10.
22. Shaikh N. An obstetric emergency called peripartum cardiomyopathy! J Emerg Trauma Shock. 2010;3(1):39–42.
23. Bern S, Weinberg G. Local anesthetic toxicity and lipid resuscitation in pregnancy. Curr Opin Anaesthesiol. 2011;24(3):262–7.

Anesthesia-Related Complications in Obstetrics and Gynecology

Seema Nahid, Hayat Elfil, Eynas Abdalla, Gisha Mathew, and Santhosh Gopalakrishnan

Abstract Striving to ensure every effort to provide a secure safe environment and well-being of mother and baby to start their happy and healthy journey together. Over the past three decades, mortality from general anesthesia in obstetrics has decreased.

Factors influencing the choice of the appropriate anesthetic technique include the type of surgery, patient factors (comorbidities, emergencies), and the effects of anesthesia on the fetus. A high maternal mortality rate associated with general anesthesia in obstetrics was related to the risk of aspiration and airway management. Regional anesthesia is preferred to minimize fetal drug exposure, reduce the need for airway management, and provide some degree of postoperative analgesia. Over time, the method has been improved to reduce the potentially harmful effects and complications caused by various anesthetic procedures.

Neuraxial techniques have gained popularity with advancements in obstetric anesthesia and replaced general anesthesia primarily because of their intense focus on safety and widely utilized options in operative procedures for vaginal delivery. Approximately 1–2% of obstetric patients require non-obstetric procedures during pregnancy that require general anesthesia due to the nature of the procedure and patient factors. However, 6% of cesarean sections still require general anesthesia and tracheal intubation, and it is essential to remember that any intervention may come with unwanted side effects.

Keywords Post-dural puncture headache (PDPH) · Combined spinal epidural (CSE) · Local anesthesia systemic toxicity (LAST) · Cerebrospinal fluid (CSF) · General anesthesia (GA) · Spinal epidural abscess (SEA) · Spinal epidural hematoma (SEH) · Accidental awareness under general anesthesia (AAGA) · Obstetric anesthetist association (OAA) · Difficult Airway Society (DAS)

S. Nahid (✉) · H. Elfil · E. Abdalla · G. Mathew · S. Gopalakrishnan
Hamad Medical Corporation, Doha, Qatar
e-mail: snahid@hamad.qa

N. Shaikh et al. (eds.), *Updates in Intensive Care of OBGY Patients*,
https://doi.org/10.1007/978-981-99-9577-6_10

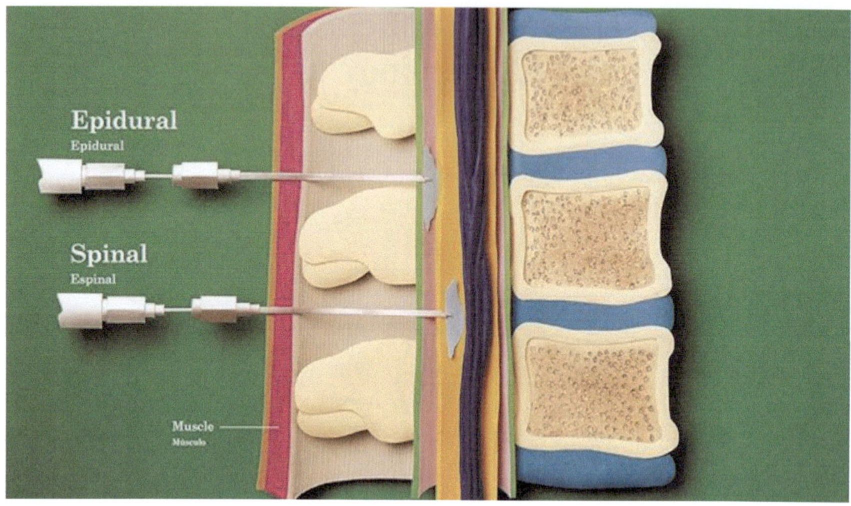

Fig. 1 Epidural and spinal anatomy

1 Introduction

The complications in obstetrics are related to the physiological and anatomical changes that occur during pregnancy and can affect the frequency with which these happen. Interventions undertaken by the anesthetist are performed emergently, frequently out of hours, with high patient expectations.

In the obstetric population, it is well recognized that neuraxial anesthesia has many advantages over general anesthesia. Although serious complications are uncommon with regional anesthesia, they must be discussed with the patient.

August Bier was the first to report the use of spinal anesthetics and identified post-dural puncture headache as one of the known complications associated with using regional anesthetics.

In obstetric anesthesia practice, the most effective and commonly used neuraxial techniques (i.e., spinal, epidural, and combined spinal epidural (CSE)) establish a high safety record and adequate record for labor analgesia and cesarean delivery anesthesia; however, transient mild neurological complications and serious life-threatening complications can occur. The most common obstetric anesthesia complications are given in Fig. 1.

2 Post-dural Puncture Headache (PDPH)

A potential complication of neuraxial anesthesia and analgesia that can occur after an accidental dural puncture during epidural needle or catheter insertion and spinal technique. It is the third most common cause of a legal claim in obstetric anesthesia.

Pregnant women are at increased risk of PDPH because of their gender, young age, and hormonal status. Additional risk factors determining the incidence include a traumatic bevel tip and a large needle gauge, a low body mass index (<35), history, and pushing during labor. In pregnant women, high estrogen levels alter cerebral responsiveness and increase vascular distension in response to hypotension.

Risk factors associated with needle characteristics are beveled orientation, the direction of the needle approach, multiple unsuccessful needle insertions, and operator experience.

The incidence of PDPH following spinal anesthesia with fine needles is approximately 1:500, compared to the risk of accidental dural puncture by a 16–17G Tuohy needle, which is approximately 1:100, and 70–80% of these patients will go on to develop PDPH [1–4].

Clinical significance with lower incidence of PDPH when using a small gauge pencil point or atraumatic noncutting bevel design (Fig. 2) (Whitacre, sprotted) [5, 6].

Normal CSF production by the choroid plexus in the ventricles is about 450–500 ml in adults, with 25 ml in the cerebral ventricles and 125 ml in subarachnoid spaces, with absorption into the venous circulation by the cranial and spinal arachnoid villi.

The pathogenesis of post-dural puncture headache (PDPH) begins with increased loss of cerebrospinal fluid through the dural hole exceeding the replacement, leading to subsequent alterations in CSF pressure dynamics. At the same time, the patient is upright and has decreased intracranial pressure and cerebral hypotension.

Loss of cerebrospinal fluid volume can cause downward traction on the dura, subdural hematoma caused by the stretch of the bridging intracerebral cortical vein, and traction on the sixth cranial nerve due to the long course and intracranial hypotension.

Diagnostic criteria for post-dural puncture headache by the International Classification of Headache Disorders [7].

A. Any headache fulfills criteria C.
B. Dural puncture has been performed.
C. Headache developed within 5 days of the dural puncture.
D. Not accounted for other ICHD diagnosis.

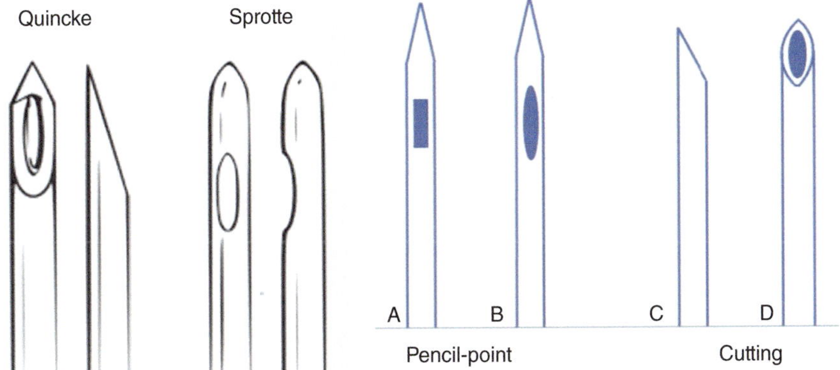

Fig. 2 Needle types

A neglected dural leak may lead to chronic headaches or neurological complications such as cranial nerve palsy and, rarely, subdural hematoma. Debilitating headaches usually develop within 48 h but can be delayed up to 14 days; classically described as frontal-occipital and postural in nature, classified as mild when daily activities are not restricted and not associated with symptoms, and respond to nonopioid analgesics, moderate when bedridden for a reasonable amount of time with concomitant symptoms that require opioid analgesia, and severe when completely bedridden and associated with symptoms restricting daily activities and refractory to conservative treatment. It is usually associated with neck stiffness, photophobia, tinnitus, and subjective hearing symptoms. It remits spontaneously after 2 weeks or after the sealing of the leak with an autologous blood patch.

Managing PDPH involves pharmacological and nonpharmacological strategies depending on the individual's functional limitations.

- Conservative management: hydration, regular analgesia (nonopioid and opioid), bed rest, caffeine, triptans, adrenocorticotrophic hormone (cosyntropin), reassurance.
- Interventional: occipital nerve block and epidural blood patch.

An epidural blood patch is considered the gold standard for treating severe PDPH. It seals the dural puncture site, preventing further CSF leaks, which allows an increase in intracranial pressure [8, 9]. It is performed under a full aseptic technique at or one space below the initial puncture site, with 10–30 ml of the patient's autologous blood injected into the epidural space. The procedure is terminated with relief of headache, fullness in the lumbar region, or radicular pain in the lower extremities. An epidural blood patch carries the risk of repeat dural tap, failure, backache, nerve damage, and meningitis. It is contraindicated in patients with systemic fever, local infection at the injection site, coagulopathy, and patient refusal. When performed after 24 h, it has a success rate between 70% and 90%; however, when the symptoms are severe, it can be performed early with a high chance of recurrence of the headache and a lower success rate. Prophylactic patching has been proven to be not beneficial. A second blood patch may be repeated where relief of symptoms is refractory, and there is a reduced likelihood of improvement.

Other potential causes of headaches other than post-dural puncture are preeclampsia, migraine, subdural hematoma, and cluster headaches, which affect roughly 40% of women in the postnatal period. The headache and its related symptoms can cause significant discomfort and suffering with a prolonged hospital stay. Early identification and diagnosis are essential to increasing productivity, reducing litigation, and minimizing medical care costs.

3 Inadequate Block for Cesarean Section

Neuraxial blocks are the most common mode of anesthesia widely practiced for cesarean sections, considering it safe and reliable, but occasional failures are known.

Failure could be related to drug, technique, or patient factors affecting the incidence of the failed block, are obesity, anatomical variations, postsurgical spine abnormalities, and stage of labor.

Failure to provide adequate analgesia/anesthesia necessitating additional measures to continue surgery is considered an inadequate block following an epidural, spinal, or combined spinal epidural (CSE) technique [10].

Clinically inadequate blocks may vary from a complete absence of sensory and motor blocks to a unilateral block or inadequate or partial block for surgical anesthesia. The inadequate or partially misplaced dose may result in a patchy block or a reduced duration of the block to last for the duration of surgery. Communication is key during surgery, as all the sensations may not be taken away initially and may be uncomfortable to continue and offer alternative analgesia.

The significant risk of an inadequate block is the need to convert regional anesthetic to general anesthesia, which occurs 1:50 times for spinal and 1:20 times for epidurals.

The most frequently quoted block height for cesarean sections is the bilateral loss of cold sensation below T4. When the block is not achieved initially and more time is needed due to time constraints in category one cesarean section, an alternative anesthetic technique should be used before surgery, general anesthetic, a second regional technique.

Inadequate blocks are managed by *R*epeat block in non-urgent situations, *R*evive block in urgent situations by alternate analgesia, including nitrous oxide, the head down position for the cephaloid spread of the drug, short-acting intravenous opioids, *R*edirected for conversion to general anesthesia when the revival of a block fails, and time constraints.

Administration of opioids before delivery crosses the placenta and causes respiratory depression in neonates. The neonatal team must be informed if these drugs are given to the mother before birth.

4 Subdural Injection

A subdural block is defined as an extensive neural block in the absence of an [11] subarachnoid puncture disproportionate to the amount of local anesthetic injected. It is the traumatically created potential space between the dura and arachnoid matter. The subdural space is bigger posteriorly, tracking anesthetics here, minimizing the anterior motor block. Anterolateral sympathetic fibers are affected, causing hypotension more than expected from an epidural and relatively less than a total spinal. When a local anesthetic that was meant for the epidural space is accidentally injected into this space, it can cause a patchy block that leads to more widespread cranial anesthesia with an action time between spinal and epidural anesthesia, which is a common way for symptoms to show up in the clinic.

- Gradual/delayed onset (10–30 min)
- Extensive sensory block with a minimal motor block

- Hypotension (more than expected with epidural and less than with spinal)
- Horner Syndrome
- Dyspnea and loss of consciousness with intracranial spread

It is relatively easy to treat with fluids and small bolus doses of vasopressors.

5 High Spinal/Total Spinal

They are different severity levels of the same process. A high spinal or regional block is the inappropriate high spread of local anesthetic affecting spinal nerves above T4. The severity of clinical features depends on the level of spinal nerves affected by the local anesthetic, compromising cardiovascular and respiratory function when untreated may ascend and progress to total spinal (Fig. 3).

Total spinal is the intracranial spread of local anesthetic resulting in loss of consciousness. Early recognition and management are mandated for optimal maternal and fetal outcomes [12, 13].

The reported incidence of high 0.001% varies from 1% (1:100), while the risk for total spinal states is approximately 0.001% (<1:100,000), according to the OAA patient information booklet.

When a high block is suspected

- Call for help.
- Stop the epidural pump if present.
- High flow of oxygen.
- Reverse Trendelenburg position to prevent the spread of local anesthetic/left lateral position for uterine displacement.

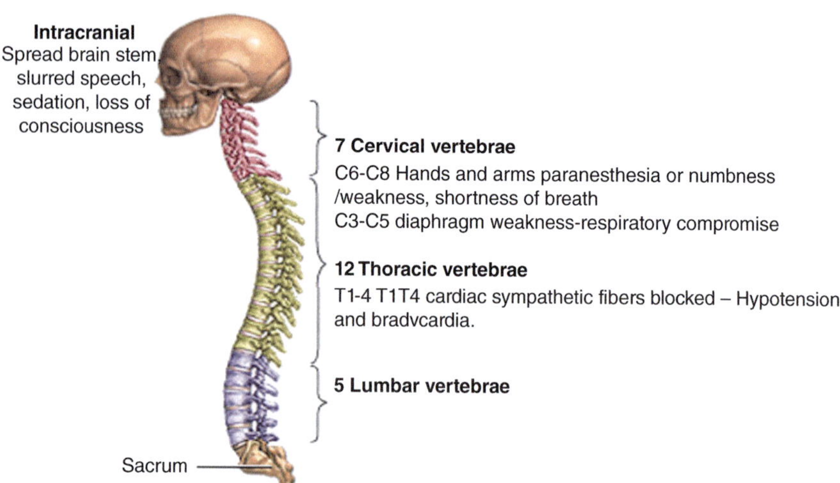

Fig. 3 Segmental clinical manifestation

- Reassure mother.
- ABC approach for assessment of patient.

Respiratory compromise and loss of consciousness with maternal collapse have been determined; maternal resuscitation is initiated and may require intubation and ventilation (Fig. 4).

- Rapid sequence induction with cricoid pressure.
- An induction agent can be used for the possibility of awareness.
- Muscle relaxants (succinylcholine, rocuronium).
- Fluids and vasopressors.
- Sedation and ventilation are to be continued until the block wears off and spontaneous ventilation resumes, which may take a few hours, depending on the local anesthetic dose.
- Once the mother is stabilized, delivery is dictated according to the level of urgency.

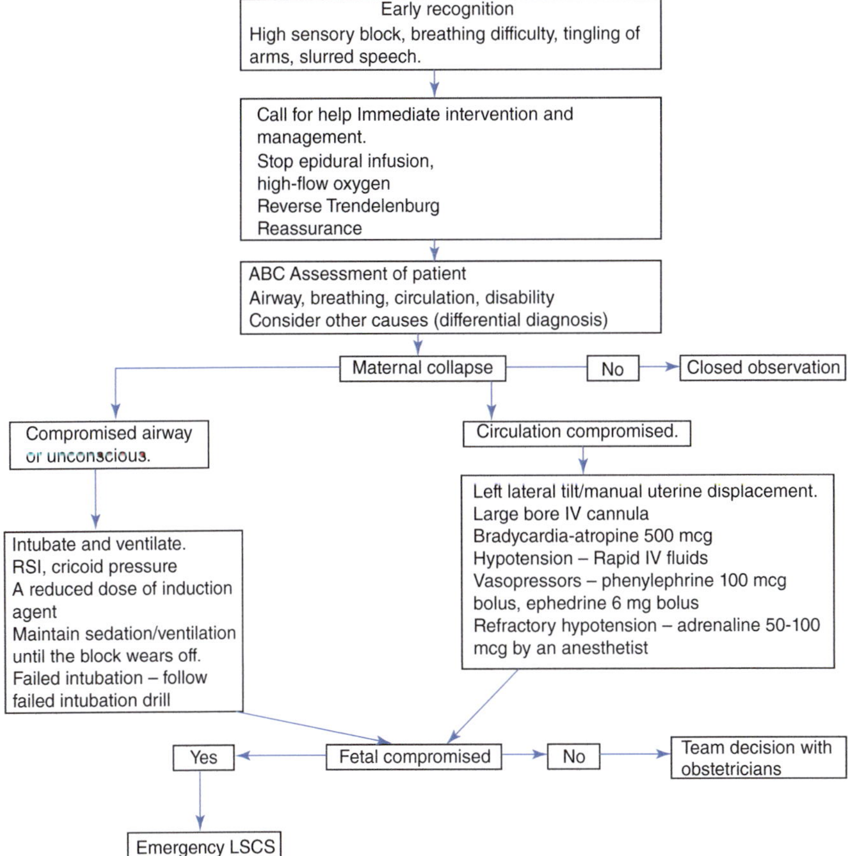

Fig. 4 Management of high spinal block

Circulatory collapse management

- Left lateral tilt for uterine displacement.
- Large bore IV cannulas.
- Bradycardia—glycopyrrolate 200–600 mcg/atropine 200–500 mcg.
- Hypotension—fluids and vasopressors.
- Phenylephrine and ephedrine in titrated doses.
- Consider diluted adrenaline if there is no response to the above (10 mcg/ml minimum dilution).
- Structured ABCD assessment to identify the compromised status and closely monitoring for maternal stabilization is considered. Delivery of the fetus is planned as per the advice of the obstetric team.
- When the high block resolves, normal vaginal delivery or elective cesarean section is not precluded.

6 Local Anesthetic Systemic Toxicity

This may occur due to an accidental intravascular injection or vascular uptake into the blood from the local spread to the systemic circulation, resulting in supratherapeutic blood and tissue levels, which can cause toxicity.

The risk of toxicity increases with the dose, the location of the injection, the comorbidities of the patient, the age extremes, and the lipophilicity of the local anesthetic. The patient risk factors associated with this condition are organ dysfunction and a high serum level of protein binding. A higher total dose and the dose-to-weight ratio with the cumulative effect of multiple injections or continuous infusions increase the possibility of LAST [14].

LAST manifests with prodromal symptoms and signs such as perioral numbness, tinnitus, agitation, confusion, and dysarthria, followed by central nervous system depression, seizures, coma, and respiratory arrest. Cardiovascular dysfunction can occur as bradycardia and hypotension, progressing to serious ventricular arrhythmias and asystole [15].

The three pillars of LAST management are seizure control, advanced cardiac life support (ACLS), and prompt administration of a 20% lipid emulsion. Early intervention to stop the administration of local anesthetic and maintain pulmonary ventilation and adequate organ perfusion with well-oxygenated blood and to avoid further acidosis (Airway, Breathing, and Circulation goal).

7 Neurological Complications

Nerve Injury Nerve injuries are common in the obstetric population, with 1:100 women reporting some form of neurological injury in the postpartum period, most of which are of obstetric etiology rather than any anesthetic cause. Three potential causes of nerve injuries by regional anesthetic techniques can result in

- Direct trauma to the nerve
- Chemical injury
- Comprehensive injury

Direct trauma to nerve tissue occurs when needles, catheters, or fluids are inserted, causing transient neuritis, which usually resolves in 3 months to 1 year. They present with paranesthesia and muscle weakness along the nerve distribution of the affected nerve [16].

Chemical injuries after inadvertent neuraxial injection of chemical substances, contaminated drug solutions or equipment with detergents, foreign substances, local preservatives, neurotoxic local anesthetics, or subarachnoid blood may result in arachnoiditis. Iatrogenic meningitis following poor aseptic technique highlights the importance of sterility during neuraxial procedures [17].

Chemical toxicity can cause cauda equina syndrome and adhesive arachnoiditis causing collagen to develop between the nerve roots and the pia arachnoid, eventually resulting in ischemia and atrophy.

Comprehensive injuries that can cause damage to the spinal cord and subsequent ischemia are rare but can be caused by spinal hematoma or epidural abscess. These comprehensive injuries are reversible when identified early and treated by surgical decompression, but late intervention can result in severe and irreversible nerve damage leading to paralysis below the lesion. Any non-resolving or progressive motor block following neuraxial block should be initially managed as comprehensive injury and urgent MRI scan to confirm the diagnosis or exclude nervous pathology.

Neuraxial procedures can commonly cause transient mild neurological complications to serious life-threatening neurological injuries. A large multicentered study by the National Audit Project (NAP) into anesthesia complications quotes the risk of permanent injury from an obstetric regional anesthetic technique as 0.2–1.2:100,000.

Paranesthesia frequently occurs during neuraxial procedures indicating that the needle or catheter has contacted nerve tissue; however, should paresthesia occur, needle advancement should be halted or redirected. If paranesthesia persists, the needle should be withdrawn.

The subarachnoid space is more vulnerable to permanent injury because of poorly myelinated nerve roots, minimal chemical irritant protection, and large amounts of potentially neurotoxic local anesthetics. Three meningeal protective layers surround nerve roots in the epidural space and are more likely to resolve over days to months. Single traumatic nerve root injuries are commonly reported; persistent paresthesia and injury are uncommon. Risk factors contributing are obesity, technical difficulties, patient movement, vertebral anomalies, severe spinal canal stenosis, and preexisting spinal diseases are predisposing factors for nerve injury.

8 Injury to the Spinal Cord, Cauda Equina

Injury to the spinal cord can occur by neuraxial needle, catheter trauma, inadvertent injection of an anesthetic solution, unintended drug, or other routes of administration (e.g., neuraxial administration of medication intended for the intravenous route) into the spinal cord or nerve [16].

Damage to conus medullaris may occur during unintentional spinal anesthesia performed at a higher lumbar interspace; however, the spinal cord ends at the body of L1 vertebrae, the intended interspace may be misidentified, and the actual interspace is cephaloid to the intended interspace sometimes by more than one interspace; thus, the clinician may initiate spinal anesthesia at a higher than mid-lumbar interspace, there increasing the risk of direct trauma to conus medullaris or direct injection into the parenchyma of the spinal cord may likely result in paraplegia.

8.1 Prevention and Management

Direct trauma to the spinal cord can be prevented by identification of the correct intervertebral space at or below the level of L3–L4 interspace to avoid injury to conus medullaris, redirecting the needle in the presence of persistent paresthesia, avoiding injection of neuraxial medication if the patient experiences severe pain, avoiding neuraxial blockade in the presence of tethered cord, severe spinal stenosis, and other spinal and spinal cord pathologies. Trauma to nerve roots can be minimized by using soft-tip flexible reinforced epidural catheters and threading the catheter not more than 6 cm into the epidural space. Every effort should be made to reduce the risk of administering the wrong medication or using the wrong route. A neurology consultation for the evaluation of all neurological complications is mandated [17].

9 Hemorrhage

9.1 Spinal Epidural Hematoma (SEH)

It is a rare, potentially serious complication of neuraxial blockade in healthy obstetric patients. The proposed reason for protection is the hypercoagulable state of pregnancy, with a relatively low incidence of spinal pathology [18]. Risk factors include hematological abnormalities (overt coagulopathy, inherited clotting dysfunction, severe thrombocytopenia, platelet function disorder), administration of antithrombotic medications, and preexisting spinal deformities (spinal stenosis). There is a greater risk of developing hematoma due to pathological processes in HELLP syndrome, hepatic or renal failure, or by medications used in modern obstetrics; therefore, increased vigilance is needed to ensure adequate time intervals between anticoagulants dose and undertaking regional anesthetic techniques. Similarly, caution must be paid with the timing of epidural catheter removal as 50% of hematomas develop at this time. The overall incidence of SEH after regional obstetric anesthesia is very low, with 1.2 per 100,000 epidurals and 0.5 per 100,000 spinal anesthetics [19].

9.2 *Intracranial Hemorrhage*

Intracranial hemorrhage (commonly subdural hematoma) is an infrequent but potentially lethal complication of a dural puncture during neuraxial anesthesia. It should be considered a differential diagnosis in patients with delayed onset of headache after dural puncture (up to 72 h) and in patients with nonpostural headaches who develop other neurological symptoms or symptoms that persist after one or two epidural blood patches.

10 Infective Complications

Iatrogenic bacterial meningitis is a rare but potentially fatal life-threatening complication of neuraxial blockade in obstetric patients, occurring after a dural puncture during the spinal or combined spinal-epidural technique or after an unintentional dural puncture during an epidural technique, with favorable outcomes when diagnosed early and treated promptly.

Adherence to strict basic aseptic technique is the most effective way to minimize the risk of neuraxial infection, along with the administration of pre-procedure antibiotic administration with known or suspected systemic bacterial infections, considering an alternate mode of anesthesia, replacing epidural catheters after unwitnessed catheter disconnections, and removing epidural catheters without delay and as clinically appropriate. Arachnoiditis has been reported after unintentional injection or blood spread into the subarachnoid or subdural space during or after an epidural blood patch [20].

Clinically present with headache, nausea, diminished reflexes, muscle spasm, sensory numbness along the appropriate dermatomes, segmental numbness, and lower extremity weakness. Signs and symptoms may be devastating if not recognized and treated early. Treatment is mainly supportive of infection control with antibiotics and analgesia. Severe and deteriorating symptoms with a decline in functional status may need expert neurological advice for further management.

10.1 Spinal Epidural Abscess

Spinal epidural abscess (SEA) is a rare complication of neuraxial blockade with reported incidence ranging from 1:1930 to 1:205,000, according to patient demographic data.

Patient risk factors related to altered immunity in pregnancy or receiving immunosuppressive therapy are identified to have low immunity predisposing for SEA. Several other procedure-related risk factors are poor aseptic technique, multiple attempts, traumatic placement, prolonged catheterizations, localized/systemic infections at the site or time of needle insertion, opioid administration without local anesthetic, and the presence of blood nidus after the traumatic neuraxial procedure. Neurological compromise from the epidural spinal abscess may result from ischemia due to mechanical compression of the spinal cord and its vasculature (thrombosis) precipitated by infection [21].

The route of infection in cases of SEA with neuraxial techniques in obstetric patients may be predominantly by the contagious spread from a nearby source of infection in which bacteria gain access to the epidural space by direct contamination from the catheter entry point via patients' skin or hair follicles, aerosolized droplets from the upper airway of medical personnel, migration of organisms along the catheter, contaminated equipment or contaminated injectables from multidose vials, traumatic neuraxial procedures, blood collection (hematoma), or hematogenous seedling. The diagnosis may get complicated in obstetric patients with abscess unrelated to neuraxial procedures from the nearby spread of bone and muscle infection, complicating the diagnosis.

Clinical presentation varies, with only a small proportion of patients presenting with the triad of symptoms of back pain, fever, and progressive focal neurological deficits with sensory loss of one or several dermatomes, lower limb weakness, and bladder dysfunction.

The diagnosis should be considered after neuraxial anesthesia in febrile patients with persistent or worsening backache, consistent radiculopathy, and focal neurological deficits. Spinal imaging confirms the diagnosis and the causative organism is isolated from the blood sample, abscess content, and epidural catheter tip.

The mainstay of management includes prompt diagnosis, immediate catheter removal, early initiation of broad-coverage antibiotics, and decompressive laminectomy as soon as the diagnosis is confirmed. A delay in diagnosis and treatment may result in permanent neurological deficits.

11 Side Effects

The sympathectomy accompanying neuraxial anesthesia results in physiological side effects caused by the local anesthetics or opioids used for the techniques.

- Cardiovascular side effects of hypotension are revived with intravenous fluid boluses of crystalloid solution and vasopressors (ephedrine 6 mg or phenylephrine 50 mcg titrated dose or infusion), and bradycardia is treated by atropine or glycopyrrolate. Avoid aortocaval compression by full lateral position of the parturient.
- Venous puncture of epidural/dural veins.
- Shivering is caused by sympathetic block-induced vasodilation and the redistribution of body heat from the core to the periphery.
- Urinary retention is a possible side effect of both neuraxial analgesia and anesthesia by local anesthetics and neuraxial opioids, causing decreased ability to sense a full bladder and void.
- Catheter breakage.
- Maternal fever has been associated with epidural analgesia.
- Backache-localized tenderness may persist for several days after a neuraxial procedure which resolves without any evidence of long-term neckache.
- Nausea and vomiting caused by drugs (opioids, methergine).
- Anaphylaxis.
- Respiratory depression (opiates).

12 General Anesthesia Complications

Historically, general anesthesia was the go-to anesthetic in obstetrics for both vaginal births and cesarean sections. Pregnancy-related physiological changes influence the approach to general anesthesia in parturients. Anatomical and physiological changes during pregnancy, issues with training, environmental factors, and human variables contribute to the higher incidence of difficult airway. Important changes related to anesthesia involve the respiratory, cardiovascular, and gastrointestinal systems. Fetal exposure to anesthetics raises concern about the risk of teratogenicity and the future behavioral environment [22].

Real-time live training opportunities have diminished over time due to a considerable decline in the use of GA for CS. Multidisciplinary team simulations are recommended to address the nontechnical aspects of managing the obstetric airway, such as inadequate or poor communication, substandard care, a lack of supervision, organizational issues, and human errors.

The Airway Assessment Mallampati scores can worsen during pregnancy and can further change during labor [23]. Respiratory changes related to pregnancy include upward displacement of the diaphragm by the uterus and an increase in the transverse diameter of the thorax, functional residual capacity (FRC) is reduced by 20% at term, and minute ventilation is increased by 50%. This decreased FRC, in addition to increased oxygen consumption, explains the consequences of rapid oxygen desaturation of the pregnant mother during apnea or airway obstruction. Anatomically, mucosal engorgement and laryngeal or pharyngeal edema contribute to the increased difficulty of tracheal intubation and excessive risk of bleeding.

Cardiac output increases by 50% at term with increased heart rate (10–20 beats per minute) and stroke volume (30–40%), describing faster induction of anesthesia with IV anesthetics.

Gastrointestinal changes include the gravid uterus displacing the stomach in a cephalad direction, increasing intragastric pressure, and the loss of protective effect of the diaphragm on the lower esophageal sphincter tone as the esophagus enters the thorax in addition to progesterone reducing the tone of the lower esophageal sphincter. Commonly pregnant women experience symptoms of gastric reflux and regurgitation. Gastric emptying is delayed at the onset of labor and when using parenteral or neuraxial opioids but remains normal in pregnancy.

Maternal arterial pressure is a key factor in fetal perfusion; hence, it is critical to avoid maternal hypotension. Maintaining adequate maternal oxygenation while giving pregnant women GA is crucial to preventing fetal hypoxemia. Placental is not autoregulated and is entirely dependent on maternal blood pressure; therefore, maternal hypotension can lead to decreased fetal oxygenation and deterioration in fetal heart rate patterns. Fetal monitoring provides information during fetal procedures or nonobstetric surgery to ensure adequate fetal perfusion and oxygenation. Before delivery, skilled, trained staff, and a defined strategy are required to hasten delivery if concerns over fetal heart rate arise.

Compared to neuraxial procedures, neonatal outcomes after GA have been shown to have a slightly lower base deficit and a higher umbilical artery pH; this is partially explained by the effects of aortocaval compression and the use of vasopressors rather than the technique itself.

Failure to intubate the trachea, the possibility of aspirating and developing aspiration pneumonitis, and accidental awareness are the most feared complications of GA.

The consequences may affect the mother and the fetus in obstetric patients, highlighting the importance of identifying risk factors (obesity, known difficult airways) and preparing adequately (fasting, stomach decompression). Although the mortality rate associated with GA in obstetrics has reduced to 60%, inadequate airway management is one of the leading causes of mortality.

Airway-related maternal mortality during obstetric GA for CS is approximately 2.3 per 100,000 and 1% after failed intubation, compared to 1 in 180,000 GA for the general population. The incidence of front-of-neck access is higher at 3.4 per 1,000,000 GA for CS compared to two per 100,000 GA for the general population.

The obstetric difficult airway guidelines algorithm published by the obstetric anesthetist association and difficult airway society (OAA/DAS). Table 1 emphasizes preinduction planning and preparation, including airway assessment, fasting, antacid prophylaxis, and the role of waking up the patient if intubation fails [22, 23].

Pregnancy-related increases in breast size combined with cricoid pressure prevent the insertion of the laryngoscope handle during laryngoscopy. The ramping head-up position during induction of GA improves airway manipulation and enhances the laryngoscopic view. In addition to pregnancy-related changes, the

Table 1 AAGA risk factors in cesarean delivery

• No sedative premedication
• High incidence of emergency procedures
• Increased cardiac output affects the uptake and distribution of volatile anesthetics
• Administration of neuromuscular blocking agents
• Low-dose induction agents
• Obesity
• Difficult airway causing prolonged time to intubate
• Avoiding opioids before delivery
• Inadequate depth of anesthesia

increased prevalence of obesity in pregnancy increases the likelihood of a difficult airway. These patients are carefully positioned with specific positioning devices, such as the Oxford Help Pillow, to increase the likelihood of successful tracheal intubation. To prevent desaturation during induction and intubation, the following measures are recommended.

- Preoxygenation with a tight fighting face mask for a minimum of 3 min to achieve an end-tidal oxygen level of 90%.
- Mask ventilation before intubation with a maximum peak inspiratory pressure of 20 cm H_2O.
- Apnoeic oxygenation via nasal cannula at 5–15 l/min.

The consensus about using an anesthetic induction agent for RSI in obstetric anesthesia includes its familiarity, availability, better suppression of airway reflexes, and reduced drug errors. There is disagreement on the routine use of short-acting opioids during obstetric GA induction; however, carefully titrated doses of opioids are given before induction in preeclampsia, maternal cardiac diseases, or neurological diseases to attenuate the hypertensive response to intubation, provide cardiovascular stability, and decrease the risk of intraoperative awareness. Maternally administered drugs with a maternal-fetal transfer are sedatives and opioids (e.g., volatile anesthetic agents, propofol, fentanyl, and remifentanil) known to cross the placenta.

Modern airway adjuvants and video laryngoscopes with Macintosh-style blades have increased the success rate of tracheal intubation in obstetric patients by providing a better direct and indirect laryngeal view. There was a minimal increase in intubation time between video and direct laryngoscopy. When there is difficulty with the airway during the laryngoscopy's first attempt, cricoid pressure must be decreased or removed earlier.

Anatomical changes in pregnancy may make tracheal intubation challenging in obstetric patients, with a higher incidence of likely failed intubation rate of 1:300 compared to 1:1000–2000 in the general population.

Approximately 1–2% of pregnant women require nonobstetric surgery during pregnancy (appendectomy, cholecystectomy, ovarian procedures, laparoscopic), potentially requiring GA as the primary anesthetic, and patients refuse anything except GA [24].

Assessing the nature of pain and the sensory level is critical for the anesthetist. Despite an anesthetist's best efforts, neuraxial blocks with inadequate anesthesia are encountered during surgery, requiring conversion to GA. If redosing the neuraxial catheter is not an option, supplementary analgesia with IV or inhaled adjuvants (opioids, ketamine, and nitrous oxide) may be needed. Conversion to GA may be necessary if the analgesia dose used is insufficient [25].

It is essential to balance the risk of converting to GA against the risk of not converting at any given time. Understanding the complexity of conversion in hemodynamically unstable patients and in unarousable patients with reduced ability to maintain airway reflexes should be considered during induction of GA.

A maximum number of two attempts are recommended. If the first attempt at intubation fails, continue ventilation with a face mask or high-flow humidified nasal oxygen and communicate with the team. The second attempt should be by the senior anesthetist using a different laryngoscope, considering the removal of cricoid pressure. The third attempt should be made rarely by senior and additional anesthetists as airway swelling can develop rapidly, and progress to a critical situation (CICO) cannot intubate/cannot oxygenate in a pregnant woman [26].

Following unsuccessful intubation, failed intubation is declared with priority.

To establish and maintain oxygenation by face mask or second-generation supraglottic airway devices (SAD) and follow failed intubation algorithm. Having two airway management expert anesthetists at this stage is always preferred.

Maternal well-being is the most crucial factor once oxygenation is established; several factors influence the final decision to proceed with the anesthetic or wake up, ensuring safety, good ventilation, and appropriate depth of anesthesia while the decision is invariably made during a stressful time [4], with human factors and situational awareness playing a significant role. If the decision is to wake up the woman, a planned safe delivery is formulated with an obstetric team, including regional anesthesia and awake tracheal intubation with a flexible bronchoscope.

Maternal well-being is the most important factor once oxygenation is established; several factors influence the final decision to proceed with the anesthetic or wake up, ensuring safety, good ventilation, and appropriate depth of anesthesia while the decision is invariably made during a stressful time, with human factors and situational awareness playing a significant role. If the decision is to wake the woman, a planned safe delivery is formulated with an obstetric team, including regional anesthesia and awake tracheal intubation with a flexible bronchoscope.

The preferred technique is controlled ventilation using neuromuscular agents, second-generation SAD as a rescue airway device and volatile anesthetics agents. Regurgitation and pulmonary aspiration risk are reduced by aspirating the gastric tube through SAD and minimizing fundal pressure at delivery [4].

If the oxygenation attempt fails and the CICO scenario develops, this is managed by surgical cricothyroidotomy; however, if cardiac arrest develops before the baby is delivered, a perimortem CS is carried out and completed within 5 min of cardiac arrest.

A critical incident report form should be filled out, and the incident should be included in the patient's medical records. She should be counseled with information communication should the woman require GA in the future.

13 Accidental Awareness Under General Anesthesia

Accidental consciousness under general anesthesia occurs when a patient becomes conscious during the procedure and subsequently has a recall of cognizant events during surgery. The general incidence of awareness for all types of surgeries is 1:19,000. It is significantly higher during general anesthesia for cesarean delivery compared to the general population [27].

The general incidence of awareness in obstetric procedures under GA for all procedures was 1:1200. Still, for cesarean delivery, it was 1:670 as per the fifth National Audit Project done by the Royal College of Anesthetists over the period of the anesthetist. AAGA has prolonged and severe psychological sequelae (anxiety state or nightmares) in about 21% of patients. Empathy and physiological support are crucial in patients with AAGA.

Several factors are thought to increase the risk of unintentional awareness during cesarean delivery. Most general anesthetics for cesarean deliveries are performed in an emergency, necessitating rapid sequence induction and using neuromuscular blocking drugs masking the physical signs of inadequate anesthesia depth (Table 1).

Pregnancy-related physiological changes can mask signs of inadequate depth of anesthesia, and because of the increased cardiac output, intravenous induction drugs have quicker onset and offset times. Due to the nature of the emergency category, one cesarean section requires surgery to start soon after tracheal intubation because it is safe for the mother. This means insufficient time to build a high concentration of volatile agents to ensure adequate depth of anesthesia. BIS monitoring in conjunction with clinical signs can assist in adjusting anesthetic depth.

Obesity is a risk factor for an obstetric population. Increased volume of distribution during pregnancy and patient body weight drug volume may be insufficient for the distribution (neuromuscular blocking drugs), making tracheal intubation more challenging and time-consuming and raising the chance of awareness.

14 Aspiration

Mendelson first described in 1946 a woman who died of airway obstruction due to solid material. Pregnancy-induced hormonal and physical changes increase the risk of aspiration during pregnancy and labor. These include increased intragastric pressure due to a gravid uterus, reduced lower esophageal sphincter tone as an effect of increased progesterone, and delayed gastric emptying during labor. Delayed gastric emptying may be exaggerated by opioid analgesia during labor. The incidence of gastric aspiration is 2 in 10,000 GA [28].

Unfasted obstetric patients have a lower pH and greater volume with a high risk of aspiration; however, 50% of fasted patients have a residual gastric volume of 25 ml. Consideration is given to prevent aspiration and altering the pH of gastric fluid so that subsequent complications of aspiration are reduced.

Antiacid prophylaxis is commonly administered orally or intravenously to increase the pH of gastric contents and reduce the risk of pulmonary injury in the event of aspiration. Difficult airway society recommends rapid sequence induction for all obstetric procedures requiring general anesthesia to reduce the risk of aspiration [29].

It is important to consider the risk of aspiration during tracheal extubation and intubation. Patients are extubated fully awake with the return of airway reflexes and woken up in head up or left lateral position to reduce the risk of gastric regurgitation into the lungs.

15 Cardiac Arrest in Pregnancy

Maternal cardiac arrest is rare, complicating 1 in 20,000–30,000 pregnancies caused by various medical, surgical, and obstetric causes. Maternal collapse is defined as an acute event involving the cardiorespiratory system and/or central nervous system, resulting in a reduced or absent consciousness (and potentially cardiac arrest and death) at any stage in pregnancy and up to 6 weeks after birth. Pregnancy increases the risk to the mother and fetus and the mother's ability to adapt to illness. Resuscitation of the mother is performed with minor adjustments related to anatomical and physiological changes of pregnancy. Early and effective resuscitation by a well-coordinated multidisciplinary team of obstetricians, anesthesiologists, midwives, and neonatologist minimizes maternal and neonatal morbidity and mortality and improves outcomes. The focus should be on the mother although another potential life is at stake. Important anatomical and physiological changes in pregnancy affecting resuscitation are aortocaval compression syndrome which leads to decreased venous return and cardiac output by 30–40%, leading to hypotension; hence, manual displacement of the uterus to the left is important while resuscitation. Delivery of the fetus improves venous return and cardiac output and facilitates chest compressions making ventilation easier. Tachycardia is an early sign of blood loss which can get masked by concealed bleeding and hypotension, underestimated blood loss (exceeding 30–35% of blood volume), causing a delay in intervention.

Maternal resuscitation is the priority, primarily emphasizing airway, breathing, circulation (ABC), and maternal well-being. In women over 20 weeks of gestation, if there is no response to cardiopulmonary resuscitation (CPR) within 4 min of maternal collapse, perimortem cesarean section (PMCS) should be undertaken to assist maternal resuscitation. This should be achieved within 5 min of maternal collapse.

Primary ABC airway assessment with 15°–30° left lateral tilt or manual displacement of the gravid uterus to the left relieves compression on the inferior vena cava, optimizing sufficient venous return without significantly impacting the effectiveness of chest compressions [30].

No modifications are needed in positioning or dosage for defibrillation. Defibrillation does not increase the risk to the fetus, but the fetal monitor needs to be removed prior to defibrillation.

The secondary survey requires modification to the optimal alignment of the larynx and difficulty in intubating, placing the mother in a sniffing position to facilitate intubation. Consider rapid sequence intubation during resuscitation to prevent the risk of aspiration. With the progress of pregnancy, soft tissue oropharyngeal edema increases with an increase in the Mallampati classification (Mallampati III), making mask ventilation and intubation challenging and higher the chances of failed intubation. The airway is more prone to injury and trauma from attempted intubation, causing bleeding, increased swelling, and soft tissue edema. Pre-oxygenation is essential because of the increased risk of hypoxemia during pregnancy due to changes in lung dynamics. Ventilation is difficult due to diaphragmatic splinting by the gravid uterus; hence, early endotracheal intubation is recommended and monitored by capnography.

Immediately after maternal stabilization, fetal heart sounds are assessed immediately by evaluating fetal heart sounds. Placental disruption or insufficiency, maternal hypoxia, hypovolemia, and hypotension can all result in fetal hypoxia. Fetal demise can be minimized by maintaining adequate perfusion and oxygenation to the placenta.

Causes of maternal cardiac arrest include direct pregnancy complications and preexisting disease (Table 2).

Table 2 Obstetric and non-obstetric causes of cardiac arrest in pregnancy

Obstetric causes	Non-obstetric causes
Hemorrhage (17%)	Pulmonary embolism (19%)
Pregnancy-induced hypertensive disorders (16%)	Infection/sepsis (13%)
Idiopathic peripartum cardiomyopathy (8%)	Stroke (5%)
Anesthesia complications (2%)	Myocardial infarction
Anaphylaxis	Congenital/rheumatic heart diseases/prosthetic valves
Amniotic fluid embolism (1.7 per 10,000 deliveries)	Drugs and toxins
	Trauma
	4 H and 4 T

16 Trauma in Pregnancy

Trauma can complicate any pregnancy and is the most common nonobstetric cause of morbidity and mortality in pregnancy. The first evaluation step is airway, breathing, and circulation in pregnant trauma patients. The second survey follows the first primary survey and initial maternal stabilization.

17 Hemorrhage

Obstetric hemorrhage contributes to 25% of maternal deaths in pregnancy. The most common causes are intrapartum and postpartum, while antepartum is also prevalent. The causes of antepartum hemorrhage are abruption of the placenta, placenta previa, and uterine rupture. It is underestimated due to clinical difficulties in accurately estimating blood loss or concealed bleeding in uterine and abdominal cavities or the retroperitoneal space.

A pregnancy-induced hypervolemic physiological state prepares a pregnant woman for hemorrhage with a greater risk of blood loss from a gravid uterus; consequently, pregnant patients can experience massive blood loss prior to manifesting significant changes in vital signs. Failure to detect and treat hemorrhage early can result in maternal and fetal death [31]. Rapid evaluation and initiating appropriate resuscitation can enhance the patient's prognosis (Fig. 5).

Postpartum hemorrhage is defined as abnormal bleeding manifesting signs of hypovolemia or total blood loss of >500 ml after vaginal delivery or >1000 ml after cesarean section. PPH remains one of the leading causes of preventable maternal mortality (Table 3).

Postpartum hemorrhage is the most common form of life-threatening obstetric hemorrhage, estimated at 1–5% of deliveries. It is underestimated due to clinical difficulties in accurately estimating blood loss or concealed bleeding in uterine and abdominal cavities or retroperitoneal space. A timely, accurate diagnosis and intervention (drugs, surgical) reduces maternal mortality and admission to the intensive care unit. PPH is classified as primary and secondary with different etiologies (Table 4).

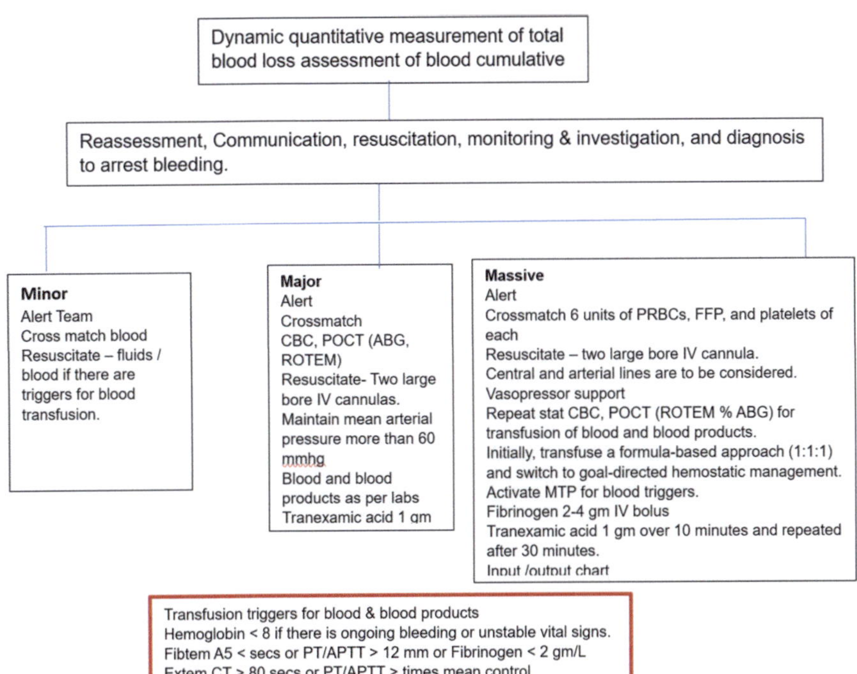

Fig. 5 Management of PPH

Table 3 Classification of hemorrhage

• Minor obstetric hemorrhage 500–1000 ml blood loss with no evidence of clinical shock
• Major obstetric hemorrhage of more than 1000 m`l blood loss or with evidence of clinical shock
• Massive hemorrhage: uncontrolled hemorrhage of more than 1500 ml or acute loss requiring transfusion of more than four units PRBCS or suspicion/evidence of coagulopathy due to hemorrhage

Table 4 Classification and etiology of PPH

Primary PPH—occurring within 24 h after vaginal delivery or Cesarean section	*Secondary PPH*—occurs between 24 h and 12 weeks postpartum
Etiology—4 Ts	*Etiology*
• Tone	• Retained tissues
• Tissue	• Gestational trophoblastic disease
• Trauma	• Inherited coagulation defects
• Thrombin	• Endometritis

18 Embolism

Embolism is the common cause of acute hemodynamic and respiratory collapse in pregnancy, contributing to approximately 20% of maternal deaths. The majority of embolic patients may be asymptomatic. The common emboli are thrombus and amniotic fluid that can enter the pulmonary circulation resulting in ventilation/perfusion (V/Q) mismatch and hypoxia and, consequently, cardiac arrest. Rapid assessment and initiation of resuscitative measures reduce morbidity and mortality [32].

Due to venous stasis, hypercoagulability, and vascular injury (Virchow's triad), the risk of thromboembolism rises five- to tenfold during pregnancy. Other risk factors include previous thromboembolism history, advanced maternal age, obesity, multiple parity, and a sedentary lifestyle.

The aim of treatment for pulmonary embolism in pregnancy is to maintain adequate oxygenation and circulation. In addition to supportive care, heparin is started before a definitive diagnosis. Pregnancy is a relative contraindication to thrombolytic therapy.

Amniotic fluid embolism is a systemic inflammatory response to anaphylactoid reaction initiated by foreign debris from amniotic fluid that enters maternal circulation. It is not a common complication associated with a high mortality rate, with 50% of patients dying within 1 h of onset. It commonly occurs immediately following delivery. Risk factors include difficult labor, ruptured membranes, trauma, placental abruption, ruptured uterus, multiparity, and advanced maternal age. It typically presents with maternal respiratory distress, hypotension, shock, pulmonary edema, seizures, confusion, and coma, progressing to disseminated intravascular coagulation (DIC) and multisystem organ failure. Treatment is supportive with the goal of maintaining oxygenation and circulation to minimize long-term sequelae.

19 Disseminated Intravascular Coagulation

Disseminated intravascular coagulation is a potentially life-threatening complication in pregnancy. Normal hemostasis is maintained by a balance between coagulation factors and inhibitors, as well as thrombus formation and lysis. In DIC, systemic activation of the coagulation cascade disrupts normal hemostasis.

Instead of local typical local reaction to vascular bed damage, the body begins to uncontrollably form and lyse clots throughout the system resulting in consumptive coagulopathy and hemorrhage. Platelets are destroyed with fibrin plugs deposition in a small vessel leading to ischemia. Common triggers for DIC are placental abruption, intrauterine fetal death, amniotic fluid embolism, septic shock, and transfusion reactions. Diagnosis of DIC platelet count and fibrinogen levels are focused on.

Suspicion of DIC is high when the platelet count and fibrinogen levels are low, needing further evaluation. Treatment is to focus on the underlying etiology and eliminate the trigger. If the hemorrhage is extensive, replacement of platelets, clotting factors, fibrinogen, and red blood cells is needed.

20 Eclampsia

Eclampsia is the continuum of hypertensive disorders of pregnancy. Risk factors include teenage pregnancy, family predisposition, twin gestation, molar pregnancy, and obesity. Preeclampsia is new onset hypertension presenting after 20 weeks of gestation with or without proteinuria or involvement of one or more maternal organ systems or fetus. Eclampsia is preeclampsia with added seizure activity. Commonly presents with headache, nausea, vomiting, edema, epigastric pain, visual disturbances, hypertension, hyperreflexia, and seizure [33]. Eclampsia is considered in any patient with 20 weeks or more of gestation with seizure. Initial management is to secure airway and intravenous access with magnesium sulfate as the drug of choice for eclamptic seizures. Blood test to evaluate end-organ damage and look for signs of HELLP (Hemolysis, EL elevated liver enzymes, and LP low platelet count). Antihypertensives medications are recommended to be considered if blood pressure is persistently elevated 150/100 mmHg with features of preeclampsia or not. The blood pressure must be maintained and not lowered too much to prevent placental hypoperfusion and fetal compromise. Common serious life-threatening complications include pulmonary edema and cerebrovascular accident necessitating ICU admission. Fluid management plays an essential role.

21 Cardiac Diseases in Pregnancy

Pregnancy with increased cardiac output and blood volume dramatically impacts patients with preexisting cardiac diseases with increased demand on the heart. In addition to the increased volume, the hypercoagulable state of pregnancy increases the risk of thromboembolic events. The presence of artificial cardiac valves and stenotic lesions further increases the risk in pregnancy.

22 Conclusion

Physiological changes of pregnancy occur in all organs caused by hormonal and mechanical factors, and increasing incidence of obesity, medical conditions, and altered physiological response to neuraxial anesthesia affect the approach to anesthesia, increasing the likely risk of complications highlighting the importance of vigilance, early detection, and fastidious attention in the management of anesthesia-related obstetric complications.

With significant advances in obstetric anesthesia practice, regional anesthesia is the most common method of providing anesthesia to pregnant women due to its high safety profile. To reduce aortocaval compression and cardiovascular compromise in patients beyond 18–20 weeks of gestation, they should be positioned supine with a 15°–30° left lateral tilt.

While general anesthesia is generally avoided in pregnant patients, it remains the method of choice in certain circumstances. Video laryngoscopy should be used as the first line of laryngoscopy to maximize the success rate of intubation during Rapid Sequence Intubation and minimize the risk of failed intubation, aspiration, and awareness in obstetric practice. General anesthesia establishes a reversible stage III surgical anesthesia stage with a goal to provide hypnosis/unconsciousness, amnesia, analgesia, and muscle relaxation as appropriate for the procedure as well as an autonomic and sensory block of responses to noxious surgical stimulus. Converting regional blocks to GA is a critical skill, and anesthetists need to balance the risk of converting unnecessary GA Vs. The risk of not converting to GA and the patient requiring GA when in a precarious condition.

Pregnant women's medical, obstetric history and airway assessment are evaluated to assess the risk and develop a safe anesthesia plan for obstetric/nonobstetric surgery. There are risks and benefits associated with both types of anesthetics.

Obstetric anesthesia-related complications range a span complication from transient nerve injury to life-threatening complications; hence, the anesthesiologist must explain the risk and document any neurological symptoms present during pregnancy.

References

1. Smith EA, Thorburn J, Duckworth RA, et al. A comparison of 25 G and 27 G Whitacre needles for caesarean section. Anaesthesia. 1994;49:859–62.
2. Van de Velde M, Teunkens A, Hanssens M, et al. Post dural puncture headache following combined spinal epidural or epidural anaesthesia in obstetric patients. Anaesth Intensive Care. 2001;29:595–9.
3. Paech M, Banks S, Gurrin L. An audit of accidental dural puncture during epidural insertion of a Tuohy needle in obstetric patients. Int J Obstet Anesth. 2001;10:162–7.
4. Morley-Forster PK, Singh S, Angle P, et al. The effect of epidural needle type on postdural puncture headache: a randomized trial. Can J Anaesth. 2006;53:572–8.
5. Vakharia SB, Thomas PS, Rosenbaum AE, et al. Magnetic resonance imaging of cerebrospinal fluid leak and tamponade effect of blood patch in postdural puncture headache. Anesth Analg. 1997;84:585–90.
6. Grant R, Condon B, Hart I, et al. Changes in intracranial CSF volume after lumbar puncture and their relationship to post-LP headache. J Neurol Neurosurg Psychiatry. 1991;54:440–2.
7. Headache Classification Subcommittee of the International Headache Society (IHS). The international classification of headache disorders, 3rd edition (beta version). Cephalalgia. 2013;33:629–808.
8. Boezaart AP. Effects of cerebrospinal fluid loss and epidural blood patch on cerebral blood flow in swine. Reg Anesth Pain Med. 2001;26:401–6.
9. Kroin JS, Nagalla SK, Buvanendran A, et al. The mechanisms of intracranial pressure modulation by epidural blood and other injectates in a postdural puncture rat model. Anesth Analg. 2002;95:423–9.

10. Bogod D. Pain during caesarean section. Br J Obstet Gynaecol. 2016;123:753.
11. Clive B. Collier accidental subdural injection during attempted lumbar epidural block may present as a failed or inadequate block: radiographic evidence. Reg Anesth Pain Med. 2004;29(1):45–51.
12. Cook TM, Counsell D, Wildsmith JA. Major complications of central neuraxial block: report on the Third National Audit Project of the Royal College of Anaesthetists. Br J Anaesth. 2009;102(2):179–90.
13. Poole M. Management of high regional block in obstetrics. Update in Anaesthesia. http://www.e-safeanaesthesia.org/e_library/13/High_regional_block_in_obstetrics_Update_2009.pdf.
14. Butterworth JF IV, Walker FO, Lysak SZ. Pregnancy increases median nerve susceptibility to lidocaine. Anesthesiology. 1990;72:962.
15. Moller RA, Datta S, Fox J, et al. Effects of progesterone on the cardiac electrophysiologic action of bupivacaine and lidocaine. Anesthesiology. 1992;76:604.
16. Saifuddin A, Burnett SJ, White J. The variation of position of the conus medullaris in an adult population. A magnetic resonance imaging study. Spine (Phila Pa 1976). 1998;23:1452.
17. Broadbent CR, Maxwell WB, Ferrie R, et al. Ability of anaesthetists to identify a marked lumbar interspace. Anaesthesia. 2000;55:1122.
18. Rosero EB, Joshi GP. Nationwide incidence of serious complications of epidural analgesia in the United States. Acta Anaesthesiol Scand. 2016;60:810.
19. Vandermeulen EP, Van Aken H, Vermylen J. Anticoagulants and spinal-epidural anesthesia. Anesth Analg. 1994;79:1165.
20. Rice I, Wee MY, Thomson K. Obstetric epidurals and chronic adhesive arachnoiditis. Br J Anaesth. 2004;92:109.
21. Darouiche RO. Spinal epidural abscess. N Engl J Med. 2006;355:2012.
22. Hawkins JL, Chang J, Palmer SK, Gibbs CP, Callaghan WM. Anesthesia-related maternal mortality in the United States: 1979–2002. Obstet Gynecol. 2011;117:69–74.
23. Kovacheva VP, Brovman EY, Greenberg P, Song E, Palanisamy A, Urman RD. A contemporary analysis of medicolegal issues in obstetric anesthesia between 2005 and 2015. Anesth Analg. 2019;128:1199–207.
24. Tolcher MC, Fisher WE, Clark SL. Nonobstetric surgery during pregnancy. Obstet Gynecol. 2018;132:395–403.
25. Mushambi MC, Kinsella SM, Popat M, et al. Obstetric Anaesthetists' Association and Difficult Airway Society guidelines for the management of difficult and failed tracheal intubation in obstetrics. Anaesthesia. 2015;70:1286–306.
26. Brien KO, Conlon C. Failed intubation in obstetrics. Anaesth Intensive Care Med. 2013;14:315–9
27. Helsehurst N, Ells LJ, Simpson H, Batterham A, Wilkinson J, Summerbell CD. Trends in maternity obesity incidence, rates, demographic predictors and health inequalities in 38,821women over a 15 year period. Br J Obstet Gynaecol. 2007;114:187–94.
28. Mendelson CL. The aspiration of stomach contents into the lungs during obstetric anesthesia. Anesthesiology. 1946;7:694–5.
29. Rout CC, Rocke DA, Gouws E. Intravenous ranitidine reduces the risk of acid aspiration of gastric contents at emergency cesarean section. Anesth Analg. 1993;76:156–61.
30. Ueland K, Novy MJ, Peterson EN, Metcalfe J. Maternal cardiovascular dynamics. IV. The influence of gestational age on the maternal cardiovascular response to posture and exercise. Am J Obstet Gynecol. 1969;104:856.
31. Committee on Practice Bulletins-Obstetrics. Practice Bulletin No. 183: Postpartum hemorrhage. Obstet Gynecol. 2017;130:e168.
32. Leung AN, Bull TM, Jaeschke R, et al. An official American Thoracic Society/Society of Thoracic Radiology clinical practice guideline: evaluation of suspected pulmonary embolism in pregnancy. Am J Respir Crit Care Med. 2011;184:1200.
33. Pritchard JA, Cunningham FG, Pritchard SA. The Parkland Memorial Hospital protocol for treatment of eclampsia: evaluation of 245 cases. Am J Obstet Gynecol. 1984;148:951.

Ovarian Hyperstimulation Syndrome

Seema Nahid, Lolwa Alansari, Firdos Ummunnisa, Umm E Amara, Neelima Ramireddy, and Thoraya Almarzooqi

Abstract The challenge of taking a baby home without impairing women's health and quality of life remains the main outcome of reproductive techniques. It is the cost of our attempts to disrupt nature's precise equilibrium designed to ensure single oocyte ovulation is OHSS. Prevention of this syndrome is intrinsically more desirable than treatment.

OHSS is characterized by an exaggerated response to fertility drugs with stimulation of ovarian granulosa cells in gonadotropin-stimulated ovaries leading to swollen and painful ovaries, fluid accumulation in the abdomen, and in severe cases, potential complications such as kidney failure, blood clots, or even death.

The primary risk factor for OHSS is the use of high doses of gonadotropin hormones to stimulate the ovaries leading to the development of OHSS, consecutively there are also secondary risk factors that can increase the likelihood of developing OHSS. Early diagnosis and treatment significantly reduce mortality and multi-organ dysfunction.

A cascade of pathophysiological events brought on by ovarian overproduction of vasoactive mediators results in increased vascular permeability and clinical symptoms of life-threatening OHSS.

S. Nahid (✉)
Department of Anesthesia, Hamad Medical Corporation, Doha, Qatar
e-mail: snahid@hamad.qa

L. Alansari · T. Almarzooqi
Women's Wellness and Research Center, Hamad Medical Corporation, Doha, Qatar

F. Ummunnisa
University of Missouri, Kansas, MO, USA

U. E Amara
Apollo Institute of Medical Sciences and Research, Hyderabad, Telangana, India

N. Ramireddy
Hamad Medical Corporation, Doha, Qatar

N. Shaikh et al. (eds.), *Updates in Intensive Care of OBGY Patients*,
https://doi.org/10.1007/978-981-99-9577-6_11

With an understanding of the disease and careful attention to fluid and electrolyte management, respiratory support, infection control, and thromboembolism prophylaxis OHSS can effectively manage and protect the threatened lives of critically ill patients.

Recognizing high-risk individuals prior to treatment, choosing treatments that respect safety, managing infertility, and performing ovarian stimulation during therapy are primary preventative principles.

Few specific preventive strategies regarding the length of infertility, treatment timelines, and the development of minimal risk management procedures with consideration for alternative infertility treatments like insulin resistance drugs, ovarian drilling, and natural cycle in vitro fertilization should be considered.

Keywords Ovarian hyperstimulation syndrome (OHSS) · Follicle-stimulating hormone (FSH) · Luteinizing hormone (LH) · Abdominal compartment syndrome (ACS)

1 Definition

OHSS is a rare iatrogenic, potentially fatal complication occurring in the luteal phase or during early pregnancy after ovulation induction (provoking ovulation in anovulatory) or after ovulation stimulation (in ART), suggesting exaggerated and unpredictable patient response. It constitutes multiple ovarian cystic enlargements and increased vascular capillary permeability subsequently, fluid shifts from intravascular space to third space, causing ascites, pleural effusion, and rarely pericardial effusion. Severe life-threatening variations may be associated with thromboembolic risk, hepatic, renal, cardiac, and pulmonary impairment, and hemodynamic and electrolyte disturbances. The third-space sequestration caused by a widespread capillary leak is one of the main signs of ovarian hyperstimulation syndrome.

While ovulation stimulation stimulates the ovaries to produce mono-follicular development, prediction, and prevention are challenging due to the restricted range of responses that might range from no response to an exaggerated or unpredictable response [1].

Commonly HCG is used as a surrogate for luteinizing hormone for oocyte maturation, induction, and ovulation. HCG treatment causes a prolonged luteotropic effect due to its long half-life of >24 h, characterized by the formation of numerous corpora lutea and supraphysiological levels of progesterone and estradiol E2. This persistent luteotropic effect could lead to the onset of OHSS.

In rare cases, spontaneous forms of OHSS have been documented to be associated with abnormally high supraphysiological production of HCG in multiple pregnancies, hydatidiform mole [2].

2 History

This syndrome has been known since gonadotropins were used first to induce ovulation in 1943 was in 1943 following the use of gonadotropins for ovulation induction, and the first major fatal cases were was published in 1951 by Gotzche and Figueroa, necessitating laparotomies, ovariotomies, puncture or suturing of ruptured cysts, and catastrophic side effects like oliguria and renal failure that resulted in death.

3 Incidence

The incidence of OHSS is ill-defined by a large variation in the degree and grade of OHSS. Golan et al. and Novot and co-workers first classified OHSS into three categories: mild, moderate, and severe. The incidence of mild OHSS may vary between 8% and 23% (in gonadotropin-stimulated IVF cycles) with minimal clinical relevance. Moderate varying between <1% and 7%, and the prevalence of severe form reported is small between 0.1% and 2% [3].

Iatrogenic OHSS continues to be a severe issue with potentially fatal outcomes, high morbidity, and a mortality rate of 1/45,000–500,000.

Future prospective registries will strive to accurately capture the incidence of all fertility procedures and their significant complications.

4 Pathogenesis

The human natural cycle is designed to recruit a single dominant follicle from which a fertilized oocyte emerges. Antral follicles that failed to reach dominance are destined for atresia, which occurs before mid-cycle LH surge, which assures the formation of only a single corpus luteum in each cycle and explains the rarity of spontaneous OHSS. During the development of the corpus luteum in a normal menstrual cycle, a significant amount of vasoactive mediators are produced. These vasoactive mediators include vascular endothelial growth factors, angiotensin II, and a variety of interleukins.

When the secondary corpus luteum with luteotropic effect merges with endogenous HCG while pregnancy is achieved, providing ongoing stimulation of the corpus luteum gives rise to OHSS [4].

Generally, in ovarian stimulation, multiple follicles are stimulated to grow and develop in the ovaries using medications. The goal is to stimulate the growth of a sufficient number of mature follicles containing the eggs that will be retrieved for fertilization. However, in some cases, excessive stimulation results in the development of OHSS.

The renin-angiotensin system (RAS) plays an important role in ovarian physiology. Angiotensin II intervenes in the production of steroid synthesis and follicle production and maturation, ovulation, and follicular atresia.

5 Natural Cycle OHSS

Spontaneous mid-cycle LH surge is characterized by three phases rapidly ascending limb of 14 h duration, the plateau of 14 h descending phase of 20 h.

The parallel FSH surge is of low amplitude. Serum E2 levels peak at the onset of the LH surge and then decline rapidly. Serum progesterone levels rise 12 h before the LH surge, continue to rise for an additional 12 h, and then plateau until follicular rupture 36 h after the LH surge onset. Follicular rupture is associated with a second rise in progesterone and a fall in estrogen as the luteal pattern of ovarian steroidogenesis is attained [5].

In non-IVF patients, low-dose stimulation protocol resulting in mono-follicular ovulation prevents OHSS regardless of HCG dose; however, in ART, when multi-folliculogenesis is required the risk of OHSS is the concern. Physiological regulatory mechanisms are stretched with the release of vasoactive molecules reaching the threshold resulting in exaggerated local inflammation, which leads to the onset of OHSS symptoms.

The two main pathophysiologies proposed in developing and establishing OHSS are inflammation and increased capillary permeability. This increased vascular permeability causes a change in extracellular fluid equilibrium with the fluid shift into extravascular third space, causing ascites, pleural and pericardial effusion, and hemoconcentration. Cardiac preload fails due to hypovolemia caused by fluid shifts and inferior vena cava compression from increasing intraperitoneal ascitic pressure.

The underlying pathophysiology of OHSS is increased capillary permeability with resultant third-space fluid accumulation. The sequestration of abnormal amounts of fluid in cavities (abdominal cavity, pleural cavity and pericardial sac) is responsible for specific problems [6].

Falling cardiac preload reduces cardiac output, leading to decreased renal perfusion. Decreased renal perfusion increases proximal tubule salt and water reabsorption, leading to decreased urinary sodium excretion and oliguria. The proximal sodium reabsorption and consequently diminished exposure of the distal tubule to sodium impairs sodium–hydrogen/potassium exchange in the distal tubule causing hyperkalemic acidosis [7].

The main factors produced by the ovaries and implicated in ovarian hyperstimulation syndrome are the renin-angiotensin system (RAS) and cytokines (interleukin-2 and -8) [8].

Other modulators of ovarian origin also play a role, in addition to the ovarian and systemic renin-angiotensin systems, in the development of the syndrome. OHSS also produces a hypercoagulable state, possibly due to a combination of hemoconcentration and high-level ovarian steroids.

6 Pathophysiology

The primary hypothesis for the development of OHSS is a disruption in the regulation of inflammation, such as during the ovulation process, causing local proinflammatory factors in the ovary, which results in increased capillary leakage and transmission of vasoactive inflammatory mediators in the systemic circulation, peritoneal cavity, and other compartments. Severe forms cause an extravascular third compartment fluid shift, arteriolar vasodilatation, and systemic symptoms. Possible association between arterial vasodilation and capillary leakage since arterial dilatation causes the development of interstitial edema by raising the capillary surface area and capillary hydrostatic pressure.

The pathological hyper response to ovarian gonadotropin stimulation and excessive ovarian sensitivity are the causes of OHSS. In ovulation-stimulated cycles, HCG triggers ovulation stimulation and, given its long half-life and luteotropic activity, initiates OHSS. When pregnancy is achieved, endogenous HCG synthesis augments and replaces the triggered dose resulting in OHSS.

6.1 Potential Biochemical Mediators

The key components involved in the pathophysiology of OHSS are potential mediators produced by the ovary causing illness: cytokines histamine, serotonin, RAS, and estrogen.

The ovary secretes renin-angiotensin as a homeostatic response to hypovolemia, and HCG influences it as a potential risk factor for OHSS. The renin-angiotensin system, or RAS, is crucial to ovarian physiology because it regulates steroid synthesis, follicle development and maturation, ovulation, and follicular atresia. Along with mediators of ovarian origin, the systemic and ovarian renin-angiotensin systems contribute to ovarian hyperstimulation syndrome.

Estrogen is a marker of the ovary, but it is not the hormone that causes ovarian hyperstimulation syndrome.

Allergic cytokine and histamine response may be related to the pathophysiological alterations associated with OHSS, reflecting an overactive inflammatory response, raising the possibility of hyperactive ovarian mast cells in OHSS. Increased levels of VEGF in the plasma, serum, and follicular fluid are associated with the OHSS cascade, which VEGF mediates (Fig. 1).

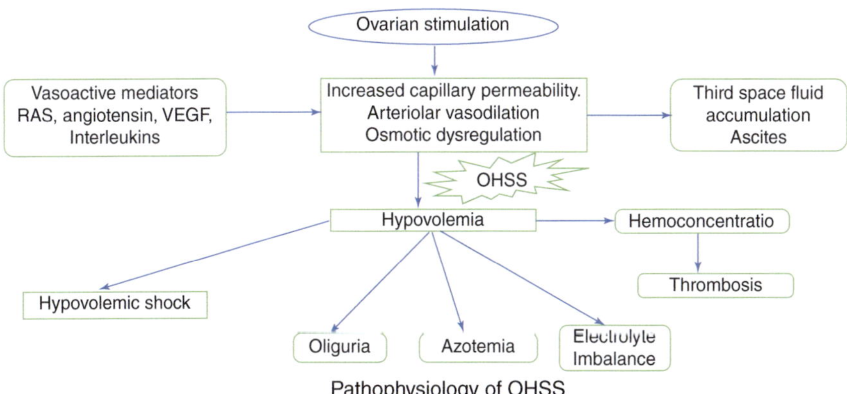

Fig. 1 The pathophysiology of OHSS

7 Immunological Aspects

In controlled stimulation, IL-10 levels are within normal range, limiting the ovarian-related inflammatory response.

Immunological dysregulation during follicular phases (folliculogenesis, ovulation/luteinization) intensifies ovarian-related inflammatory response in inherently low production of IL 10 and changes in the ovary contributing to OHSS-related events, thereby increasing the risk of OHSS.

Women with inherent genetic immune system disorder may exhibit increased inflammatory response exemplified by hypersensitivity/allergy and decreased/altered anti-inflammatory response.

8 Genetic Aspects of OHSS

Various gene mutations have been identified in cases of recurrent and spontaneous OHSS.

Smits et al. discovered a heterozygous FSH receptor gene mutation in a patient exhibiting spontaneous [9] OHSS. Four mutations in recurrent OHSS were identified in Exon, ten of the follicles stimulating hormone FSH receptor [10].

The development of spontaneous OHSS is attributed to the aberrant functioning and abnormal sensitivity to trophoblastic HCG to mutant FSH receptors causing recruitment and follicular growth. HCG further stimulates these processes by inducing follicular luteinization and releasing vasoactive molecules, which account for the onset of this syndrome.

A nonphysiological interaction between ovarian FSH receptors and pregnancy-derived HCG or supraphysiological abnormally high HCG levels, such as in multiple or molar pregnancies, and normal FSH receptors led to the development of spontaneous OHSS [11].

Genes specific to vasoactive molecules could also be candidates susceptible to the development of iatrogenic OHSS.

9 Primary Risk Factors

The primary risk factor for OHSS is the use of high doses of gonadotropin hormones to stimulate the ovaries leading to the development of OHS consecutively; other risk factors that can increase the likelihood of developing OHSS and come to the surface once controlled ovarian stimulation has started (high estradiol levels and previous episodes of OHSS).

9.1 Before Treatment

- Young age is the main risk factor, and those under the age of 30 are at a higher risk of getting OHSS than older patients who have a lower risk due to poor response to controlled ovarian hyperstimulation (COH).
- Women with low BMI body mass index are at increased risk of developing OHSS due to increased sensitivity of ovaries to fertility medications.
- Polycystic ovarian syndrome (PCOS) is a risk factor for ovarian hyperstimulation syndrome. With a narrow therapeutic range of more than ten follicles and hormonal imbalance of luteinizing hormone/follicle-stimulating hormone (LH/FSH) ratio of more than two in PCOS, they are at elevated risk of OHSS. The pathophysiology of OHSS is greatly influenced by higher levels of circulating follicle-stimulating hormone. Lower circulating FSH levels after coasting were linked to improved outcomes.
- Incomplete forms of PCOS:
  - High number of resting follicles >10 follicles of 4–10 mm in each ovary.
  - Luteinizing hormone/follicle-stimulating (LF/FSH) ratio >2.
  - Hyperandrogenism.
- Allergies—Individuals with an allergic propensity are at high risk of OHSS.
- Previous history of OHSS.

9.2 At Risk During Stimulation of OHSS

- Serum estradiol levels >3000/4000 pg/ml—In clinical practice, a rising serum E2 level and the number of oocytes or follicles retrieved are used to track and start preventative measures. In patients at risk of OHSS, serum estradiol assay is a crucial indicator for determining and implementing preventive strategies such as coasting. Serum estradiol levels of more than 6000 pg/ml were associated with a higher incidence of severe OHSS, nearly 80%.
- Follicle number >20–25 in both ovaries—Follicular size is also a factor that can contribute to the development of OHSS (ovarian hyperstimulation syndrome) during ovarian stimulation for IVF or other ART. The risk is higher with a follicle size of 15 mm or larger.
- Ovarian volume as a risk factor for OHSS ultrasound was used to measure the initial ovarian volume in women receiving reproductive treatment who later developed OHSS. By Danninger and colleagues, less than 10% of patients experienced OHSS with ovarian volumes under 10 ml, whereas 23.5% did so with volumes more than 10 ml.

- Higher follicle counts and oocyte collections are frequently related to an increased risk of OHSS. Recovery of more than 30 oocytes has a sensitivity of 83%, a specificity of 67%, and a positive predictive value of 23%.
- Women with high anti-Mullerian hormone (AMH) levels are at higher risk of developing OHSS.

9.3 Other Risk Factors

Other risk factors associated with are as follows:

- Higher inhibin levels produced during ovarian stimulation activate endothelium and increase capillary permeability. The C-reactive protein marker shows a systemic inflammatory response, which rises as a risk factor for OHSS.
- Vascular endothelial growth factor (VEGF) production is exaggerated during the early luteal phase of controlled ovarian hyperstimulation. It is greater than the ability of VEGF-binding proteins and receptors to neutralize it. Vascular endothelial growth factor (VEGF) >200 pg/ml is significant.

10 Forms, Classification, and Grading Schemes

Many classification systems have been proposed based on the time of onset, the severity of a patient's symptoms, signs, laboratory results, and radiological signals over the past 25 years. The classification of OHSS is intended to assist clinicians in deciding whether the patient should be managed supportively or intensively, medically, or surgically, at home or in the hospital.

10.1 Early (<10 Days After Ovulation Triggering Injection of HCG) [12]

Three to 7 days after hCG administration.
Related to intensity of ovarian response.
Severe forms.

10.2 Late Forms (>10 Days After Ovulation Triggering Injection of HCG)

Twelve to 17 days after the hCG administration.
Related to fetal hCG secretion.
A mild but prolonged form.

11 Clinical Classification

11.1 Mild OHSS

Abdominal discomfort and distension (Grade 1).
Grade 1 plus nausea, vomiting, diarrhea, and 5–12 cm of ovaries.

11.2 Moderate OHSS

Grade 2 and ultrasonic evidence of ascites (grade 3).

11.3 Severe OHSS

Moderate OHSS plus clinical evidence of ascites and/or hydrothorax or dyspnea (grade 4) and all of the above plus hemoconcentration, coagulation abnormalities, diminished renal perfusion (grade 5).

The most popular classification system is that of Golan, and two more refinements were later introduced: "Critical OHSS" and "Group C Severe OHSS," which describe life-threatening clinical entities (severe reduction in circulating volume, severe hemoconcentration, multiple organ failure (kidney, liver, and heart), and thromboembolic symptoms). In the current classification of Golan, both are classified as grade 6.

The severity of OHSS manifestations varies, necessitating classification to analyze and assess the disease severity, plan appropriate clinical care, manage the condition, and study epidemiology. This classification enables researchers to create universal standards and preventive measures.

Golan et al. in 1989 [13] the classification system OHSS and eliminating hormones, including introducing ultrasound evidence. Golan defined the grading scheme:

Grade 1: abdominal discomfort and distension—Mild
Grade 2: nausea, vomiting, and enlarged ovaries to 5–12 cm—Mild
Grade 3: ultrasound evidence of ascites—Moderate OHSS
Grade 4: respirators symptoms (dyspnea and tachypnea) with clinical evidence of hydrothorax/ascites—severe
Grade 5: hemoconcentration, oliguria, increased blood viscosity, coagulation abnormalities, hypotension, and hypoperfusion—severe
Grade 6: life-threatening clinical entities and thromboembolic symptoms—Critical OHSS and Group C Severe OHSS (Table 1)

Table 1 Classification of OHSS by Golan et al. [13]

Grade	Mild	Moderate	Severe
1	Abdominal distension and discomfort		
2	Criteria of grade 1 + nausea, vomiting, and/or diarrhea. Ovaries enlarged 5–12 cm		
3		Criteria of mild OHSS + echographic signs of ascites	
4			Criteria of moderate OHSS + clinical signs of ascites and/or hydrothorax and respiratory distress
5			All the above + changes in blood volume and viscosity, hemoconcentration, coagulation disorder and decreased renal output and function
6			Life threatening form

12 Clinical Manifestations of OHSS

OHSS has a wide clinical presentation with varied severity from a mild form with an increase in the size of ovaries which is usually self-limiting but requires careful observation, to advanced moderate and severe disease forms attributing to cystic ovaries resulting in life-threatening complications requiring hospitalization, intensive care monitoring, and expert multidisciplinary management.

12.1 Mild OHSS

Mild OHSS commonly occurs after ovulation or after oocyte retrieval manifesting as lower abdominal pain, diarrhea, nausea, vomiting, and diarrhea. Mild ovarian hyperstimulation symptoms are predicted consequences of administering HCG after exogenous gonadotropin stimulation; they are typically self-limited and respond to support interventions.

The development of ascites together with hemoconcentration, renal hypoperfusion, oliguria, and the propensity for thromboembolic events clinically signaled by a triad of worsening symptoms, hemoconcentration, and decreased serum albumin concentration marking the progression of OHSS to moderate or severe OHSS.

12.2 Severe OHSS

Severe OHSS presents with progressive pain, rapid weight gain, and tense ascites accompanied by hemodynamic instability (orthostatic hypotension), respiratory difficulty (tachycardia), oliguria, hypercoagulability with thromboembolic sequelae, and hepatic impairment. Hyperoestrogenemia has a role in the pathogenesis of intractable nausea and vomiting, deserving timely diagnosis.

Increased abdominal pressure is treated as secondary abdominal compartment syndrome (ACS). ACS is defined as persistently elevated intraabdominal hypertension that leads to compromised end-organ function.

Increased vascular permeability with marked arterial dilatation is subsequent to circulatory dysfunction presenting as ascites as a first sign of OHSS. Large cystic ovaries may compress the ureter and result in hydro ureter resulting in critical end-organ failure.

Extravasation of protein-rich exudate from the vascular compartment to extra-vascular peritoneal, pleural, and pericardial third-space result is associated with volume depletion, hemoconcentration, hypovolemia, and anasarca.

12.3 Critical OHSS

12.3.1 Circulatory Effects

Circulatory effects include contraction of vascular volume, hypotension, tachycardia, low central venous pressure, high cardiac output, low peripheral resistance, and increased vascular stasis constituting thromboembolic phenomenon and coagulation impairment.

12.3.2 Thrombosis

The loss of serum causes hemoconcentration, which increases blood viscosity and the concentration of circulating coagulation components, which is a key element in increasing the risk of thrombosis. Generalized increases in the risk of thrombosis in women undergoing ovarian stimulation are potentially dehydrated and laid up in bed with general malaise.

Intrinsic changes in the blood clotting mechanism are evident in the presence of thrombocytosis, elevated coagulation factors, and endogenous antifibrinolytics. Symptoms of OHSS are exaggerated by an increase in von Willebrand factor resulting in thrombosis in atypical parts of the body or in the lung or brain embolism [14].

12.3.3 Respiratory

Dyspnea due to pulmonary compromise may affect lung function and critical respiratory issues because of the combination of lung restriction due to abdominal pressure from enlarged ovaries and tense ascites, hydrothorax and pericardial effusions, thromboembolic occurrence leading to pulmonary embolus and intraperitoneal increase in capillary permeability leading to ARDS. The potentiality of pleural effusion is almost universal in critical OHSS and is usually not always bilateral.

12.3.4 Renal

Impaired renal perfusion secondary to hypoperfusion or hypovolemia, reduced glomerular filtration induces sodium and water reabsorption, manifesting as oliguria, hyponatremia, and hyperkalemia.

Patients with critical often demonstrate initial hypernatremia due to intravascular dehydration. Still, dilutional hyponatremia frequently develops as the syndrome begins to resolve and massive volumes of extravascular fluids are returned to the circulation.

12.3.5 Hepatic

Liver function tests, such as transaminase and alkaline phosphatase, are frequently elevated with hypoalbuminemia and hypogammaglobulinemia, and gross edema persisting for up to 2 months in moderate OHSS.

13 Clinical Manifestation of OHSS in Patients Not Receiving Ovulation-Inducing Drugs

- Intrauterine life hyperstimulation

  Berezowski et al. reported intrauterine hyperstimulation in a female fetus with big cystic ovaries and considerably elevated maternal serum beta HCG levels at 35 weeks of pregnancy. Following delivery, both the maternal serum beta HCG level and the fetal ovarian volume naturally decrease. Lack of knowledge about this condition leads to unplanned pregnancies ending, neonatal surgery, and female castration.
- Preterm ovarian hyperstimulation

  Preterm neonates physiologically secrete large amounts of estradiol stimulating ovaries to produce large ovarian cysts causing temporary stimulation of external and internal genitalia with spontaneous regressing a few weeks after delivery without surgical intervention.
- Gonadotrophic adenoma ovarian hyperstimulation [15]

  Gonadotroph adenoma has been associated with spontaneous ovarian hyperstimulation [4, 5]. Patients exhibit symptoms that mimic ovarian hyperstimulation, including ovarian enlargement, high estradiol levels, elevated FSH, mildly elevated LH, headache, and galactorrhea. Pituitary magnetic resonance imaging

(MRI), which reveals a pituitary adenoma, and computer tomography are used to confirm the diagnosis.

- Ovarian hyperstimulation in spontaneous pregnancy

  Between 8 and 14 weeks of pregnancy is when spontaneous OHSS manifest. The initially developed corpus luteum does not cause OHSS. It is the formation of the secondary corpus luteum, a critical mass of luteinized granulosa cells, or a mutation of the follicle-stimulating hormone receptor to chronic gonadotropin. Vasoactive mediators are released due to massive luteinization of enlarged stimulated ovaries, which causes OHSS [16].

  Multiple gestations, polycystic ovaries, hyperemesis gravidarum, polycystic ovarian syndrome, familial, transient gestational thyrotoxicosis, and hydatidiform mole have been associated with excessive, abnormally high endogenous chronic gonadotropin 11 and 16 production during pregnancy (hyperreactio luteinalis).

Frequently, ovarian cancer is misdiagnosed, which might lead to laparotomy, castration, renal insufficiency, and other life-threatening consequences.

14 OHSS in Patients Related to Intake of Ovulation-Inducing Drugs (Iatrogenic OHSS)

Follicular enlargement and recruitment occur in cases of iatrogenic OHSS when the ovary is stimulated by exogenous FSH or clomiphene citrate, followed by administration of gonadotropin-releasing hormone (GnRH) [17].

14.1 OHSS In Vitro Fertilization Programs

In vitro fertilization, centers execute many IVF cycles with the common use of GnRH agonist (GnRH) for pituitary desensitization with exogenous gonadotropin injection resulting in OHSS.

Concerns for OHSS are raised by an increase in the number of women getting ovulation induction or enhancement (OI/OE) with gonadotropins and its use over 3 consecutive months. When the diagnosis is delayed, possible oophorectomy might be warranted.

14.2 Patients at Risk of Iatrogenic OHSS

According to the European Society of Human Reproduction and Embryology (ESHRE), polycystic ovarian syndrome (PCOS), more than ten resting follicles in each ovary, young age, low BMI, hypergonadism, and prior history of OHSS are early indicators of patients at risk before ovarian stimulation.

Higher gonadotropin dose, rapidly rising blood estradiol levels, more than 25 small or intermediate-sized follicles, and using exogenous HCG for ovulation

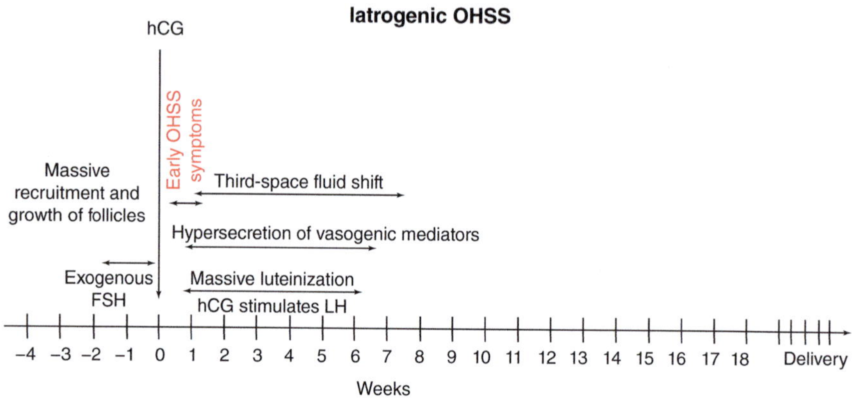

Fig. 2 Onset of early and late OHSS [17]

induction and luteal phase support, multiple pregnancies are all risk factors for OHSS in patients during stimulation or after oocyte pick up.

The manifestation of OHSS requires luteinization. Low doses of gonadotropins should be given to at-risk women to reduce granulosa/luteal cell mash. Pregnancy increases the duration and severity of OHSS [18].

With two distinct risk factors, early and late OHSS can occur. The early form appears 3–7 days after hCG administration, reflecting the degree of ovarian stimulation and severity. The increase in hCG surge related to pregnancy or numerous gestational sacs results in late-onset OHSS, manifesting as mild, protracted symptoms 12–17 days after hCG administration (Fig. 2).

14.3 Clinical Manifestations of Iatrogenic OHSS

It exhibits a wide range of clinical symptoms varying from mild illnesses that require close observation, mostly self-limiting, to moderate and severe life-threatening diseases requiring hospitalization, intensive care monitoring, and expert management. Three categories and six degrees of OHSS severity are used to classify OHSS [17].

14.4 Clinical Manifestations of Mild Iatrogenic OHSS

The onset of symptoms occurs after ovulation or oocyte retrieval with transient lower abdominal discomfort, nausea, vomiting, diarrhea, and abdominal distension.

After ovulation or egg extraction in ART cycles, symptoms such as temporary lower stomach pain, nausea, vomiting, diarrhea, and abdominal distension begin to manifest. Progression of illness is recognized when symptoms persist or worsen.

14.5 Clinical Manifestations of Severe Iatrogenic OHSS

Combined with ovarian enlargement, abdominal distension, persistent nausea and vomiting, respiratory distress, and progressive oliguria, severe pain with these accompanying symptoms and signs of hemodynamic instability can be diagnosed as severe OHSS in a patient receiving ovulation induction agents.

14.6 OHSS in Singleton and Twin Pregnancies

Lyons et al. first hypothesized the risk of developing severe OHSS and increased occurrence related to multiple pregnancies.

It is widely recognized that hCG injection contributes to the onset of ovarian hyperstimulation syndrome. Early onset OHSS is triggered by hCG treatment for ovulation induction, whereas late-onset OHSS form is by developing pregnancy.

Several steps can be taken to lower the incidence of OHSS, such as oocyte retrieval following HCG treatment, but cancel embryo transfers and cryopreservation (freeze) of all embryos.

14.7 Spontaneous to Iatrogenic OHSS

OHSS can appear in two different ways: spontaneously or as a familial condition associated with pregnancy. Although these two manifests at different times, they share the same pathophysiological sequences of massive recruitment and growth of ovarian follicles, extensive luteinization provoked by HCG, and over-secretion of vasogenic molecules by luteinized corpora. FSH receptor mutations are implicated in the development of spontaneous OHSS. The risk factor in developing iatrogenic OHSS is mutation or polymorphism in the FSH gene receptor (Fig. 3).

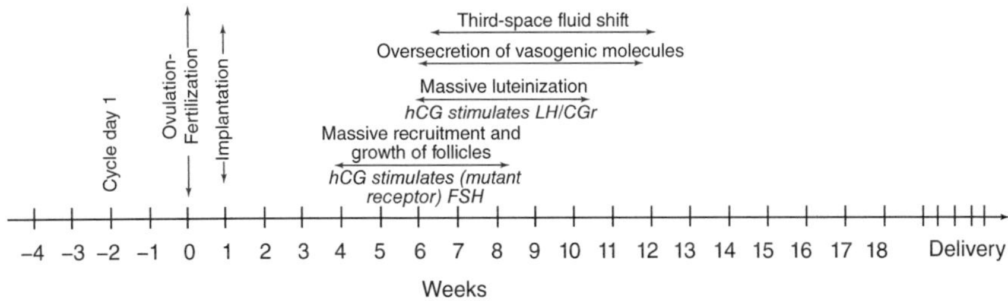

Fig. 3 Spontaneous OHSS [7]

14.8 Clinical Manifestation of Complications of OHSS

Certain complications may manifest as the initial symptom of OHSS and be challenging to identify because the symptoms may be concealed.

The complications of OHSS include:

14.8.1 Ovarian Torsion

Risk is about 1 per 5000 stimulations with greater susceptibility in early pregnancy after hyperstimulation and OHSS. It manifests as sudden extreme abdominal pain due to an increase in ovarian size and softening of a ligament.

When the regression to normal ovarian size is not accomplished, the risk of torsion continues beyond the treatment cycle and may be triggered by exercise or intense activities. Ovarian necrosis may result because of delayed diagnosis [19].

14.8.2 Ovarian Hemorrhage

It presents with severe abdominal pain, distension, hypotension, severe pallor, and ascites. In OHSS, ovarian hemorrhage occurs due to ovarian rupture or intraovarian hemorrhage and may get precipitated by abdominal trauma or bimanual examination. Ovaries become large tense, and edematous, with multiple cysts filled with blood.

Symptoms associated with severe OHSS can mask ovarian rupture. Ultrasonography and repeat hemoglobin level assessment will help in diagnosis.

14.8.3 Thromboembolism

OHSS is a potentially life-threatening risk factor attributed to transient changes in coagulation factors, hemoconcentration, and increases the risk of thrombosis because of increased blood viscosity, immobility due to pain, and venous compression of occluded vessels by enlarged ovaries and ascites [20]. Identification of associated thrombophilia disorders, obesity significantly increases mortality.

In severe OHSS, evidence suggests that tissue factor in the coagulation pathway is elevated while tissue factor pathway inhibitor is lowered. Hemoconcentration allows prolonged exposure of circulating factors to the endothelial surface, increasing the effect of local damage. Circulatory factors affect the endothelial surface making it more stimulating thrombus formation.

Thrombosis is the formation of clots within the vessel and emboli resulting from the movement of clots in smaller vessels resulting in the occlusion of smaller vessels carrying a crucial risk of pulmonary embolism and episodes of tissue hypoperfusion. Ventilation scan with or without perfusion confirms the diagnosis of PE.

Doppler ultrasound imaging and magnetic resonance angiography are used for diagnosis and the start of treatment before the onset of lethal complications.

Improved outcome with anticoagulation therapy remains the mainstay of treatment in high-risk strategy patients. A multidisciplinary expert team approach to early diagnosis and rapid intervention remains cornerstones for enhancing patient safety and reducing mortality.

15 Additional Risk Factors

A greater risk of thromboembolism exists in women having assisted conception if they have concurrent thromboembolic disorders, obesity, pregnancy, or a history of thromboembolic disease.

Women with recognized risk factors ought to be given appropriate thromboprophylaxis consideration at the start of treatment and continued throughout pregnancy.

Early mobilization or graduated compression stockings and thromboprophylaxis may be used in the prevention of thrombosis after risk assessment using a scoring system [21].

15.1 Hepatic Complications

In mild to severe OHSS, liver impairment has been documented. Impaired liver functions persist for longer periods and revert to normal with a resolution of the syndrome.

An early diagnosis of this condition and an urgent exploratory laparotomy will help to save these patients' lives.

Gastrointestinal symptoms such as intractable nausea and vomiting may be the initial presentation; failing to suspect such a condition result in the later presentation of these patients with cerebrovascular accidents.

15.2 Renal Complications

Impaired renal functions in severely hypovolemic cases and prerenal failure will be heralded by oliguria, raised blood urea, and creatinine, followed by anuria, hyperkalemia, and uremia. Temporary failure of the transplanted pelvic kidney has been reported due to pressure from enlarged ovaries.

The signs of acute renal failure, such as hyperkalemia and metabolic acidosis, can appear in critical OHSS, occasionally necessitating sometimes dialysis.

Reduced renal perfusion following hypovolemia stimulates renal tubules to increase water reabsorption in proximal tubules producing oliguria and renal impairment.

15.3 Respiratory Complications

Chest tightness, a dry cough, and dyspnea are common symptoms of pulmonary impairment from hydrothorax or pulmonary edema ARDS. Blood gases, lung function, a chest X-ray, or chest ultrasound are used to confirm the diagnosis.

An increased amount of pleural fluid can cause respiratory compromise, characterized by a decreased tidal volume and hypoxia.

Avoiding hydration is the most effective strategy for preventing pulmonary edema; however, when it occurs, careful diuresis in an intensive care setting is mandatory.

15.4 Cardiac Complications

The diagnosis of pericardial effusion and cardiac tamponade by echocardiography, a rare but potentially lethal condition, necessitates pericardiocentesis.

The most serious possibility is cardiac tamponade, characterized by decreased cardiac output; however, emergency pericardiocentesis is reserved for those identified.

15.5 Sepsis

Patients identified with critical OHSS were found to have plasma immunoglobulin levels deficiency, especially IgG and IgA, which suggests that transcapillary exudation into the third space is the etiology of low plasma protein levels. Presumably related to immunodeficiency, the incidence of infection in such patients is high [22].

C-reactive protein (CRP) is a biological marker of systemic inflammation produced by the liver and reflects the systemic inflammatory response. This substantiates the role of systemic inflammation in the pathophysiology of ovarian hyperstimulation syndrome (OHSS) and is a risk factor for OHSS in ovarian stimulation [23].

16 Clinical Symptoms

Lower abdominal discomfort, nausea, vomiting, diarrhea, respiratory distress, oliguria, anuria, and rapid weight gain.

Paraclinical signs: Enlarged ovaries, ascites, pleural effusion (right > left), thromboembolism, pericardial effusion.

16.1 Biological Findings

Electrolyte imbalance, hypovolemia, hemoconcentration, leukocytosis, low creatinine clearance, elevated liver enzymes, hypercoagulability, hypoalbuminemia.

16.2 Laboratory Findings

Elevated liver enzymes, elevated hematocrit >45%, leukocytosis (white blood cell count >15,000), electrolyte imbalance (hyponatremia 135 hyperkalemia >5.0 mEq/l), renal impairment (serum creatinine >1.2 mg/dl and creatinine clearance 50 ml/min), and low serum albumin 30 g/l are common in women with severe OHSS.

17 Management

17.1 Outpatient Management

The goal of the outpatient regimen is to minimize the progression of illness and consequences through careful monitoring and efficient management. The outpatient strategy focuses on the luteal phase management of OHSS, the severity of illness, and available facilities.

A predictable pattern of symptoms progression over the luteal phase allows for close monitoring and early intervention. At the time of oocyte retrieval and super ovulatory cycles, high-risk women are identified using a variety of clinical risk indicators and are given verbal and written advice. When super ovulatory cycles with five or more preovulatory follicles are canceled or converted to IVF, the development of OHSS is rare.

Vigilant monitoring and early outpatient intervention can serve as a safe and effective method of managing symptoms, attenuating the course of the illness, and minimizing complications for both the women and their pregnancies.

A patient handout describing the progression from mild to severe OHSS, instructions for monitoring and symptoms relief at each stage, and description of worsening signs and symptoms that necessitate contact with the clinic. Follow up with a blood test and an ultrasound examination every 48 h and consult instructions at any sign of complication with careful monitoring of the fluid chart and the abdominal circumference.

17.2 Inpatient Management

Criteria for hospitalization: Any sign of severe OHSS, Hemoconcentration >45%.

Follow-up: Fluid chart, vitals monitoring, ultrasound for ascites volume and ovarian size, complete blood picture for leukocytosis, electrolytes, coagulation profile, renal and liver functions (albumin and total proteins).

17.3 Medical Management

17.3.1 Fluid Administration

To maintain diuresis, intravascular colloid pressure, and electrolyte balance, the major principal treatment strategy is to continue intravascular hydration with intravenous ringer lactate or sodium chloride 0.9% (saline) of 1500–3000 ml in the first 24 h and subsequently determined according to urine output.

17.3.2 Plasma Expanders

HES hydroxyethyl starch 6% solution in isotonic sodium chloride is administered gradually. A maximum daily dose of 33 ml/kg, or 250–500 ml, is recommended to prevent lung congestion.

17.3.3 Albumin Administration

Albumin administration is reserved for confirmed hypoalbuminemia because of cost, severe albumin overload, impaired renal function, overall viral contamination, and viral hepatitis.

The daily dose of between 25 and 75 g (100–300 ml) per day, according to the total volume of ascitic fluid drained and severity of hypoalbuminemia.

17.3.4 Anticoagulants

Heparin or low molecular weight heparin is used as an anticoagulant in patients with clinical evidence of the thromboembolic phenomenon, hypercoagulability, history of thromboembolic events, uncorrected hemoconcentration 48 h after IV fluid administration, congenital or acquired thrombophilia diseases, or both.

Low-dose aspirin is one method for preventing thromboembolic problems in obese or long-term immobilized patients (Fig. 4).

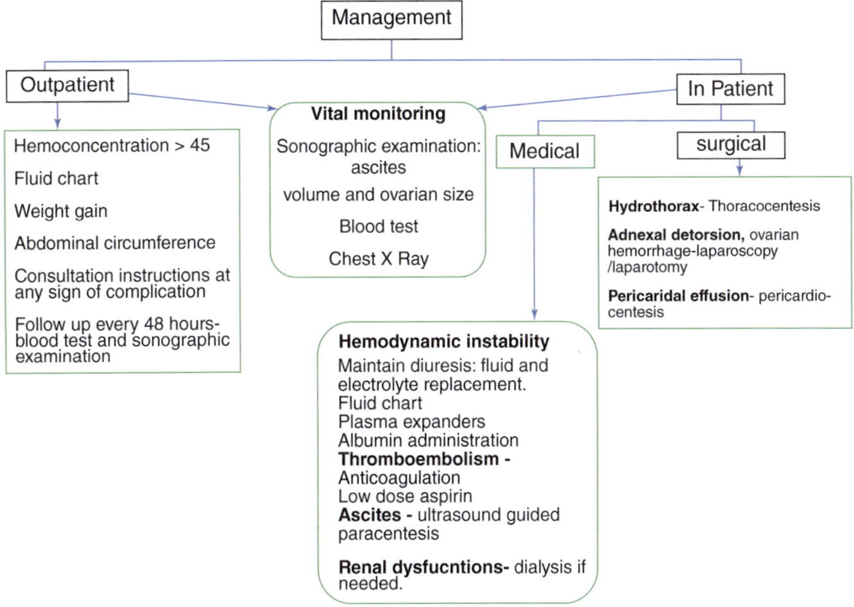

Fig. 4 Management strategies

17.4 Surgical Management

Paracentesis is a modality of treatment for life-threatening OHSS that does not respond to conventional therapy. The desire for symptomatic relief, dyspnea, tense ascites, oliguria, increasing creatinine, and hemoconcentration refractory to medical treatment are indications for paracentesis. In patients with stable hemodynamics, it can be done transvaginal or transabdominal under ultrasound guidance.

Thoracocentesis might be considered if pulmonary symptoms worsen after conservative treatment options or present with pleural effusion and respiratory compromise. Mechanical ventilation may be indicated if ARDS develops [24].

A conservative management strategy can be used to treat ovarian hemorrhage or cyst rupture in OHSS; however, emergency surgical detorsion is required to treat ovarian torsion [25].

Rarely in cases of critical stage OHSS complicated by renal failure, ARDS, thromboembolism, and multi-organ failure, life-saving termination of pregnancy may be carried out as a last option.

18 Prevention

Several attempts are made to prevent OHSS, an iatrogenic condition that can be fatal in young, healthy women desiring fertility and demanding active management to prevent complications.

The primary goal of infertility management should be to reduce the risk of ovarian hyperstimulation syndrome (OHSS) by identifying high-risk situations and adhering to established safety protocols when selecting a treatment and carrying out ovarian stimulation.

Prior to treatment, it is important to identify known risk factors to focus on high-risk patient groups and develop appropriate preventative measures, including the necessity of ovarian stimulation, duration of infertility, and treatment timelines.

Development of procedures with minimal risk that can be managed by timelines for the treatment.

Consideration for alternative infertility treatments—tubal ligation, ovarian drilling by electrocautery, laser vaporization, insulin resistance reducing drugs, natural cycle in vitro fertilization.

A preventive strategy during treatment in women with identified risk factors for OHSS requires the pertinent choice of drug combination for ovarian stimulation and the adjustment of individualized low-dose step-up regimens by careful monitoring.

Primary prevention is the identification of causing and predisposing factors, the disease's etiology, and monitoring of ovarian response to gonadotropins. The gold standard for ovulation monitoring is the combination of an ultrasound and a serum estradiol E2 assay. Secondly, avoid or control such factors as a preventive strategy.

Secondary prevention requires early identification methods and intervention to minimize the probability of OHSS in high-risk patients. Late-onset OHSS is related to HCG levels and probably the number of ovarian cells capable of producing unidentified ovarian mediators under the influence of HCG (Fig. 5).

It is intervened on two different levels. The first was accomplished by reducing the HCG dose used to induce ovulation, cryopreservation, and supplementing

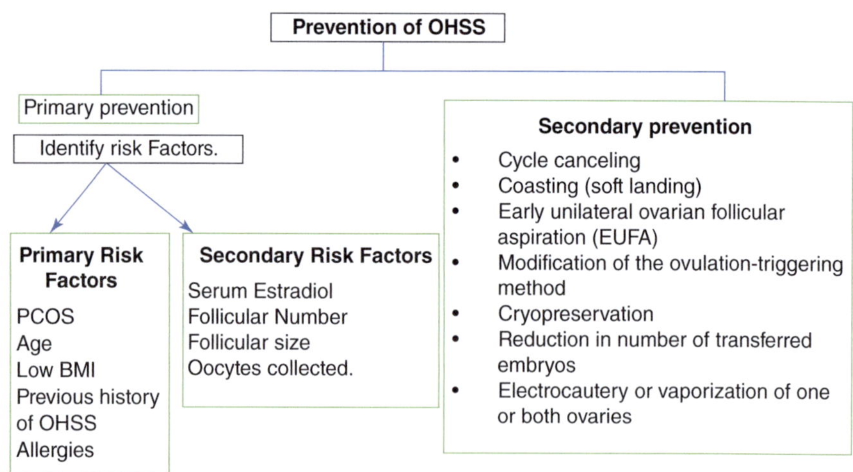

Fig. 5 Preventive strategies

during the luteal phase. Inducing luteolysis, EUFA, coasting, and electrocautery comprise the second level. The effectiveness of the combined use of both approaches in subsequent follow-ups produces the best results.

In non-IVF patients, low-dose stimulation protocol results in mono-follicular ovulation and completely prevents OHSS regardless of the HCG dose. When multi-folliculogensis is required for ART, the risk of OHSS is a concern [4].

Apart from canceling, none of the approaches are efficient, but the below-mentioned methods decrease the incidence in patients at high risk of OHSS.

18.1 Canceling the Cycle

The only way to eliminate the risk of OHSS is to withhold HCG when estrogen levels are too high and cancel the cycle at risk. All other methods decrease the risk or severity of OHSS.

18.2 Coasting

Coasting is described as a popular and effective method of reducing OHSS, but it does not eliminate it. First described in hyperstimulated cycles [26] and applied first in IVF cycles by Sher et al. in 1993 [27, 28].

The term "coasting" is described as withholding or significantly reducing the dose of gonadotropins in patients at risk for developing severe OHSS.

This method assumes that E2 levels reached during HCG administration predict the risk for OHSS. Coasting acts probably by apoptosis of granulosa cells and a reduction in their functional capacity to produce vasoactive factors such as vascular endothelial growth factors VEGF [29].

Three advantages of coasting are it rescues the cycle and does not abandon the cycle, enables the transfer of fresh embryos, and finally, no supplementary procedure or gonadotropin medical therapy is involved; however, it is associated with a reduced oocyte collection rate and especially when the coasting period is prolonged [30, 31].

The proposed consensus for coasting is considered when >20 follicles are developing, serum estradiol levels exceed 3500 pg/ml, and the diameter of the largest follicle reaches 18 mm.

The administration of HCG should be delayed until the estradiol level drops below 3000 pg/ml. Still, the coasting duration should be limited to <4 days because the number of oocytes and pregnancy rate drops considerably after a long interval. HCG administration is postponed until the patient's serum E2 levels decrease to a safer zone.

18.3 Early Unilateral Ovarian Follicular Aspiration

Due to the invasiveness of the procedure, it is used less frequently. Aspiration of granulosa cells from one ovary could cause intraovarian hemorrhage, reducing the risk of developing severe OHSS by limiting the synthesis of ovarian OHSS mediators.

18.4 Modifying the Methods of Ovulation Triggering

HCG is a well-known promoter to initiate a complex cascade that leads to the development of OHSS. Reduction in HCG dose or triggering ovulation with recombinant human (rh) LH or endogenous LH surge is a different approach to reducing the incidence of OHSS. Further clinical studies are needed to establish the value of these approaches.

The unique advantage offered by combining an initial gonadotropin flare-up followed by pituitary downregulation and complete luteolysis can significantly reduce the likelihood of OHSS occurring.

18.5 Administration of Glucocorticoids

Further studies are necessary to determine whether glucocorticoids, used as an anti-inflammatory, are a beneficial treatment for OHSS prophylaxis due to limited evidence supporting their use.

18.6 Cryopreservation of All Embryos

Giving HCG to retrieve oocytes and subsequently cryopreserving all embryos is an alternative to canceling the cycle. On the other hand, the possibility that thawed embryos could be successfully replaced in a later cycle without compromising the chance of pregnancy is one of the many benefits of maintaining many of the advantages of an IVF cycle.

But there is insufficient evidence to support cryopreservation on a routine basis or the elective freezing of all embryos to eliminate the possibility of OHSS. Both of these approaches would involve freezing embryos before they are implanted.

However, the risk of secondary exacerbation of early OHSS is avoided, and late OHSS is avoided in high-risk patients in terms of severity and duration. This is because endogenous HCG induces late OHSS. Early OHSS is not prevented.

18.7 Electrocautery or Laser Vaporization of One or Both Ovaries

The major risk factor in PCOS for OHSS is the unpredictable ovarian response. Destruction of follicles at the ovary's surface using wedge resection or repeated punctures utilizing laparoscopic ovarian electrocauterization is one method of treating PCOS.

Endocrine effects with this treatment include a reduction in serum LH and serum androgens with improvement in ovulation and conception; however, these methods may develop postoperative adhesions and loss of ovarian tissue [32].

Because it is invasive, this approach should only be used in severe cases of OHSS in patients with PCOS and as a last resort.

18.8 Reduction in the Number of Transferred Embryos

Late-onset OHSS may be induced or aggravated by rising HCG produced by early pregnancy. It might be hypothesized that lowering the number of transferred embryos could be an effective preventive approach for high-risk patients because HCG secretion is higher in multiple pregnancies and increases the severity of OHSS.

Identifying individuals likely to experience a hyper response to standard stimulation treatments would allow for modification of their care and avoidance [33, 34].

Recognizing high-risk individuals prior to treatment, choosing treatments that respect safety, managing infertility, and performing ovarian stimulation during therapy are primary preventative principles.

Prevention of the illness is preferable to treatment on an individual basis, but this objective, unfortunately, remains elusive. A successful preventative strategy aims at preventing hospitalizations and reducing OHSS complications [35]. The options of oocyte retrieval, fertilization, and cryopreservation of embryos can be given to patients at risk of OHSS in vitro fertilization cycle.

The conversion of superovulation cycles to in vitro fertilization cycles is the American perspective's preferred method of preventing OHSS. Higher birth rates and other risk factors, such as multiple pregnancies, can be controlled, even though it raises treatment costs.

GnRH agonist was used as an effective alternative to HCG in high-risk ART patients with an imminent threat of OHSS. It offers more physiological ovulation stimulus mimicking LH and FSH surge eliciting gonadotropins' pituitary secretion, which can be utilized for triggering oocyte maturation and ovulation.

19 Conclusion

OHSS is an iatrogenic condition that may be life-threatening when applying controlled ovarian hyperstimulation. The key recommendations are that gonadotropin therapy for ovulation induction should only be used when all other options have been exhausted following prolonged therapy. The subjective discomfort and potentially significant objective changes associated with this illness are profoundly traumatic for the patient and their spouse. Despite the possibility of life-threatening complications, fatal instances are uncommon.

All women develop some degree of ovarian hyperstimulation; however, this should not be confused with the clinical condition known as OHSS (ovarian hyperstimulation syndrome). The same patient can experience spontaneous OHSS multiple times, either due to iatrogenic causes or as a flare-upside effect of gonadotropins. Early recognition of primary risk factors, young age, and low BMI is mandatory.

The most popular clinical classification system of OHSS is that of Golan, classified into three categories: mild, moderate, and severe, based on the severity of symptoms and the degree of ovarian enlargement. Later two refinements were introduced: “Critical OHSS” and “Group C Severe OHSS,” which describe life-threatening clinical entities.

The severity of the illness dictates management. A successful preventative strategy aims at preventing hospitalizations and reducing the severity of illness and OHSS complications individually.

Use friendly stimulation regimens that target the treatment of a single ovarian follicle when gonadotropin stimulation for ovulation is necessary but not preferred and can be replaced with safer alternatives (recLH, endogenous GnRH surge). Clinically severe OHSS is eliminated with GnRH availability, a single mid-cycle dose causes a preovulatory LH/FSH surge leading to oocyte maturation in women undergoing ovarian stimulation for IVF or induction ovulation in vivo.

Milder stimulation regimes should replace the principle of ART, obtaining as many good-quality oocytes as possible. The consideration of friendly IVF providing fewer oocytes and embryos does not reduce the chance of potential embryo implantation, thus maintaining a high pregnancy rate.

Patients in high-risk situations should know their options for canceling, coasting, or freezing future replacements. At the first sign of OHSS, the patient must be informed and hospitalized at the first sign of deterioration. Patients with diagnosed OHSS need expert management and follow-up. Admission to the intensive care unit may be necessary when critical OHSS develops.

Primary prevention depends on two main requirements:

First, the etiology of the disease must be known, while casual and predisposing factors should be identified. Second, avoid or manipulate such factors as part of the preventive strategy.

Secondary prevention requires knowledge of the pathophysiology mechanism of the disease, availability of early detection methods, and means to intervene and correct the pathophysiological changes. The effect of combining methods that act at two different levels (1 and 2) should be assessed [36].

Monitoring during the cycle with a careful adaptation of the daily dose of gonadotropin administered for ovarian stimulation to ovarian response results in non-IVF and IVF procedures, leading to a decreased incidence of OHSS.

References

1. Brinsden PR, Wada I, Tan SL, et al. Diagnosis, prevention and management of ovarian hyperstimulation syndrome. Br J Obstet Gynaecol. 1995;102:767–72.
2. Check JH, Choe JK, Nazari A. Hyperreactio luteinalis despite the absence of a corpus luteum and suppressed serum follicle stimulating concentrations in a triplet pregnancy. Hum Reprod. 2000;15:1043–5.
3. Navot D, Bergh PA, Laufer N. Ovarian hyperstimulation syndrome in novel reproductive technologies: prevention and treatment. Fertil Steril. 1992;58:249–61.
4. Smits G, Olatunbosun OA, Delbaere A, et al. Spontaneous ovarian hyperstimulation syndrome caused by a mutant follitropin receptor. N Engl J Med. 2003;349:760–6.
5. Homburg R, Howies CM. Low dose FSH therapy for anovulatory infertility associated with polycystic ovary syndrome: rationale, reflections and refinements. Hum Reprod Update. 1999;5:493–9.
6. Whelan JG III, Vlahos NF. The ovarian hyperstimulation syndrome. Fertil Steril. 2000;73:883–96.
7. Navot D, Levine Z, Klein J. Severe ovarian hyperstimulation syndrome. In: Gardner DK, editor. Textbook of assisted reproductive techniques. 2nd ed. London: Taylor & Francis; 2004. p. 805–16.
8. Navot D, Margalioth EJ, Laufer N. Direct correlation between plasma renin activity and severity of the ovarian hyperstimulation syndrome. Fertil Steril. 1987;48:57–61.
9. Montanelli L, Delbaere A, Di Carlo C, et al. A mutation in the follicle-stimulating hormone receptor as a cause of familial spontaneous ovarian hyperstimulation syndrome. J Clin Endocrinol Metab. 2004;89:1255–8.
10. Delbaere A, Smits G, De Leener A, et al. Understanding ovarian hyperstimulation syndrome. Endocrine. 2005;26:285–90.
11. Suzuki S. Comparison between spontaneous ovarian hyperstimulation syndrome and hyperreactio luteinalis. Arch Gynecol Obstet. 2004;269:227–9.
12. Papanikolaou EG, Tournaye H, Verpoest W, et al. Early and late ovarian hyperstimulation syndrome: early pregnancy outcome and profile. Hum Reprod. 2005;20:636–41.
13. Golan A, Ron-El R, Herman A, et al. Ovarian hyperstimulation syndrome: an update review. Obstet Gynecol Surv. 1989;44:430–40.
14. Ogawa S, Minakami H, Araki S, et al. A rise of the serum level of von Willebrand factor occurs before clinical manifestation of the severe form of ovarian hyperstimulation syndrome. J Assist Reprod Genet. 2001;18:114–9.
15. Vochem M. Ovarian hyperstimulation syndrome in preterm infants. Z Geburtsh Neonatol. 2002;4:156–60.
16. Delbaere A, Smits G, Olatunbosun O, et al. New insights into the pathophysiology of ovarian hyperstimulation syndrome. What makes the difference between spontaneous and iatrogenic syndrome? Hum Reprod. 2004;3:486–9.
17. The Practice Committee of the American Society for Reproductive Medicine. Ovarian hyperstimulation syndrome. Fertil Steril. 2003;5:1309–14.
18. Al-Shawaf T, Grudzinskas JG. Prevention and treatment of ovarian hyperstimulation syndrome. Best Pract Res Clin Obstet Gynaecol. 2003;2:249–61.
19. Littman ED, Rydfors JR, Milki AA. Exercise induced ovarian torsion in the cycle following gonadotrophin therapy: case report. Hum Reprod. 2003;8:1641–2.

20. Rogolino A, Coccia ME, Fedi S, et al. Hypercoagulability, high tissue factor and low tissue factor pathway inhibitor levels in severe ovarian hyperstimulation syndrome: possible association with clinical outcome. Blood Coagul Fibrinolysis. 2003;3:277–82.
21. Scottish Intercollegiate Guidelines Network (SIGN). Section 2: Risk factors for venous thromboembolism. In: Prophylaxis of venous thromboembolism. Scottish Intercollegiate Guidelines Network; 2002. www.sign.ac.uk/guidelines/fulltext/62.
22. Tukamizawa S, Shibahara H, Taneichi A, et al. Dynamic changes of the immunoglobulins in patients with severe ovarian hyperstimulation syndrome: efficacy of a novel treatment using peritoneo-venous shunt. Am J Reprod Immunol. 2002;47:25–30.
23. Orvieto R, Chen R, Ashkenazi J, et al. C-reactive protein levels in patients undergoing controlled ovarian hyperstimulation for IVF cycle. Hum Reprod. 2004;19:357–9. Clinical diagnosis.
24. Brower RG, Matthay MA, Morris A, et al. The acute respiratory distress syndrome network: ventilation with lower tidal volumes as compared with traditional tidal volumes for acute lung injury and the acute respiratory distress syndrome. N Engl J Med. 2000;342:1301–8.
25. Chew S, Ng SC. Laparoscopic treatment of a twisted hyperstimulated ovary after IVF. Singapore Med J. 2001;42:228–9.
26. Rabinovici J, Kushnir O, Shalev J, et al. Rescue of menotrophin cycles prone to develop ovarian hyperstimulation. Br J Obstet Gynaecol 1987;94:1098–102.
27. Urman B, Pride SM, Yuen BH. Management of overstimulated gonadotrophin cycles with a 3 and by Figuerona-Casass in 1958 controlled drift period. Hum Reprod 1992;7:213–17.
28. Sher G, Salem R, Feinman M, et al. Eliminating the risk of life-endangering complications following overstimulation with menotropin fertility agents: a report on women undergoing in vitro fertilization and embryo transfer. Obstet Gynecol 1993;81:1009–11.
29. Tozer AJ, Iies RK, Iammarrone E, et al. Characteristics of populations of granulosa cells from individual follicles in women undergoing 'coasting' during controlled ovarian stimulation (COS) for IVF. Hum Reprod. 2004;19:2561–8.
30. Rizk B. Prevention of OHSS. In: Rizk B, editor. Epidemiology, pathophysiology, prevention and management of ovarian hyperstimulation syndrome. Cambridge: Cambridge University Press; 2005. p. 264–94.
31. Rizk B, Grace J, Mulekhar M. Coasting is effective for abolishing the risk of OHSS but possibly decreases the quality of oocytes and pregnancy rates. Is that the price we pay? Fertil Steril. 2006; in press.
32. Tozer AJ, Al-Shawaf T, Zosmer A, et al. Does laparoscopic ovarian diathermy affect the outcome of IVF-embryo transfer in women with polycystic ovarian syndrome? A retrospective comparative study. Hum Reprod. 2001;16:91–5.
33. Koike T, Minakami H, Araki S, et al. Severity of ovarian hyperstimulation syndrome: its relation to number of conceptuses. Int J Fertil Womens Med. 2004;49:36–42.
34. De Neubourg D, Mangelschots K, Van Royen E, et al. Singleton pregnancies are as affected by ovarian hyperstimulation syndrome as twin pregnancies. Fertil Steril. 2004;82:1691–3.
35. Fluker MR, Copeland JE, Yuzpe AA. An ounce of prevention: out-patient management of the ovarian hyperstimulation syndrome. Fertil Steril. 2000;73:821–4.
36. Isik AZ, Vicdan K. Combined approach as an effective method in the prevention of severe ovarian hyperstimulation syndrome. Eur J Obstet Gynecol Reprod Biol. 2001;97:208–12.

COVID-19 Infection in Obstetrical Patients Requiring Intensive Care: An Update

Sarah Salameh and Muna Al Maslamani

Abstract Women who are pregnant and who have COVID-19 infection have unique challenges from both a medical and non-medical perspective. In a post-pandemic society, there are new considerations for prenatal and postnatal care in addition to infection control measures, physiologic changes in the pregnancy, and fetal needs. Pregnant women were discovered to be at much higher risk for intensive care unit (ICU) admission, invasive ventilation, extracorporeal membrane oxygenation (ECMO), and death than non-pregnant women. Risk persisted even when age, race/ethnicity, and underlying medical conditions were taken into account. Additionally, preterm birth, stillbirth, and postpartum hemorrhage have all been linked to higher obstetrical problems when comorbidity with COVID-19 infection exists. When presenting at an age over 35, with obesity, chronic hypertension, chronic lung disease, gestational diabetes, and pre-eclampsia, obstetric patients are especially susceptible to complications. Therefore, it is recommended that serious COVID-19 obstetric patients be managed by a multidisciplinary team, with the team having a thorough understanding of how to manage the ongoing COIVD-19 and pre-existing disorders. For COVID-19-infected patients who are not pregnant, the target oxygen saturation is 92%. Aiming for a higher objective of 95% is advised by the Society for Maternal-Fetal Medicine (SMFM), and if this is not attained with supplementary oxygen or with growing demand, intensive care admission should be considered. High-flow nasal cannula (HFNC) is a viable therapy when adequate oxygenation cannot be attained by conventional oxygen support and indications for endotracheal intubation are not imminent. The critically ill obstetric patient population can often benefit from mechanical ventilation strategies used in non-pregnant people with some notable exceptions. While permissive hypercapnia may be employed in the situation of acute respiratory distress syndrome (ARDS), it is typically advised not to exceed 60 mmHg. This is in contrast to pregnancy-specific hypocapnia, which is preferred to minimize fetal academia and oxygen dissociation

S. Salameh · M. Al Maslamani (✉)
Center for Disease Control (CDC)/Infectious Disease Department, Hamad Medical Corporation, Doha, Qatar
e-mail: MALMASLAMANI@hamda.qa

N. Shaikh et al. (eds.), *Updates in Intensive Care of OBGY Patients*,
https://doi.org/10.1007/978-981-99-9577-6_12

changes. The Food and Drug Administration (FDA) recently approved intravenous tocilizumab for the management of COVID-19 in hospitalized patients taking systemic corticosteroids and requiring mechanical ventilation, NIV, or supplementary oxygen. The NIH currently advises preventive dosage heparin in hospitalized patients who need mechanical ventilation, comparable to those on HFNC or NIV, for both pregnant and non-pregnant people (unless contraindicated). Gestational age, preterm risk, risk of a serious disease for the mother, and risk of an unsettling fetal state should be balanced against each other while fetus delivery is taken into account.

Keywords COVID-19 · Corticosteroids · ECMO · High-flow nasal cannula · Higher risk · Fetus · Intensive care unit · Pregnancy · Tocilizumab · Ventilation

1 Introduction

COVID-19 infection in pregnant females poses unique challenges from both medical and non-medical perspectives. In addition to the changing landscape of prenatal and postnatal care in a post-pandemic society, there are infection control precautions, maternal physiologic changes and fetal requirements to consider. In general, critical care management in obstetrical patients is similar to that in the non-pregnant adult. However, there are important differences with regard to ventilation, pharmacologic interventions, and issues related to fetal monitoring and delivery.

While the preponderance of pregnant persons infected with SARS-CoV-2 virus appears to be asymptomatic, symptomatic presentation in the pregnant individual represents a risk for progression to severe COVID-19 disease [1, 2]. A large surveillance study conducted by the Centers for Disease Control and Prevention (CDC) included over 400,000 symptomatic persons of reproductive age. In comparison with non-pregnant individuals, pregnant persons were found to be at significantly increased risk for intensive care unit (ICU) admission, invasive ventilation, extracorporeal membrane oxygenation (ECMO) and death. Risk remained after adjustment for age, race/ethnicity, and underlying medical conditions [3]. Moreover, comorbidity with COVID-19 infection has been associated with increased obstetrical complications, particularly preterm birth, stillbirth, and postpartum hemorrhage [1, 4, 5].

2 Recognizing the High-Risk Patient

Factors identified as predisposing to severe COVID-19 disease in non-pregnant individuals may similarly contribute to severity in pregnant or recently pregnant individuals [6–10]. Obstetrical patients are particularly vulnerable to complications when presenting at age above 35 years, with obesity, chronic hypertension, chronic lung disease, gestational diabetes, and pre-eclampsia [6, 11]. In managing critical COVID-19 obstetrical patients, a multidisciplinary team approach is thus recommended, with expertise to address pre-existing and ongoing pathologies.

Upon presentation, features of COVID-19 infection can sometimes overlap with symptoms of normal pregnancy, such as dyspnea, fatigue, nausea, and vomiting. In the absence of fever, recognizing a symptomatic pregnant person at risk may therefore be problematic [1]. Furthermore, in pregnant and parturient patients suspected of hypertensive disease, clinical features and complications may mimic those of severe COVID-19. These include headache, cerebrovascular insult, and seizures. Laboratory derangements in HELLP (hemolysis, elevated liver enzymes, and low platelets) syndrome can be similarly misleading [12–14]. Moreover, when evaluating the degree of COVID-19 severity, certain lab parameters such as C-reactive protein (CRP) and D-dimer may be difficult to interpret as they are frequently altered at baseline in the normal pregnancy [15, 16].

Several classification systems for COVID-19 disease severity are available that may be used for triaging patients. These include the National Institutes of Health (NIH) [17] and WU classifications [18] that are primarily based on data from non-pregnant individuals. In their latest guidelines, the International Society of Infectious Disease in Obstetrics and Gynecology (ISIDOG) suggests a critical care admission for patients fulfilling any one of the following criteria; pregnant patients with severe disease, i.e., respiratory rate ≥30/min, resting oxygen saturation $SaO_2 < 94\%$, arterial blood oxygen partial pressure (PaO_2)/oxygen concentration (FiO_2) ≤ 300 mmHg, pregnant patients with oxygen requirement and comorbidities or pregnant patients with critical disease including shock with organ failure, respiratory failure requiring mechanical ventilation or refractory hypoxemia requiring ECMO [19].

In an internally validated model, Kalafat et al. have recently proposed a clinically useful prediction model for determining risk for ICU admission and maternal death. The “miniCOMIT” tool uses pertinent baseline characteristics available at disease onset; namely maternal age, body mass index (BMI), and diagnosis in the third trimester. An expanded “fullCOMIT” tool utilizes BMI, lower respiratory symptoms, and biomarkers (neutrophil to lymphocyte ratio and serum CRP) which are also frequently available. Characterization into “high risk” by either tool is associated with shorter interval to ICU admission (log-rank test $P < 0.001$, both), higher maternal death (5.2% vs. 0.2%; $P < 0.001$), and pre-eclampsia (5.7% vs. 1.0%; $P < 0.001$). In both models, obesity was found to be an independent predictor of severe COVID-19, further emphasizing obesity as a risk factor for a future targeted approach [20].

3 Oxygenation and Ventilatory Support

Target oxygen saturation for non-pregnant COVID-19 infected patients is 92% [21]. The Society for Maternal-Fetal Medicine (SMFM) recommends aiming for a higher target of 95% and to consider intensive care admission if this is not achieved with supplemental oxygen or with escalating requirements [22]. Other experts have emphasized a range of acceptable saturation (92%–96%) as long as fetal status is reassuring particularly at preterm gestational ages [23]. Alternatively, blood gas measurements aimed at achieving greater than 70 mmHg partial pressure of oxygen can be used for guidance. This relatively higher oxygenation target may be justified by an increased functional pulmonary shunt due to an increased cardiac output, particularly in the latter weeks of pregnancy, which may exacerbate hypoxemia at similar degrees of lung consolidation compared to non-pregnant COVID-19 patients [24, 25].

When sufficient oxygenation cannot be achieved by conventional oxygen support and indications for endotracheal intubation are not imminent, high-flow nasal cannula (HFNC) is a reasonable therapy [11]. Nasal blockage associated with pregnancy does not appear to be a barrier to HFNC which provides alveolar recruitment and allows FiO_2 to be titrated more accurately [26, 27]. Furthermore, evidence from clinical trials conducted pre-COVID-19, support the use of HFNC with findings of greater ventilator-free days and lower 90-day mortality or reduced rates of intubation and ICU mortality in the HFNC groups compared to noninvasive positive pressure ventilation (NIV) depending on the study [28, 29]. This may be particularly useful in pregnant persons at increased risk of aspiration due to decreased esophageal sphincter tone and increased abdominal pressure [11, 30]. Progression to higher (>60%) FiO_2 requirements and increased inspiratory effort may lend to a trial of NIV with close clinical monitoring [31].

In a large multi-centric international study (COVIDPREG), 8% of pregnant individuals hospitalized with COVID-19 during the study period were admitted to ICU and their data retrospectively analyzed [32]. Conventional oxygenation, HFNC and NIV were used as the sole technique in 41 (22%), 55 (29%), and 18 (10%) of patients, respectively, whereas 73 (39%) of patients were intubated. Around one-third of patients required multi-modal oxygenation. Risk factors for intubation in this study were obesity, pregnancy-related complications, advanced term of pregnancy and NIV use. In a multivariant analysis, cause-specific hazard ratio for extent of CT scan abnormalities greater than 50% was found to be 2.69 (95% CI (1.30–5.60) $P < 0.01$).

Strategies for mechanical ventilation in non-pregnant individuals are generally applicable to the critically ill obstetrical patient group with notable differences [11]. Whereas pregnancy-specific hypocapnia is desirable to prevent fetal acidemia and oxygen dissociation shifts; in the setting of acute respiratory distress syndrome (ARDS) permissive hypercapnia may be used and is generally advised not to exceed 60 mmHg [11, 33]. Moreover, goals for oxygen saturation and oxygen partial pressure are likewise more liberal in an attempt to ensure adequate fetal oxygenation [11, 30].

Prone positioning is a key management strategy of moderate-to-severe ARDS due to COVID-19 supported by the Surviving Sepsis Campaign panel [21]. Awake prone positioning can be used in non-mechanically ventilated patients with persistent hypoxemia on HFNC for whom endotracheal intubation is not indicated. Furthermore, prone positioning is also recommended by the NIH guidelines in mechanically ventilated patients with refractory hypoxemia [34]. In pregnant persons, proning may be achieved with padding above and below the gravid uterus [11, 33]. This, however, may present with difficulties in fetal monitoring and that should be balanced with gains in oxygenation [32, 33, 35].

In patients with refractory hypoxemia, evaluation and referral for ECMO is often considered to advance care [31]. It is important to note that pregnancy is not a contraindication for such escalation of care [22]. Furthermore, similar criteria for respiratory failure should apply when considering referring pregnant and postpartum women for ECMO [22, 36, 37]. In a cohort study analyzing the Extracorporeal Life Support Organization Registry that included adult women supported on VV-ECMO with COVID-19, survival outcomes and ECMO-related complications were apparently more favorable in the pregnant/peripartum group [38]. In comparison with a propensity score-adjusted non-pregnant adult female cohort, pregnant or peripartum women were more likely to survive to hospital discharge (84% vs. 51.5%; overlap propensity score–weighted OR, 1.18; 95% CI, 1.10–1.27) and suffered fewer ECMO-related renal complications (overlap propensity score-weighted OR, 0.90; 95% CI, 0.84–0.97). Physiologic changes in angiotensin II, progesterone, and increased nitric oxide during pregnancy are hypothesized to improve renal perfusion and explain lower rates of injury [38, 39]. Other reports have similarly supported favorable efficacy and safety outcomes for ECMO in this patient group [40, 41]. Importantly, if patients are considered for ECMO, involving intensivists, cardiothoracic surgeons, obstetricians, maternal-fetal medicine specialists, and neonatologists may enable individualization of care [11]. ECMO in and of itself is not an indication for delivery, and decision for early delivery should be taken as part of a multidisciplinary discussion with the patient or surrogate decision-maker [22].

4 Pharmacological Agents in COVID-19

4.1 Corticosteroids

In the recovery trial, administration of an oral or intravenous dexamethasone regimen compared to standard of care reduced mortality among COVID-19 patients requiring supplemental oxygen or mechanical ventilation [42]. This benefit was not seen among patients off respiratory support and may be due to the absence of a hyper-inflammatory state early in the disease [34, 42]. Use of corticosteroids in pregnancy should take into account possibility of fetal exposure with potential deleterious neurocognitive and neuroendocrine effects [43]. On the other hand, administration of glucocorticoids in patients with imminent preterm delivery is merited for fetal lung maturity as it is known to improve neonatal outcomes [44]. To address this issue, alternative regimens using oral prednisolone, intravenous hydrocortisone, or intravenous methylprednisolone are variably advocated by the Royal College of Obstetricians and Gynecologists (RCOG), and other experts in the event pharmacologic induction of fetal lung maturity are not required at the time of respiratory decompensation due to COVID-19 infection [43, 45]. These non-fluorinated glucocorticoids are metabolized by placental enzymes minimizing the amount crossing the placenta and subsequent fetal harm [46, 47]. If induction of fetal lung maturity is indicated, an intra-muscular dexamethasone regimen may be administered for this purpose, followed by a non-fluorinated alternative at the dose recommended for COVID-19 to complete a total of 10 days or until discharge, whichever is sooner [43, 44]. Alternatively, the SMFM recommends using dexamethasone as the sole agent while adjusting the dose and duration according to the situation at hand [22].

4.2 *Immune-Modulating Agents*

A proportion of patients with severe COVID-19 infection demonstrate an exaggerated inflammatory response postulated to be a form of cytokine release syndrome or cytokine storm. Elevated inflammatory markers including CRP, D-dimer, ferritin, and inteleukin-6 have been associated with critical COVID-19 disease and form the basis for recommending interleukin-6 receptor antagonists including tocilizumab and sarilumab to ameliorate such response [34, 48]. Intravenous tocilizumab recently received approval by the Food and Drug Administration (FDA) for the treatment of COVID-19 in hospitalized adults who are receiving systemic corticosteroids and require supplemental oxygen, NIV, mechanical ventilation, or ECMO [49]. The benefit from tocilizumab use in COVID-19 is most evident in patients with worsening hypoxia and significant systemic inflammation. In the RECOVERY trial, mortality benefits were observed regardless of the level of respiratory support and were found additional to the benefits achieved with corticosteroids [50]. Additional studies further provide evidence supporting improved outcomes with tocilizumab use [51–55]. Data on the efficacy and safety of such agents in pregnancy, however, is comparatively scarce. In a Spanish review including 12 pregnant women who received tocilizumab for severe COVID-19 disease; all pregnancies resulted in live births. The median gestational age at admission was 27.7 weeks, and somatometric values were reportedly normal for all newborns with favorable follow-up at 14 and 28 days. The majority of women were discharged prior to delivery with improved COVID-19 outcomes. Of note, secondary infections due to immune suppression have been detected, which raises the importance of considering potential serious complications and close clinical monitoring [56]. In a more extensive review of tocilizumab use in pregnancy and lactation, including 610 pregnant women with largely non-COVID-19 indications, no serious safety signals were detected. The authors, however, acknowledged significant limitations in drawing conclusions with regard to the full spectrum of potential adverse effects [57]. The NIH currently advises joint decision-making to inform pregnant individuals of potential risks and benefits of tocilizumab use. Sarilumab, another monoclonal interleukin-6 receptor antibody, is even less well-studied in pregnancy [34].

A different group of immune-modulators, namely the Janus kinase (JAK) inhibitors baricitinib and tofacitinib, have also shown improved COVID-19 clinical outcomes. Baricitinib has similarly received FDA approval for the treatment of hospitalized COVID-19 patients requiring supplemental oxygen, noninvasive ventilation (NIV), mechanical ventilation, or extracorporeal membrane oxygenation (ECMO) [49]. Although an NIH recommendation for use of Baricitinib or tofacitinib in combination with dexamethasone in hospitalized patients with evidence of inflammation and increasing oxygen needs exists, special considerations for shared decision-making in pregnant individuals also applies. Factors such as maternal COVID-19 severity, comorbidities, and gestational age should be taken into account, with reference to ongoing registries and available safety data [34].

4.3 *Remdesivir*

Remdesivir is a nucleotide analog antiviral which has demonstrated some benefit in preventing progression to severe disease. Use of this agent is therefore most appealing in the non-critically ill population during early course of the disease [58–60]. Some experts, however, suggest adding remdesivir for the potential benefit in immune compromised patients on HFNC or NIV to control viral replication while others may consider its use in patients recently started on mechanical ventilation [34].

The use of remdesivir in pregnancy has not been extensively studied. Evidence from prior use in Ebola and Marburg disease has not shown fetal toxicity [61]. Compassionate use of remdesivir in COVID-19 infection among hospitalized pregnant and postpartum women with hypoxia revealed high recovery rates and low incidence of serious adverse effects [62]. Data from other studies however do raise concern regarding risk for hepatotoxicity in the pregnant population [63, 64].

4.4 *Prevention of Venous Thromboembolism*

Risk for venous thromboembolism (VTE) is known to increase in pregnancy and even more so in the postpartum period, with predisposition likely compounded by underlying pro-thrombotic genetic states [65, 66]. It is not yet clear whether COVID-19 infection further increases this risk [34]. With regard to VTE prevention during COVID-19 illness, the majority of evidence is in non-pregnant individuals and guidelines continue to evolve. The NIH currently recommends prophylactic dose heparin (unless contraindicated) in hospitalized patients who require mechanical ventilation, similarly to those on HFNC or NIV, for both pregnant and non-pregnant individuals [34]. Evidence for these recommendations largely comes from the REMAP-CAP/ACTIV-4a/ATTACC and inspiration trials [67, 68]. Although a randomized controlled trial suggested clinical benefit of therapeutic over prophylactic heparin in non-critically ill patients [69], the same was not demonstrated in the critically ill population [67]. Furthermore, the inspiration trial provided evidence that intermediate-dose prophylactic anticoagulation in intensive care patients does not result in significant improvement in composite venous or arterial thrombosis, requirement for ECMO or mortality within 30 days compared with standard-dose prophylactic anticoagulation [68]. Moreover, the NIH recommends that low-molecular weight heparin (LMWH) and unfractionated heparin (UFH) be used for the duration of hospitalization only [34]. The RCOG similarly recommends prophylactic dose LMWH for patients on HFNC, CPAP, noninvasive and invasive ventilation, however for all pregnant women who have been hospitalized and had confirmed COVID-19 infection, the RCOG recommends thromboprophylaxis for 10 days following hospital discharge, with consideration for extension in women with significant ongoing morbidity [45]. Some experts advocate utilizing CRP or D-dimer measurements to guide anticoagulation [70]. In critically ill pregnant patients who are started on therapeutic anticoagulation without confirmed thrombosis, the SMFM recommends using UFH due to its short half-life and reversibility with protamine sulfate. UFH is particularly useful in patients with imminent delivery and can be adjusted according to activated partial thromboplastin time or anti-Xa monitoring [22].

5 Delivery of Fetus

In critically ill pregnant patients, early delivery may be considered for optimization of care. Various maternal or fetal indications for delivery may arise over the hospital course. The ability to respond to dynamic changes is best attuned with input from each maternal-fetal medicine, neonatology, obstetrics anesthesia, and the patient whenever possible [11]. Moreover, a set-up in preparation for delivery should take into account the feasibility of delivery in the ICU setting versus transfer to a labor and delivery ward.

Gestational age and risk of prematurity are factors which should be balanced with risk of worsening maternal respiratory status and critical illness or a non-reassuring fetal condition. Criteria suggested for refractory maternal hypoxia include $PaO_2 < 60$ mmHg while receiving 100% inspired FiO_2, or PaO_2 to FIO_2 ratio of <150 unresponsive to measures such as increases in positive end expiratory pressure (PEEP), recruitment of lung volumes, prone positioning, and/or deep sedation with chemical paralysis [71, 72]. Fetal cardiotocography may be considered an additional "vital sign" reflecting both maternal and fetal well-being and response to therapy [71, 73].

In pregnancies at 32–34 weeks of gestation or beyond, the decision for delivery is generally well-supported. Corticosteroids should be administered, when possible, prior to delivery as indicated for fetal lung maturity. In patients with viable pregnancies and up to 32 weeks of gestation, the decision to deliver should take into account criteria for maternal worsening as well as neonatal resuscitation [71, 74]. In the COVIDPREG study, most deliveries conducted in the ICU occurred in intubated patients due to maternal respiratory decline. Notably, significant improvement in

PaO_2 to FIO_2 ratio and driving pressure were noted post-delivery, with a trend towards decreasing plateau pressure and improving respiratory system compliance [32]. Changes in these parameters provide evidence to support early delivery in improving maternal oxygenation. Overall, in this large study, maternal and neonatal mortality rates appeared to be low; however, complications tended to increase with invasiveness of maternal ventilatory support [32].

6 Conclusion

Pregnant women with COVID-19 infection are at higher risk for ICU admission, invasive ventilation, ECMO, and death than non-pregnant women. Comorbidity with COVID-19 infection can lead to higher obstetrical problems, so a multidisciplinary team approach is recommended. The recommendation in the management of critical COVID-19 obstetric patients is to target oxygen saturation of 92%. High-flow nasal cannula (HFNC) is a viable therapy when adequate oxygenation cannot be attained by conventional oxygen support. The FDA has approved intravenous tocilizumab for the management of COVID-19 in hospitalized patients taking systemic corticosteroids and requiring mechanical ventilation, NIV, or supplementary oxygen. The NIH advises preventive dosage heparin in hospitalized patients who need mechanical ventilation.

References

1. Allotey J, Stallings E, Bonet M, Yap M, Chatterjee S, Kew T, Debenham L, Llavall AC, Dixit A, Zhou D, Balaji R, Lee SI, Qiu X, Yuan M, Coomar D, Sheikh J, Lawson H, Ansari K, van Wely M, van Leeuwen E, et al. Clinical manifestations, risk factors, and maternal and perinatal outcomes of coronavirus disease 2019 in pregnancy: living systematic review and meta-analysis. BMJ. 2020,370.m3320. https://doi.org/10.1136/bmj.m3320.
2. Yanes-Lane M, Winters N, Fregonese F, Bastos M, Perlman-Arrow S, Campbell JR, Menzies D. Proportion of asymptomatic infection among COVID-19 positive persons and their transmission potential: a systematic review and meta-analysis. PLoS One. 2020;15(11):e0241536. https://doi.org/10.1371/journal.pone.0241536.
3. Zambrano LD, Ellington S, Strid P, et al. Update: characteristics of symptomatic women of reproductive age with laboratory-confirmed SARS-CoV-2 infection by pregnancy status—United States, January 22-October 3, 2020. MMWR Morb Mortal Wkly Rep. 2020;69(44):1641–7.
4. Villar J, Ariff S, Gunier RB, Thiruvengadam R, Rauch S, Kholin A, et al. Maternal and neonatal morbidity and mortality among pregnant women with and without COVID-19 infection: the INTERCOVID multinational cohort study. JAMA Pediatr. 2021;175:817–26. https://doi.org/10.1001/jamapediatrics.2021.1050.
5. Allotey J, Stallings E, Bonet M, et al. Update to living systematic review on COVID-19 in pregnancy. BMJ. 2022;377:o1205. https://www.ncbi.nlm.nih.gov/pubmed/35636775.
6. Knight M, Bunch K, Vousden N, et al. Characteristics and outcomes of pregnant women admitted to hospital with confirmed SARS-CoV-2 infection in UK: national population based cohort study. BMJ. 2020;369:m2107.

7. Centers for Disease Control and Prevention. Underlying medical conditions associated with high risk for severe COVID-19: information for healthcare providers. https://www.cdc.gov/coronavirus/2019-ncov/hcp/clinical-care/underlyingconditions.html. Accessed 1 Mar 2022.
8. Centers for Disease Control and Prevention. Science brief: evidence used to update the list of underlying medical conditions that increase a person's risk of severe illness from COVID-19. https://www.cdc.gov/coronavirus/2019-ncov/hcp/clinical-care/underlying-evidence-table.html. Accessed 1 Mar 2022.
9. Centers for Disease Control and Prevention. Risk for COVID-19 infection, hospitalization, and death by age group. https://www.cdc.gov/coronavirus/2019-ncov/covid-data/investigations-discovery/hospitalization-death-by-age.html. Accessed 16 June 2022.
10. Jamieson DJ, Rasmussen SA. An update on COVID-19 and pregnancy. Am J Obstet Gynecol. 2022;226(2):177–86. https://doi.org/10.1016/j.ajog.2021.08.054.
11. Levitus M, Shainker SA, Colvin M. COVID-19 in the critically ill pregnant patient. Crit Care Clin. 2022;38(3):521–34. https://doi.org/10.1016/j.ccc.2022.01.003.
12. Futterman I, Toaff M, Navi L, Clare CA. COVID-19 and HELLP: overlapping clinical pictures in two gravid patients. AJP Rep. 2020;10(2):e179–82. https://doi.org/10.1055/s-0040-1712978.
13. Mendoza M, Garcia-Ruiz I, Maiz N, Rodo C, Garcia-Manau P, Serrano B, Lopez-Martinez RM, Balcells J, Fernandez-Hidalgo N, Carreras E, Suy A. Pre-eclampsia-like syndrome induced by severe COVID-19: a prospective observational study. BJOG. 2020;127(11):1374–80. https://doi.org/10.1111/1471-0528.16339.
14. Zitiello A, Grant GE, Ben Ali N, Feki A. Thrombocytopaenia in pregnancy: the importance of differential diagnosis during the COVID-19 pandemic. J Matern Fetal Neonatal Med. 2022;35(12):2414–6. https://doi.org/10.1080/14767058.2020.1786527.
15. Hedengran KK, Andersen MR, Stender S, et al. Large D-dimer fluctuation in normal pregnancy: a longitudinal cohort study of 4,117 samples from 714 healthy Danish women. Obstet Gynecol Int. 2016;2016:3561675.
16. Hwang HS, Kwon JY, Kim MA, et al. Maternal serum highly sensitive C-reactive protein in normal pregnancy and pre-eclampsia. Int J Gynecol Obstet. 2007;98:105. [PMID: 17588579]
17. Clinical Spectrum of SARS-CoV-2 Infection. NIH COVID-19 Treatment Guidelines. National Institutes of Health. https://covid19treatmentguidelines.nih.gov/overview/management-of-covid-19/. Accessed 22 Apr 2020.
18. Wu Z, McGoogan JM. Characteristics of and important lessons from the coronavirus disease 2019 (COVID-19) outbreak in China: summary of a report of 72 314 cases from the Chinese Center for Disease Control and Prevention. JAMA. 2020;323(13):1239–42.
19. Donders F, Lonnée-Hoffmann R, Tsiakalos A, Mendling W, Martinez de Oliveira J, Judlin P, Xue F, Donders GGG, Isidog Covid-Guideline Workgroup. ISIDOG recommendations concerning COVID-19 and pregnancy. Diagnostics (Basel, Switzerland). 2020;10(4):243. https://doi.org/10.3390/diagnostics10040243.
20. Kalafat E, Prasad S, Birol P, Tekin AB, Kunt A, Di Fabrizio C, Alatas C, Celik E, Bagci H, Binder J, Le Doare K, Magee LA, Mutlu MA, Yassa M, Tug N, Sahin O, Krokos P, O'brien, P., von Dadelszen, P., Palmrich, P., … Khalil, A. An internally validated prediction model for critical COVID-19 infection and intensive care unit admission in symptomatic pregnant women. Am J Obstet Gynecol. 2022;226(3):403.e1–403.e13. https://doi.org/10.1016/j.ajog.2021.09.024.
21. Alhazzani W, Moller MH, Arabi YM, Loeb M, Gong MN, Fan E, et al. Surviving sepsis campaign: guidelines on the management of critically ill adults with coronavirus disease 2019 (COVID-19). Crit Care Med. 2020;48:e440.
22. Halscott TV, J and the SMFM COVID-19 Task Force. Management considerations for pregnant patients with COVID-19. 2021.
23. Eid J, Stahl D, Costantine MM, Rood KM. Oxygen saturation in pregnant individuals with COVID-19: time for re-appraisal? Am J Obstet Gynecol. 2022;226(6):813–6. https://doi.org/10.1016/j.ajog.2021.12.023.
24. Camporota L, Cronin JN, Busana M, Gattinoni L, Formenti F. Pathophysiology of coronavirus-19 disease acute lung injury. Curr Opin Crit Care. 2022;28:9–16. https://doi.org/10.1097/MCC.0000000000000911.

25. Camporota L, Chiumello D, Busana M, Gattinoni L, Marini JJ. Pathophysiology of COVID-19-associated acute respiratory distress syndrome. Lancet Respir Med. 2021;9:e1. https://doi.org/10.1016/S2213-2600(20)30505-1.
26. Ghafoor H, Abdus Samad A, Bel Khair AOM, Ahmed O, Khan MNA. Critical care management of severe COVID-19 in pregnant patients. Cureus. 2022;14(5):e24885. https://doi.org/10.7759/cureus.24885.
27. Pacheco LD, Saad AF, Saade G. Early acute respiratory support for pregnant patients with coronavirus disease 2019 (COVID-19) infection. Obstet Gynecol. 2020;136(1):42–5.
28. Frat JP, Thille AW, Mercat A, Girault C, Ragot S, Perbet S, et al. High-flow oxygen through nasal cannula in acute hypoxemic respiratory failure. N Engl J Med. 2015;372:2185–96.
29. Ni YN, Luo J, Yu H, Liu D, Ni Z, Cheng J, et al. Can high-flow nasal cannula reduce the rate of endotracheal intubation in adult patients with acute respiratory failure compared with conventional oxygen therapy and noninvasive positive pressure ventilation?: a systematic review and meta-analysis. Chest. 2017;151:764–75.
30. Schwaiberger D, Karcz M, Menk M, et al. Respiratory failure and mechanical ventilation in the pregnant patient. Crit Care Clin. 2016;32(1):85–95.
31. Nana M, Hodson K, Lucas N, Camporota L, Knight M, Nelson-Piercy C. Diagnosis and management of covid-19 in pregnancy. BMJ. 2022;377:e069739. https://doi.org/10.1136/bmj-2021-069739.
32. Péju E, Belicard F, Silva S, Hraiech S, Painvin B, Kamel T, Thille AW, Goury A, Grimaldi D, Jung B, Piagnerelli M, Winiszewski H, Jourdain M, Jozwiak M, COVIDPREG Study Group. Management and outcomes of pregnant women admitted to intensive care unit for severe pneumonia related to SARS-CoV-2 infection: the multicenter and international COVIDPREG study. Intensive Care Med. 2022;48(9):1185–96. https://doi.org/10.1007/s00134-022-06833-8.
33. Tolcher MC, McKinney JR, Eppes CS, et al. Prone positioning for pregnant women with hypoxemia due to coronavirus disease 2019 (COVID-19). Obstet Gynecol. 2020;136(2):259–61.
34. COVID-19 Treatment Guidelines Panel. Coronavirus disease 2019 (COVID-19) treatment guidelines. National Institutes of Health. https://www.covid19treatmentguidelines.nih.gov/. Accessed 5 Feb 2022.
35. Ray B, Trikha A. Prone position ventilation in pregnancy: concerns and evidence. J Obstet Anaesth Crit Care. 2018;8:7–9. https://doi.org/10.4103/joacc.JOACC_17_18.
36. Camporota L, Meadows C, Ledot S, et al. Consensus on the referral and admission of patients with severe respiratory failure to the NHS ECMO service. Lancet Respir Med. 2021;9:e16–7. https://doi.org/10.1016/S2213-2600(20)30581-6.
37. Combes A, Hajage D, Capellier G, et al. Extracorporeal membrane oxygenation for severe acute respiratory distress syndrome. N Engl J Med. 2018;378:1965–75. https://doi.org/10.1056/NEJMoa1800385.
38. O'Neil ER, Lin H, Shamshirsaz AA, Naoum EE, Rycus PR, Alexander PMA, Ortoleva JP, Li M, Anders MM. Pregnant and peripartum women with COVID-19 have high survival with extracorporeal membrane oxygenation: an extracorporeal life support organization registry analysis. Am J Respir Crit Care Med. 2022;205(2):248–50. https://doi.org/10.1164/rccm.202109-2096LE.
39. Cheung KL, Lafayette RA. Renal physiology of pregnancy. Adv Chronic Kidney Dis. 2013;20:209–14.
40. Barrantes JH, Ortoleva J, O'Neil ER, Suarez EE, Beth Larson S, Rali AS, et al. Successful treatment of pregnant and postpartum women with severe COVID-19 associated acute respiratory distress syndrome with extracorporeal membrane oxygenation. ASAIO J. 2021;67:132–6.
41. Clemenza S, Zullino S, Vacca C, Simeone S, Serena C, Rambaldi MP, Ottanelli S, Vannuccini S, Bonizzoli M, Peris A, Micaglio M, Petraglia F, Mecacci F. Perinatal outcomes of pregnant women with severe COVID-19 requiring extracorporeal membrane oxygenation (ECMO): a case series and literature review. Arch Gynecol Obstet. 2022;305(5):1135–42. https://doi.org/10.1007/s00404-022-06479-3.

42. Group RC, Horby P, Lim WS, et al. Dexamethasone in hospitalized patients with Covid-19. N Engl J Med. 2021;384(8):693–704.
43. Saad AF, Chappell L, Saade GR, et al. Corticosteroids in the management of pregnant patients with coronavirus disease (COVID-19). Obstet Gynecol. 2020;136(4):823–6.
44. Committee on Obstetric P. Committee Opinion No. 713. Antenatal corticosteroid therapy for fetal maturation. Obstet Gynecol. 2017;130(2):e102–9.
45. Gynaecologists RCoOa. Coronavirus (COVID-19) infection in pregnancy–version 15. 2022.
46. Beitins IZ, Bayard F, Ances IG, Kowarski A, Migeon CJ. The transplacental passage of prednisone and prednisolone in pregnancy near term. J Pediatr. 1972;81:936–45. https://doi.org/10.1016/S0022-3476(72)80547-X.
47. Blanford AT, Murphy BE. In vitro metabolism of prednisolone, dexamethasone, betamethasone, and cortisol by the human placenta. Am J Obstet Gynecol. 1977;127:264–7. https://doi.org/10.1016/0002-9378(77)90466-5.
48. Mehta P, McAuley DF, Brown M, Sanchez E, Tattersall RS, Manson JJ, HLH Across Speciality Collaboration, UK. COVID-19: consider cytokine storm syndromes and immunosuppression. Lancet (London, England). 2020;395(10229):1033–4. https://doi.org/10.1016/S0140-6736(20)30628-0.
49. Tocilizumab (Actemra) [package insert]. Food and Drug Administration. 2022. https://www.accessdata.fda.gov/drugsatfda_docs/label/2022/125276s138lbl.pdf.
50. Horby P, Lim WS, Emberson JR, et al. Dexamethasone in hospitalized patients with covid-19. N Engl J Med. 2021;384:693–704. https://doi.org/10.1056/NEJMoa2021436.
51. Ghosn L, Chaimani A, Evrenoglou T, et al. Interleukin-6 blocking agents for treating COVID-19: a living systematic review. Cochrane Database Syst Rev. 2021;3:CD013881.
52. Salama C, Han J, Yau L, et al. Tocilizumab in patients hospitalized with Covid-19 pneumonia. N Engl J Med. 2021;384(1):20–30.
53. Somers EC, Eschenauer GA, Troost JP, et al. Tocilizumab for treatment of mechanically ventilated patients with COVID-19. Clin Infect Dis. 2021;73(2):e445–54.
54. Horby P, Staplin N, Haynes R, et al. Tocilizumab in COVID-19 therapy: who benefits, and how?—authors' reply. Lancet. 2021;398(10297):300.
55. Investigators R-C, Gordon AC, Mouncey PR, et al. Interleukin-6 receptor antagonists in critically ill patients with Covid-19. N Engl J Med. 2021;384(16):1491–502.
56. Iménez-Lozano I, Caro-Teller JM, Fernández-Hidalgo N, Miarons M, Frick MA, Batllori Badia E, Serrano B, Parramon-Teixidó CJ, Camba-Longueira F, Moral-Pumarega MT, San Juan-Garrido R, Cabañas Poy MJ, Suy A, Gorgas Torner MQ. Safety of tocilizumab in COVID-19 pregnant women and their newborn: a retrospective study. J Clin Pharm Ther. 2021;46(4):1062–70. https://doi.org/10.1111/jcpt.13394.
57. Jorgensen SCJ, Lapinsky SE. Tocilizumab for coronavirus disease 2019 in pregnancy and lactation: a narrative review. Clin Microbiol Infect. 2021.
58. Beigel JH, Tomashek KM, Dodd LE, Mehta AK, Zingman BS, Kalil AC, Hohmann E, Chu HY, Luetkemeyer A, Kline S, Lopez de Castilla D, Finberg RW, Dierberg K, Tapson V, Hsieh L, Patterson TF, Paredes R, Sweeney DA, Short WR, Touloumi G, et al. Remdesivir for the treatment of Covid-19—final report. N Engl J Med. 2020;383(19):1813–26. https://doi.org/10.1056/NEJMoa2007764.
59. Ader F, Bouscambert-Duchamp M, Hites M, Peiffer-Smadja N, Poissy J, Belhadi D, Diallo A, Lê MP, Peytavin G, Staub T, Greil R, Guedj J, Paiva JA, Costagliola D, Yazdanpanah Y, Burdet C, Mentré F, DisCoVeRy Study Group. Remdesivir plus standard of care versus standard of care alone for the treatment of patients admitted to hospital with COVID-19 (DisCoVeRy): a phase 3, randomised, controlled, open-label trial. Lancet Infect Dis. 2022;22(2):209–21. https://doi.org/10.1016/S1473-3099(21)00485-0.
60. Kaka AS, MacDonald R, Linskens EJ, Langsetmo L, Vela K, Duan-Porter W, Wilt TJ. Major update 2: remdesivir for adults with COVID-19: a living systematic review and meta-analysis for the American College of Physicians Practice Points. Ann Intern Med. 2022;175(5):701–9. https://doi.org/10.7326/M21-4784.

61. Mulangu S, Dodd LE, Davey RT Jr, Tshiani Mbaya O, Proschan M, Mukadi D, Lusakibanza Manzo M, Nzolo D, Tshomba Oloma A, Ibanda A, Ali R, Coulibaly S, Levine AC, Grais R, Diaz J, Lane HC, Muyembe-Tamfum JJ, et al. A randomized, controlled trial of Ebola virus disease therapeutics. N Engl J Med. 2019;381(24):2293–303. https://doi.org/10.1056/NEJMoa1910993.
62. Burwick RM, Yawetz S, Stephenson KE, et al. Compassionate use of remdesivir in pregnant women with severe Covid-19. Clin Infect Dis. 2020;73:e3996. https://doi.org/10.1093/cid/ciaa1466.
63. Gutierrez R, Mendez-Figueroa H, Biebighauser JG, et al. Remdesivir use in pregnancy during the SARS-CoV-2 pandemic. J Matern Fetal Neonatal Med. 2022;35(25):9445–51. https://www.ncbi.nlm.nih.gov/pubmed/35168447.
64. Budi DS, Pratama NR, Wafa IA, et al. Remdesivir for pregnancy: a systematic review of antiviral therapy for COVID-19. Heliyon. 2022;8(1):e08835. https://www.ncbi.nlm.nih.gov/pubmed/35128114.
65. Pomp ER, Lenselink AM, Rosendaal FR, Doggen CJ. Pregnancy, the postpartum period and prothrombotic defects: risk of venous thrombosis in the MEGA study. J Thromb Haemost. 2008;6(4):632–7. https://doi.org/10.1111/j.1538-7836.2008.02921.x.
66. Heit JA, Kobbervig CE, James AH, Petterson TM, Bailey KR, Melton LJ 3rd. Trends in the incidence of venous thromboembolism during pregnancy or postpartum: a 30-year population-based study. Ann Intern Med. 2005;143(10):697–706. https://doi.org/10.7326/0003-4819-143-10-200511150-00006.
67. REMAP-CAP Investigators, ACTIV-4a Investigators, ATTACC Investigators, Goligher EC, Bradbury CA, McVerry BJ, Lawler PR, Berger JS, Gong MN, Carrier M, Reynolds HR, Kumar A, Turgeon AF, Kornblith LZ, Kahn SR, Marshall JC, Kim KS, Houston BL, Derde LPG, Cushman M, et al. Therapeutic anticoagulation with heparin in critically ill patients with Covid-19. N Engl J Med. 2021;385(9):777–89. https://doi.org/10.1056/NEJMoa2103417.
68. INSPIRATION Investigators, Sadeghipour P, Talasaz AH, et al. Effect of intermediate-dose vs standard-dose prophylactic anticoagulation on thrombotic events, extracorporeal membrane oxygenation treatment, or mortality among patients with COVID-19 admitted to the intensive care unit: the INSPIRATION randomized clinical trial. JAMA. 2021;325(16):1620–30. https://www.ncbi.nlm.nih.gov/pubmed/33734299.
69. Lawler PR, Goligher EC, Berger JS, et al. ATTACC Investigators, ACTIV-4a Investigators, REMAP-CAP Investigators. Therapeutic anticoagulation with heparin in noncritically ill patients with covid-19. N Engl J Med. 2021;385:790–802. https://doi.org/10.1056/NEJMoa2105911.
70. Barrett CD, Moore HB, Yaffe MB, Moore EE. ISTH interim guidance on recognition and management of coagulopathy in COVID-19: a comment. J Thromb Haemost. 2020;18:2060.
71. Rose CH, Wyatt MA, Narang K, et al. Timing of delivery with coronavirus disease 2019 pneumonia requiring intensive care unit admission. Am J Obstet Gynecol MFM. 2021;3(4):100373.
72. Meade MO, Cook DJ, Guyatt GH, et al. Ventilation strategy using low tidal volumes, recruitment maneuvers, and high positive end-expiratory pressure for acute lung injury and acute respiratory distress syndrome: a randomized controlled trial. JAMA. 2008;299:637–45.
73. Aubey J, Zork N, Sheen JJ. Inpatient obstetric management of COVID-19. Semin Perinatol. 2020;44:151280.
74. Stephens AJ, Barton JR, Bentum NA, Blackwell SC, Sibai BM. General guidelines in the management of an obstetrical patient on the labor and delivery unit during the COVID-19 pandemic. Am J Perinatol. 2020;37(8):829–36. https://doi.org/10.1055/s-0040-1710308.

ECMO in Peripartum Period: Lifesaving Therapeutic Intervention

Mogahed Ismail Hassan Hussein, Sana Saleem, Ibrahim Hasan Fawzy, Ashraf A. Molokhia, Arshad Chanda, and Nissar Shaikh

Abstract ECMO is a form of life support that can be used in the peripartum period; it involves the use of an external (outside of the body) oxygenator to oxygenate the blood. It is typically used as a last resort for patients with severe respiratory or cardiovascular failure. ECMO can be classified into two main types: veno-arterial (VA) ECMO and veno-venous. VA ECMO is used to support the function of both the heart and the lungs whereas (VV) ECMO mainly supports the lung function. It is important that healthcare providers have a clear understanding of the indications, benefits, and risks of ECMO in this setting to ensure that it is used effectively and safely. Indications for ECMO can be divided into four categories: hypoxemic respiratory failure, hypercapnic respiratory failure, cardiogenic shock, and cardiac arrest. It is crucial to remember that ECMO in pregnant patients is typically only used as a last resort because of the hazards involved, which include bleeding, infection, and blood vessel damage. The decision to use ECMO in pregnant women should be made on a case-by-case basis, considering the potential risks and benefits of the procedure. The survival rate does not appear to be affected by the indication or type of ECMO (VV or VA). The timing of ECMO assistance is crucial, and outcomes may be linked to its early use, in pregnant patients. It is important to prevent maternal hypoxia, hypercarbia, and acidosis. Referral to a specialist ECMO center with a dedicated ECMO team should be considered.

Keywords Extracorporeal life support (ECLS) · Extracorporeal membrane oxygenation (ECMO) · Peripartum period · Veno-arterial (VA) ECMO and veno-venous (VV) ECMO

M. I. H. Hussein · S. Saleem
Department of Anesthesia/SICU and Perioperative Medicine, Hamad medical Corporation, Doha, Qatar

I. H. Fawzy · A. A. Molokhia
Medical Intensive Care, Hamad Medical Corporation, Doha, Qatar

A. Chanda (✉) · N. Shaikh
Surgical Intensive Care, Hamad Medical Corporation, Doha, Qatar
e-mail: achanda@hamad.qa

N. Shaikh et al. (eds.), *Updates in Intensive Care of OBGY Patients*, https://doi.org/10.1007/978-981-99-9577-6_13

1 Introduction

Medical complications in pregnancy are on the rise as pregnant women suffer from chronic health conditions that may predispose them to cardiopulmonary complications.

Considering the increase in conditions requiring extracorporeal life support (ECLS), it is imperative that providers understand the types, indications, and limitations of extracorporeal membrane oxygenation (ECMO) [1].

ECMO is a form of life support that can be used in the peripartum period, which refers to the time around childbirth. ECMO involves the use of a machine to oxygenate the blood outside of the body and is typically used as a last resort for patients with severe respiratory or cardiovascular failure.

There are several indications for the use of ECMO in the peripartum period, including but not limited to: acute respiratory distress syndrome (ARDS), pulmonary embolism, and amniotic fluid embolism. ECMO can be used to support the mother while she recovers from these conditions or to provide oxygen to the fetus if the mother is unable to do so.

The use of ECMO in the peripartum period can be challenging, as it requires a high level of expertise and specialized equipment. It is typically only available at a few select centers with trained personnel and the necessary resources. Despite the challenges, ECMO can be a lifesaving intervention for patients with severe respiratory or cardiovascular failure in the peripartum period. Studies have shown that ECMO can improve survival rates and outcomes in these patients, particularly when used early in the course of the illness.

There are also some potential risks and complications associated with the use of ECMO, including bleeding, infection, and damage to the blood vessels. Close monitoring and careful management of these complications is essential to ensure the best possible outcomes for patients.

2 Types of ECMO

In the basic ECMO circuit, blood is removed from the venous system and passed through a membrane oxygenator, which oxygenates it before it is returned to the patient. The circuit includes a blood pump, a membrane oxygenator, tubing, a heat exchanger, and drainage and return cannula [2]. The main distinction between ECMO circuits, i.e., veno-arterial (VA) and (veno-venous) VV lies in the type of cannula used and where they are inserted [2].

ECMO can be classified into two main types: veno-arterial (VA) ECMO (Fig. 1) and veno-venous (VV) ECMO (Fig. 2). VA ECMO is used to support the function of both the heart and the lungs. Blood is taken from a vein, oxygenated by the ECMO machine, and then returned to an artery. VA ECMO is typically used in

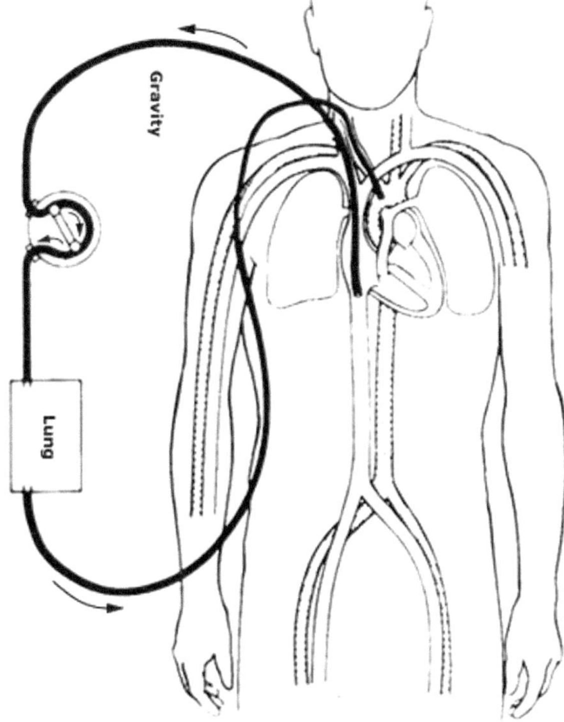

Fig. 1 Veno-Arterial (VA) ECMO. Veno-arterial (VA) ECMO for cardiac or respiratory failure by Van Meurs et al., Extracorporeal Life Support Organization, Ann Arbor 2005

patients with cardiac or respiratory failure. VV ECMO is used to support the function of the lungs only. Blood is taken from a vein, oxygenated by the ECMO machine, and then returned to a vein. VV ECMO is typically used in patients with severe respiratory failure.

VA access puts the artificial lung in parallel with the native lungs and substitutes for both heart and lung function. This technique works in a similar fashion to a standard cardiopulmonary bypass [3], allowing most of the patient's blood to move through the circuit without going through the patient's heart.

The process involves removing blood from a large vein and returning it into a large artery. Therefore, two large bore cannulas must be placed in either the neck or the groin [4].

Cannulation can be either central (blood drained directly from the right atrium and returned to the proximal ascending aorta) or peripheral (blood drained from the proximal femoral or jugular vein and returned to the axillary, or femoral artery). Cannulas can be placed by direct cut-down access to these vessels or more commonly using Seldinger Technique, via percutaneous placement of a guidewire and passage of the cannulas over the wire [5]. In a study comparing peripheral vs. central cannulation for ECMO, it was found that peripheral cannulation is preferable because central cannulation is linked to a higher risk of bleeding, higher transfusion

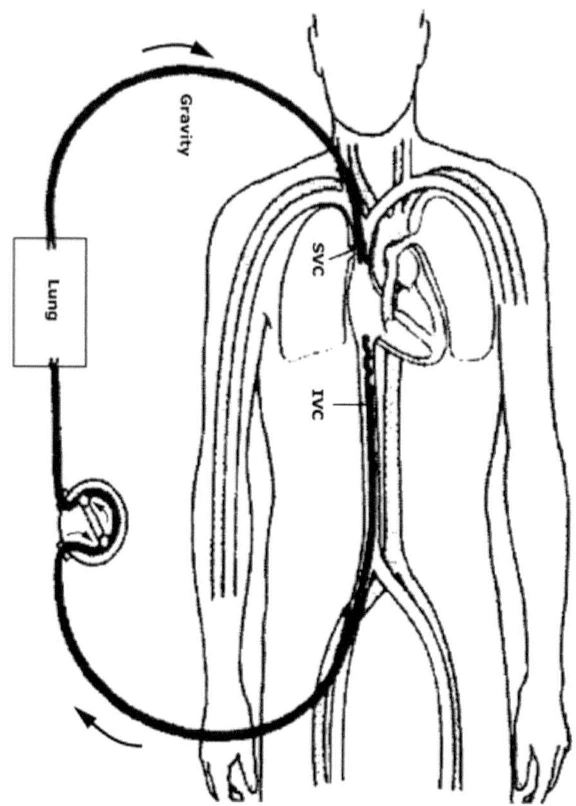

Fig. 2 Veno-Venous (VV) ECMO. Veno-arterial (VA) ECMO for cardiac or respiratory failure by Van Meurs et al., Extracorporeal Life Support Organization, Ann Arbor 2005

rates, vascular damage, and a higher rate of operation [6]. The most common method is peripheral ECMO delivered via the femoral vein +/− internal jugular vein and femoral artery. In cases of femoral arterial cannulation, due to a high risk of distal limb ischemia many centers recommend placing an ipsilateral perfusion catheter proactively [7]. Cannulation is the same as for patients who are not pregnant. However, aortocaval compression by the gravid uterus may impede femoral guide-wire advancement; therefore, it is helpful to have a cushion under the right hip to provide left uterine displacement during this process [8].

After cannulas are placed, the circuit is primed with crystalloid solution, anticoagulation is attached, and extracorporeal flow is established at 50–100 cc/kg/min. The membrane lung is ventilated with 100% oxygen. When adequate extracorporeal flow and gas exchange are achieved, the ventilator is turned down to reset settings. In many cases, the patient can be extubated, and the extracorporeal circuit takes over all respiratory and cardiac functions. As the heart and lung functions improve, the extracorporeal flow is decreased proportionately, and when heart and lung functions are fully restored, the patient is weaned from extracorporeal support and cannulas are removed [4].

2.1 Functional Mechanics

VA ECMO, as a form of partial cardiopulmonary bypass, provides 60–80% of the predicted resting cardiac output. The cardiac output provided by the ECMO circuit (i.e., ECMO blood flow) is accomplished with one of two types of pumps—centrifugal or roller. Centrifugal pumps are preload dependent and afterload sensitive [9].

Another important consideration in VA ECMO is monitoring of cerebral oxygenation. The flow of blood through VA ECMO depends on multiple modifiable factors such as Preload, Afterload, and Revolutions per minute of the pump as well as cannula length and diameter. In patients with both poor heart and lung function, oxygenated blood returning from the ECMO circuit will initially provide antegrade flow beyond the site of arterial cannulation and retrograde flow to the coronary and cerebral circulations. As heart function improves, competitive flow between patient cardiac output and the arterial cannulation may cause a distal shift in the location of blood mixing, resulting in deoxygenated blood circulating through the coronary and cerebral circulations. This phenomenon is known as North-South syndrome or Harlequin Syndrome [2, 10].

VV ECMO is designed to provide respiratory support only, without providing any cardiac support; hence, it is vital that the patient's cardiac output is sufficient to meet body requirements. The VV access puts the artificial lung in series with the native lung. For this type of ECMO, several options for cannulation exist. Most commonly, the drainage cannula is inserted into the right femoral vein and the return cannula in the right internal jugular vein. With VV cannula, more recently the physician also has an option of using special type of cannula with two lumens (a bicaval dual lumen catheter) allowing the blood to leave and enter the body in one place, benefiting the need of only one entry site instead of two [11]. In a retrospective review, dual chamber cannula was found to allow patients with greater mobilization and decreasing inflammatory responses by lessening the extent of plastic surface in contact with the blood. In case of lack of IJV access, bifemoral vein cannulation with drainage from inferior vena cava and return to right atrium is also an available option. The site of cannula can be confirmed by echocardiography or fluoroscopy.

3 ECMO in Peripartum

3.1 Indications of ECMO (Table 1)

ECMO was historically seldom used for pregnant and postpartum patients, but there is now growing interest owing to a rise in the number of complicated cases. The indications and contraindications for ECMO during pregnancy are like those for the general population. However, altered maternal physiology, maintenance of fetal well-being, and obstetric emergencies are all significant challenges that are to be

Table 1 The common indications summarized from the most common to the least as follows

Indications for ECMO during pregnancy	
1.	Acute respiratory distress syndrome
2.	Cardiac failure
3.	Cardiac arrest
4.	Peripartum cardiomyopathy
5.	Pulmonary arterial hypertension
6.	Amniotic fluid embolism
7.	Pulmonary embolism
8.	Heart disease
9.	Septic shock

considered [12]. Indications for ECMO can be divided into four categories: hypoxemic respiratory failure, hypercapnic respiratory failure, cardiogenic shock, and cardiac arrest [13].

There are several indications for the use of extracorporeal membrane oxygenation (ECMO) in peripartum period:

- Respiratory failure: ECMO can be used to support the respiratory function of the mother in cases of severe respiratory failure, such as acute respiratory distress syndrome (ARDS) or pneumonia. V-V ECMO is mostly used for acute respiratory distress syndrome (ARDS) which is typically treated with methods such as lung-protective mechanical ventilation, conservative fluid management, neuromuscular blockade to induce muscle paralysis, and prone ventilation [14]. When these methods fail, V-V ECMO may be used as an alternative to provide temporary breathing support while avoiding harmful ventilator settings, allowing the lungs time to recover.
- Cardiac failure: ECMO can be used to support the cardiac function of the mother in cases of cardiac failure, such as cardiomyopathy or myocarditis.
- Pulmonary embolism: ECMO can be used to support the respiratory function of the mother in cases of severe pulmonary embolism.
- Severe preeclampsia: ECMO can be used to support the maternal circulatory and respiratory function in cases of severe preeclampsia.
- Obstetrical emergencies: ECMO can be used in cases of obstetrical emergencies, such as placental abruption or amniotic fluid embolism, to support the maternal circulatory and respiratory function.
- Fetal distress: ECMO can be used to support the fetal circulatory and respiratory function in cases of fetal distress.

3.2 ECMO Applications in Respiratory Failure

The most common indication for veno-venous (VV) ECMO in pregnant and postpartum patients is acute respiratory distress syndrome (ARDS), accounting for up to 49% of reported cases [15, 16]. Amongst these cases, the most common etiology was found to be severe viral pneumonia (H1N1) while the minor causes included aspiration, trauma, or hypertensive disorders of pregnancy.

The prevalence of ARDS during pregnancy has been estimated as 16–70 cases per 100,000 pregnancies [17]. During pregnancy, VV ECMO is indicated in hypoxic respiratory failure with the following conditions: PaO_2/FiO_2 ratio < 80 for 6 h or PaO_2/FiO_2 ratio < 50 for 3 h. In case of hypercapnic respiratory failure, ECMO is indicated when $PaCO_2$ > 50 mmHg or (6.7 kPa) and/or pH < 7.25 on mechanical ventilation despite optimization of mechanical ventilation and despite attempts at rescue maneuvers (e.g., inhaled nitric oxide, prone positioning, neuromuscular blockade) [12]. In comparison to nonpregnant population, oxygen consumption increases 20% during pregnancy and ECMO flows must be adjusted accordingly. While an arterial oxygen saturation (SaO_2) >80% represents adequate oxygenation during ECMO support in nonpregnant adult patients, as such is not acceptable for pregnant patients. Hence the target saturation in ECMO during pregnancy is set to be >90%, with $PaCO_2$ range acceptable between 28 and 32 mmHg, pH > 7.4 Maternal hypercapnia and hypocapnia to be kept in consideration in relation to fetal hypoxemia and acidosis [12].

3.3 *ECMO Application in Cardiogenic Shock*

Cardiogenic shock may have multiple causes including post cardiotomy shock, fulminant myocarditis, and shock secondary to acute myocardial infarction. The second most common indication for ECMO overall in pregnancy reviewed to be cardiac failure (18.7%), followed by cardiac arrest (15.9%). Cardiac output increases 30–50% by the third trimester, which may reduce the capability of oxygenation during ECMO. Higher cardiac output results in more venous blood bypassing the drainage cannula and proceeding to the heart without being oxygenated. Therefore, while ECMO flow of 60–80 mL/kg/min are acceptable for nonpregnant patients, in pregnancy ECMO flows should be targeted higher than 100–120 mL/kg/min to compensate for high cardiac output. VA-ECMO is indicated in any case of inadequate tissue perfusion despite adequate intravascular volume, inotropic support, and vasoconstrictors [2, 15].

In a systematic review, peripartum patients who underwent Extracorporeal Life Support (ECLS) were separated into different time periods and observed that there were different indications for advanced support at different stages of pregnancy. Most of the cases during the antepartum period were for ARDS, while cardiac arrest was the major indication during immediate postpartum period [15].

4 Contraindications to ECMO in Peripartum

Contraindications that are identical to the general nonpregnant population to both VV and VA ECMO include:

1. Inability to tolerate anticoagulation
2. Ongoing/uncontrolled hemorrhage
3. Unwilling to receive blood products
4. Major immunosuppression (ANC < 400/mm^3)
5. Central nervous system hemorrhage acute or expanding
6. Nonrecoverable comorbidity such as major neurologic damage or malignancy

While contraindications particularly related to pregnancy include:

- Severe placental abruption: ECMO is not recommended in cases where there is a severe separation of the placenta from the uterine wall, as this can lead to severe bleeding and fetal distress.
- Placental infarction: ECMO is not recommended in cases where there is a blockage in the blood vessels that supply the placenta, as this can lead to placental infarction and fetal death.
- Multiple gestation: ECMO may not be feasible in cases where there is more than one fetus, as it may not be possible to provide adequate oxygenation to all fetuses.
- Preterm labor: ECMO may not be appropriate in cases where labor is imminent, as it may not be possible to provide adequate oxygenation to the fetus before delivery.
- Severe maternal comorbidities: ECMO may not be appropriate in cases where the mother has severe underlying medical conditions that may make her unable to tolerate the procedure.
- Severe fetal distress: ECMO may not be appropriate in cases where the fetus is in severe distress and may not be able to survive the procedure.
- Specific contraindication to VV ECMO include patient requiring home oxygen for chronic lung disease, severe acute or chronic liver disease, and patient on mechanical ventilation >10 days.

Contraindication to VA ECMO includes unrecoverable cardiac function or a patient who is not a candidate for VAD or a transplant [12]. There is no specific age contraindication; however, there is an increased risk with increasing age. Age cutoff varies with each institution [18].

5 Complications of ECMO in Pregnant Women

- Bleeding: ECMO requires the insertion of a large cannula (tube) into a vein or artery, which can cause bleeding at the insertion site.
- Infection: There is a risk of infection associated with the insertion of the cannula and with the use of ECMO, which may require the patient to be treated with antibiotics.
- Thrombosis: There is a risk of blood clots forming in the cannula or in the ECMO circuit, which can cause blockages and potentially serious complications.
- Organ damage: ECMO can cause damage to organs such as the liver, kidneys, and spleen, as well as the brain, due to a lack of oxygen and nutrients.

- Psychological effects: ECMO can be a stressful and emotionally draining experience for patients and their families, which can have psychological consequences.

It is important to note that the risks and complications of ECMO vary from patient to patient and depend on the specific circumstances of the case. It is always important for patients to discuss the potential risks and benefits of ECMO with their healthcare team before deciding whether to undergo the procedure.

6 Special Consideration in Pregnant Women

Pregnant women who require extracorporeal membrane oxygenation (ECMO) may face unique challenges and considerations due to the presence of the unborn child.

- **Delivery timing:** The timing of delivery may need to be carefully considered in pregnant women on ECMO. If delivery is necessary, it may be necessary to coordinate the timing of delivery with ECMO support.
- **Anesthesia considerations:** Pregnant women on ECMO may have increased risks associated with general anesthesia and may require special considerations for pain management and anesthesia during delivery.
- **Maternal and fetal well-being:** The primary concern in pregnant women undergoing ECMO is the safety and well-being of both the mother and the unborn child. This may require close monitoring and management of both maternal and fetal vital signs and fetal well-being.
- **Neonatal care:** If the unborn child is born during ECMO support, special neonatal care may be necessary to ensure the health and well-being of the newborn.
- **Breastfeeding:** Pregnant women on ECMO may face challenges with breastfeeding due to the presence of the ECMO circuit and potential medication use. Special considerations and support may be necessary to ensure successful breastfeeding for both the mother and the newborn.

Overall, the management of pregnant women on ECMO requires a multidisciplinary approach and close coordination between obstetric, neonatal, and ECMO teams to ensure the best outcomes for both the mother and the unborn child.

7 Evidence and Outcome of V-V ECMO AND V-A ECMO Use in Peripartum

There is limited evidence on the use of V-V ECMO in pregnant women. The use of ECMO as a rescue treatment for patients with severe heart and lung failure has grown in popularity in recent years. However, there is little information available on the use of ECMO in pregnant and postpartum women. One study conducted a review of case reports in the literature to gather information on the use of ECMO in pregnant and postpartum patients. The findings indicate that ECMO is a viable option for these patients with severe cardiopulmonary failure; however, it should be noted that the study may have a publication bias [19]. Another case series included 54 women 9 of them were pregnant, V-V ECMO was used in 8 of them, it concluded that the use of ECMO during pregnancy and childbirth has been found to have a high success rate, with 60% of mothers and fetuses surviving. This supports the use of ECMO as a rescue treatment for pregnant and postpartum women. Given that this population is generally young and healthy, ECMO has the potential to improve survival rates for both mother and fetus. Thus, it should be considered as a viable option for women with reversible forms of heart and lung failure during the peripartum period [20].

In a review that was published in 2017, the authors searched for literature on the use of ECMO in pregnant patients and found 41 cases of VV-ECMO support and only four cases of VA-ECMO support. The survival rates for mother and fetus were 77.8% and 65%, respectively, which primarily reflect outcomes from VV-ECMO as there are only a limited number of reported cases of VA-ECMO. The impact of VA-ECMO on the blood flow in the uterus is not well understood, but continuous fetal monitoring is recommended if this form of support is needed in a viable pregnancy. In cases of VA-ECMO patients should be always kept in a lateral position, especially after 20 weeks of pregnancy as lying on the back can compress the inferior vena cava and aorta, interfering with blood flow. This is less of a concern for VV-ECMO as most patients will have a single dual-lumen cannula in the right jugular vein [21].

The survival rate does not appear to be affected by the indication or type of ECMO (VV or VA). The timing of ECMO assistance is crucial, and outcomes may be linked to its early use, especially in pregnant patients. It is important to prevent maternal hypoxia, hypercarbia, and acidosis. Referral to a specialist ECMO center with a dedicated ECMO team should be considered, either directly or after rescue implementation by a mobile ECMO team [22].

8 Conclusion

It is important to note that the use of ECMO in pregnant women is generally considered to be a last resort due to the risks associated with the procedure, including bleeding, infection, and damage to the blood vessels. The decision to use ECMO in pregnant women should be made on a case-by-case basis, considering the potential risks and benefits of the procedure.

References

1. Leonard SA, Main EK, Carmichael SL. The contribution of maternal characteristics and cesarean delivery to an increasing trend of severe maternal morbidity. BMC Pregnancy Childbirth. 2019;19(1):1–9.

2. Squiers JJ, Lima B, DiMaio JM. Contemporary extracorporeal membrane oxygenation therapy in adults: fundamental principles and systematic review of the evidence. J Thorac Cardiovasc Surg. 2016;152(1):20–32. https://doi.org/10.1016/J.JTCVS.2016.02.067.
3. Types of ECMO | Extracorporeal Membrane Oxygenation | ECLS. https://www.elso.org/ecmo-resources/types-of-ecmo.aspx. Accessed 11 Jan 2023.
4. Bartlett RH, Gattinoni L. Current status of extracorporeal life support (ECMO) for cardiopulmonary failure. Minerva Anestesiol. 2010;76(7):534–40.
5. Chamogeorgakis T, Lima B, Shafii AE, et al. Outcomes of axillary artery side graft cannulation for extracorporeal membrane oxygenation. J Thorac Cardiovasc Surg. 2013;145(4):1088–92.
6. Kanji HD, Schulze CJ, Oreopoulos A, Lehr EJ, Wang W, MacArthur RM. Peripheral versus central cannulation for extracorporeal membrane oxygenation: a comparison of limb ischemia and transfusion requirements. Thorac Cardiovasc Surg. 2010;58(8):459–62.
7. Vallabhajosyula P, Kramer M, Lazar S, et al. Lower-extremity complications with femoral extracorporeal life support. J Thorac Cardiovasc Surg. 2016;151(6):1738–44.
8. Ngatchou W, Ramadan ASE, Van Nooten G, Antoine M. Left tilt position for easy extracorporeal membrane oxygenation cannula insertion in late pregnancy patients. Interact Cardiovasc Thorac Surg. 2012;15(2):285.
9. Chung M, Shiloh AL, Carlese A. Monitoring of the adult patient on venoarterial extracorporeal membrane oxygenation. Sci World J. 2014;2014:393258.
10. Al Hanshi SAM, Al Othmani F. A case study of Harlequin syndrome in VA-ECMO. Qatar Med J. 2017;2017(1):39.
11. Bermudez CA, Rocha RV, Sappington PL, Toyoda Y, Murray HN, Boujoukos AJ. Initial experience with single cannulation for venovenous extracorporeal oxygenation in adults. Ann Thorac Surg. 2010;90(3):991–5.
12. Wong MJ, Bharadwaj S, Galey JL, Lankford AS, Galvagno S, Kodali BS. Extracorporeal membrane oxygenation for pregnant and postpartum patients. Anesth Analg. 2022;135(2):277–89.
13. Chaves RC d F, Rabello Filho R, Timenetsky KT, et al. Extracorporeal membrane oxygenation: a literature review. Rev Bras Ter Intensiva. 2019;31(3):410.
14. Peek GJ, Mugford M, Tiruvoipati R, et al. Efficacy and economic assessment of conventional ventilatory support versus extracorporeal membrane oxygenation for severe adult respiratory failure (CESAR): a multicentre randomised controlled trial. Lancet. 2009;374(9698):1351–63.
15. Naoum EE, Chalupka A, Haft J, et al. Extracorporeal life support in pregnancy: a systematic review. J Am Heart Assoc. 2020;9(13):e016072.
16. Robertson LC, Allen SH, Konamme SP, Chestnut J, Wilson P. The successful use of extracorporeal membrane oxygenation in the management of a pregnant woman with severe H1N1 2009 influenza complicated by pneumonitis and adult respiratory distress syndrome. Int J Obstet Anesth. 2010;19(4):443.
17. Duarte AG. ARDS in pregnancy. Clin Obstet Gynecol. 2014;57(4):862–70.
18. Harnisch LO, Moerer O. Contraindications to the initiation of veno-venous ecmo for severe acute respiratory failure in adults: a systematic review and practical approach based on the current literature. Membranes (Basel). 2021;11(8):584.
19. Brodie D. ECMO in pregnancy and the peripartum period. Qatar Med J. 2017;2017(1):43.
20. Webster CM, Smith KA, Manuck TA. Extracorporeal membrane oxygenation in pregnant and postpartum women: a ten-year case series. Am J Obstet Gynecol Mfm. 2020;2(2):100108.
21. Pacheco LD, Saade GR, Hankins GDV. Extracorporeal membrane oxygenation (ECMO) during pregnancy and postpartum. Semin Perinatol. 2018;42(1):21–5.
22. Fiore A, Piscitelli M, Adodo DK, et al. Successful use of extracorporeal membrane oxygenation postpartum as rescue therapy in a woman with COVID-19. J Cardiothorac Vasc Anesth. 2021;35(7):2140.

Infections in Obstetrics and Gynecology: An Intensive Care Perspective

Jameela Al Ajmi, Umme Nashrah, and Umm E Amara

Abstract Community and hospital-acquired infections are increasingly reported in obstetric and gynecological patients (OBGY). The healthcare-associated illness that has the greatest global impact on patient safety is surgical site infection (SSI). It has been linked to considerable morbidity, mortality, lengthened hospital stays, and increased hospital costs. The infection in uterus, fallopian tubes, and surrounding pelvic tissues are called pelvic inflammatory disease (PID). STIs like chlamydia or gonorrhea, which are sexually transmitted infections, are typically to blame. Among the most prevalent infections during pregnancy are urinary tract infections. Every pregnant woman should undergo a urine test to check for bacteria, and then receive antibiotic treatment if necessary. Prenatal care must include preventive antibiotics because recurrent infections are frequent. UTIs can occur up to 8% of the time in expectant women. One of the crucial aspects of prenatal treatment is maternal vaccination. Maternal protection against illnesses caused by organisms, such as influenza, pneumococcus, hepatitis, and meningococcus infections, is provided via vaccination. Obstetricians and gynecologists are required to regularly examine pregnant patients' immunization status during prenatal care.

Keyword Antibiotics · Healthcare-associated infection (HAI) · Immunization · Infection · OBGY · Pelvic inflammatory disease · Sexually transmitted infection · Surgical site infection · Urinary tract infections

---

J. Al Ajmi
Executive Director Infection Control, Hamad Medical Corporation, Doha, Qatar

U. Nashrah
Deccan College of Medical Sciences, Hyderabad, Telangana, India

U. E Amara (✉)
Apollo Institute of Medical Sciences and Research, Hyderabad, Telangana, India

N. Shaikh et al. (eds.), *Updates in Intensive Care of OBGY Patients*,
https://doi.org/10.1007/978-981-99-9577-6_14

1 Surgical Site Infection (SSI)

Surgical site infection (SSI) represents the most common healthcare-associated infection affecting patient safety worldwide. It has been associated with significant morbidity, mortality, increase hospital length of stay and hospitalization cost. The risk of SSI following lower section cesarean section (LSCS) increases eight folds compared to normal vaginal births and is one of the commonest complications with a reported incidence of 3–20% and the rates continue to raise globally [1].

Factors associated with the increased risk of SSIs include longer use of antibiotics, antibiotic-resistant pathogens diabetes mellitus, alcoholism, obesity, and immunosuppression [2]. The obstetrical risk factors for increased SSI are obstetrics, post-LSCS including, obesity, high parity, prolonged labor, emergency LSCS, premature rupture of membranes (PROM), chorioamnionitis and no regular follow-up in antenatal period. The frequently isolated organisms are *staphylococcus aureus, enterococcus spp., and Escherichia coli*, respectively [2]. In the USA, the SSI rate following hysterectomy is around 2.7%, two-thirds of these SSIs were superficial incisional infections, including vaginal cellulitis, 1.1% were deep and organ-space SSIs including vaginal cuff abscess, peritonitis, and pelvic abscess [3].

1.1 Risk Factors for SSI

There are various risk factors associated with SSI in OBGY (Obstetrics and gynecological) patients, knowing these risk factors will help to improve and optimize the prevention and control measures to reduce SSI; these factors are classified into patient related, preoperative, intraoperative, and postoperative.

1.2 Microbiology of SSI

The microbes from female genital or gastrointestinal tract contaminate the sterile amniotic fluid and uterus, thus causing and spreading infection, the most common causative pathogens isolated are *Staphylococcus aureus*, coagulase-negative staphylococci, *Enterococcus* spp., *Escherichia coli*., and Proteus mirabilis [4, 5]. The Gram-negative bacilli, enterococci, group B hemolytic streptococci, and anaerobes are frequently isolated from SSI post-gynecological procedures. There can be ascending infection bacterial vaginosis, *Neisseria Gonorrhoeae*, *Chlamydia trachomatis,* or mycoplasma genital infection following transvaginal or transcervical procedures [6].

1.3 Signs and Symptoms for SSI

SSI can cause redness, fever, pain, tenderness, warmth, or swelling and delayed healing; other signs and symptoms are based on the types of SSI:

1.4 Laboratory Test and Imaging Studies

Wound swab for Gram staining and culture is the standard to identify pathogens. Signs and symptoms for SSI are ambiguous and vague in the early phase, the local ultrasonography, computerized tomography, or magnetic resonance imaging studies along with the laboratory workup (complete blood count, erythrocyte sedimentation rate (ESR), C-reactive protein (CRP), and procalcitonin levels) can detect SSI earlier [7].

1.5 Prevention of SSI

SSIs can be prevented by the strict implementation of infection prevention control measures to reduce the risk of bacterial contamination and improve the quality of patient care. Prevention requires a multidisciplinary team approach focusing on patient and procedure-related risk factors [8]. As per the different international guidelines to reduce SSI, the measures should be taken in pre-, intra-, and postoperative periods and are summarized in Table 1 [2].

1.6 Preoperative Measures

Preoperative strategies are mostly focused on controlling and preventing patient related risk factors. Lifestyle modification such as smoking cessation, loss of weight in obese patients, adequate glycemic control, optimizing hemoglobin level, and good nutrition have been shown to reduce the incidence of SSI. Certain pre-emptive measures such as detecting drug-resistant staphylococcus aureus (MRSA) preoperatively and treating it has reduced SSIs significantly. Other prophylactic measures used preoperatively include bathing with 4% chlorhexidine solution which showed a significant reduction in the incidence of SSIs in a 10-year analysis of patient data done in the USA. Savage et al. [9] concluded the same results when using chlorhexidine bath preoperatively in abdominal hysterectomy surgeries. Generally, it is not fully proven whether bathing preoperatively (night before or just before surgery) with either soap or chlorhexidine can effectively decrease the incidence of skin and soft tissue infections, but as a general recommendation, that bathing with either of the above-mentioned preparations within 6–12 h preoperatively (once or twice)

Table 1 Prophylactic antibiotics for obstetrics and gynecology surgery [13]

Indication	Antibiotics	comments
Cesarean section	Cefazolin 2 g or cefuroxime 1.5 g	If penicillin-allergic, then clindamycin 400 mg IV + gentamycin 5 mg/kg
Abdominal hysterectomy	IV cefazolin 2 g or cefuroxime 1.5 g + metronidazole 500 mg or co-amoxiclav 1.2 g	If penicillin-allergic, then clindamycin 400 mg IV + gentamycin 5 mg/kg
Vaginal hysterectomy	IV cefazolin 2 g or cefuroxime 1.5 g + metronidazole 500 mg or co-amoxiclav 1.2 g	If penicillin-allergic, then clindamycin 400 mg IV + gentamycin 5 mg/kg
Perineal procedures	IV cefuroxime 1.5 g + metronidazole 500 mg or co-amoxiclav 1.2 g, followed by oral co-amoxiclav 625 mg 8-hourly for 5 days	If penicillin-allergic, then gentamycin 5 mg/kg + Metronidazole 500 mg, followed by oral clindamycin 300–460 mg 6-hourly for 5 days
MRSA-positive patients	IV teicoplanin 400 mg IV OR vancomycin + gentamycin 5 mg/kg	

IV intravenous, *MRSA* methicillin-resistant *Staphylococcus aureus*

should be routinely done in non-minor abdominal interventions [10]. If hair must be removed then clipping followed by covering cream is superior to shaving, as the latter is thought to cause small skin tunnels and encourages the already existing skin flora to relocate causing infections [11]. Maintaining normal body temperature and blood sugar levels in all patients (diabetic or non-diabetic) is recommended; however, no adequate data or studies have been published to support that with a high level of evidence [12].

Antimicrobial prophylaxis: Prophylactic antibiotics are one of the core components of SSI bundle to prevent SSI post-surgery. In practice, administration of first-generation cephalosporins is recommended if anaerobes are suspected then coverage is recommended accordingly (Table 1). It is crucial and frequently missed to deliver the antimicrobial coverage an hour before the intervention to achieve proper plasma and tissue amounts of the drug before starting surgery and after and to administer second dose if surgery duration is exceeding the first dose effective coverage duration.

1.7 Intraoperative Factors

Proper surgical technique maintains aseptic precautions, skin antisepsis with bacteriostatic agents such as chlorhexidine, hand decontamination with antiseptics agents such as chlorhexidine or povidone before surgery and wearing personal protective equipment will help to minimize transmission of skin microflorae and reduce risk of SSI post-surgery. Alcohol is considered superior in preparing skin at the beginning of surgery. According to the NICE guidelines, chlorhexidine should be added when mucosal surfaces are involved in surgery [2, 3].

1.8 Postoperative Factors

Surgical wound infections should be suspected in the first 30 days after intervention or 12 months after surgeries involving implants. Data suggests that such infection incidence can vary from 12% to 84% after discharge. Even after discharging, it is recommended to change dressing in a sterile manner [14].

1.9 Management of Surgical Site Infection

Treatment with antimicrobials combined with source control surgery if needed is the cornerstone in the management, penicillin with clavulanic acid preparations is the first-choice antibiotic, or metronidazole with cephalosporin together, as these regimens cover most of the common pathogens that cause surgical skin and soft tissue infections (*staphylococcus aureus* and anaerobes).

When encountering penicillin allergic patient (moderate to severe allergy), other agents should be considered as a safe and effective second-line agents (such as vancomycin and clindamycin) or based on the local antibiograms or microbiological cultures attained.

2 Pelvic Inflammatory Diseases

Pelvic inflammatory disease (PID) is an infection of the upper female genital tract, including the uterus, fallopian tubes, and adjacent pelvic structures. It is usually caused by a sexually transmitted infection (STI), like chlamydia or gonorrhea [15], or *Gardnerella vaginalis* (which causes bacterial vaginosis) *Haemophilus influenza, Mycoplasma hominis, Ureaplasma Urealyticum*, anaerobes can be causative organism (*Pepto coccus* and *Bacteroides*). Infection with chlamydia or gonorrhea may be initially difficult to differentiate in symptoms; however, gonorrhea presents with more loud and acute complaints compared to chlamydia. An estimated 10–20% of untreated chlamydial or gonorrheal infections progress to PID [16].

Prompt identification and management has a major impact on alleviating the stressing symptoms of the disease, as a consensus, that effectively treating those infections will significantly reduce the incidence of spouse infection rate, also will effectively reduce the incidence of the disease progressing to chronic infection or translocation to other cavities and organs, PID if left untreated will lead to fertility-related complications specially those related to the fallopian tube, which will affect the physiological pathway of conception and implantation leading to challenges in achieving pregnancy even with IVF (in vitro fertilization) trials [17].

In many instances of Pelvic Inflammatory Disease (PID), the condition arises due to the acquisition of infections in the vaginal or cervical region, typically stemming from sexually transmitted pathogens in the early stages of infection. During the second stage, these microorganisms ascend directly from the vagina or cervix to the upper genital tract, triggering inflammation in these structures.

Improper antibiotic treatment has the potential to disrupt the balance of the natural flora in the lower genital tract, leading to an overgrowth of vaginal flora organisms that ascend. Sexual intercourse may contribute to the ascent of infection through rhythmic uterine contractions during orgasm, and bacteria can also be transported along with sperm into the uterus and fallopian tubes.

Various microbial and host factors play a role in influencing inflammation in the upper genital tract, affecting the subsequent degree of scarring that may develop. Initially affecting the mucosa, infection of the fallopian tubes can rapidly progress to transmural inflammation. This inflammatory process, seemingly mediated by complement, may intensify with subsequent infections, extending to uninfected parametrial tissues, such as, the bowels [18].

The infection can spread through the release of purulent materials from the fallopian tubes or through the lymphatic system, reaching beyond the pelvic area. This extension can lead to the development of acute peritonitis and acute perihepatitis, a condition known as Fitz-Hugh-Curtis syndrome. In this discussion, we will explore the clinical aspects of Pelvic Inflammatory Disease (PID), including how it is managed therapeutically [18].

2.1 *Signs and Symptoms of PID*

During the early stages of PID, a patient might not notice any symptoms. However, as the infection progresses, they may experience pain in the lower abdomen and pelvis, increased bleeding during their period, bleeding between periods, discomfort during sex, fever, chills, pain or difficulty during urination, vomiting or the sensation of nausea, and abnormal cervical or vaginal discharge [19].

It is important to note that some of these symptoms can overlap with other serious medical conditions such as appendicitis, ectopic pregnancy, and endometriosis, which may lead to confusion in diagnosis. Recognizing the potential for serious reproductive complications associated with PID, there is a recommendation for a low threshold criterion for diagnosis and treatment to prevent further complications [19].

2.2 *Diagnosis*

Assess the abdomen for tenderness, by physical examination. In sexually active women, a vaginal secretions examination is performed to check for the presence of bacterial vaginosis (BV). Microscopy of the vaginal secretions, known as a wet mount, is examined for the presence of leukocytes, clue cells, and trichomonads.

Table 2 Outpatient antibiotic regimen for cervicitis [21]

One dose cefixime 400 mg
Plus
Azithromycin 1 g PO one dose only
Plus
Metronidazole 500 mg PO × 2 daily duration of 7 days for bacterial vaginosis and *Trichomonas vaginalisis*

Pelvic ultrasonography is a useful tool to rule out symptomatic ovarian cysts, while computed tomography is employed to rule out appendicitis.

The World Health Organization (WHO) recommends a syndromic management approach for PID diagnosis. This means that if patients present with lower abdominal pain and exhibit cervical motion tenderness, lower abdominal tenderness, or uterine/adnexal tenderness during pelvic examination, they are treated promptly without the need for additional time-consuming and costly laboratory tests [20].

The Centers for Disease Control and Prevention (CDC) provides diagnostic criteria to enhance the specificity of PID diagnosis. These criteria include an oral temperature greater than 101 °F (38 °C), abnormal cervical or vaginal mucopurulent discharge, the presence of white blood cells on saline microscopy of vaginal secretions, an elevated erythrocyte sedimentation rate, an elevated C-reactive protein, and laboratory documentation of cervical infection with *Neisseria gonorrhoeae* or *Chlamydia trachomatis*.

2.3 *Treatment*

The choice of antibiotic treatment should be aimed at addressing infections caused by *Chlamydia trachomatis*, *Neisseria gonorrhoeae*, *Trichomonas vaginalis*, and bacterial vaginosis (BV), which are common causes of cervicitis. A short course of an oral antibiotic regimen, as outlined in Table 2, has proven to be highly effective (89%) in bringing about the resolution of histologic endometritis.

2.4 *Mild to Moderate PID*

For women who are diagnosed with inflammation in the lower genital tract and pelvic organ tenderness but don't have a mass, it often indicates a mild to moderate infection that can be safely treated on an outpatient basis. According to the recommendations from the Centers for Disease Control and Prevention (CDC), clinicians have flexibility in choosing extended spectrum cephalosporins like ceftriaxone, ceftizoxime, and cefotaxime as alternatives to cefoxitin.

Table 3 CDC updated recommended oral regimens—2007 [2, 22]

Ceftriaxone 250 mg IM as one dose
Plus
Doxycycline 100 mg PO × 2 daily for 14 days combined with Metronidazole 500 mg PO × 2 daily for 14 days if indicated
Or
Cefoxitin 2 g IM as one dose and Probenecid 1 g PO together in one dose
Plus
Doxycycline 100 mg PO × 2 daily for 14 days combined with Metronidazole 500 mg PO × 2 daily for 14 days if indicated
Or
Other third generation cephalosporin administered orally (e.g., ceftizoxime or cefotaxime)
Plus
Doxycycline 100 mg PO × 2 daily for 14 days With Metronidazole 500 mg PO × 2 daily for 14 days if indicated

The recommended treatment plans also provide the option for clinicians to enhance anaerobic coverage by including oral metronidazole in addition to doxycycline, as outlined in Table 3.

2.5 Severe PID

Women experiencing severe pelvic inflammatory disease (PID) typically require hospitalization and inpatient parenteral therapy. The decision for hospitalization is based on several criteria [23].

1. Cases where surgical emergencies like appendicitis cannot be ruled out.
2. Hospitalization is recommended if the patient is pregnant.
3. When there's no clinical improvement with oral antibiotic therapy.
4. When patient faces challenges in following or tolerating an outpatient oral regimen.
5. If patient is severely ill, including nausea, vomiting, or high fever, needs hospitalization.
6. Tubo-ovarian abscess.

For hospitalized patients, radiological imaging such as pelvic ultrasonography or computed tomography is recommended to assess for other potential causes or the presence of a tubo-ovarian abscess. Surgical intervention may be required in addition to antibiotic treatment, especially for larger abscesses (e.g., those 10 cm or greater in diameter). Approximately 30% of abscesses measuring 7–9 cm and only 15% of those 4–6 cm in diameter may necessitate surgery.

In cases where patients continue to have persistent fever, leukocytosis, and show no improvement with antibiotic treatment within 48–72 h, surgical drainage may be considered. This drainage can be performed through methods such as laparotomy, laparoscopy, or image-guided percutaneous routes [24].

Table 4 Inpatient parenteral antibiotic regimens for the treatment of severe pelvic inflammatory disease and tubo-ovarian abscess

Recommended regimen:
1. **Ceftriaxone: 1 g intravenously every 12 h** Plus either: Metronidazole: 500 mg intravenously every 6 h Or Clindamycin: 900 mg intravenously every 8 h
2. **Alternative regimens:** Ertapenem: 1 g intravenously daily Or Piperacillin/tazobactam: 3.375 g intravenously every 6 hours Or Ticarcillin/clavulanate: 300 mg/kg/day intravenously in divided doses every 4 h Or Ampicillin/sulbactam: 3 g intravenously every 6 h
3. **Alternative Regimen for Penicillin-Allergic Patients** Levofloxacin: 500 mg orally once daily for 14 days Or Ciprofloxacin: 400 mg intravenously every 12 h Plus Metronidazole: 500 mg intravenously every 6 h

Note: Intravenous antibiotics can be switched to oral antibiotics after 48–72 h of therapy or based on clinical judgment
When Chlamydia is positive, azithromycin or doxycycline should be added
Patients allergic to penicillin, culture for quinolone-resistant *Neisseria gonorrhoeae* is necessary if quinolones are used

2.6 Antibiotic Coverage for Anaerobic Bacteria Associated with PID

For patients dealing with severe pelvic inflammatory disease (PID), the treatment involves antibiotic regimens that effectively cover both Gram-negative aerobic and anaerobic bacteria. While the antibiotics mentioned earlier exhibit moderate activity against anaerobic bacteria, an ideal outpatient treatment for PID involves a combination therapy. This typically includes an extended-spectrum cephalosporin along with doxycycline or azithromycin. Clindamycin has also been utilized in combination therapy for PID, given its effectiveness against anaerobes and its ability to reach relatively high concentrations in experimental abscesses [25]. For individuals with a penicillin allergy, a recommended alternative is a combination of a quinolone (such as ciprofloxacin or levofloxacin) and metronidazole. In these cases, testing for *Neisseria gonorrhoeae* by culture is crucial to determine susceptibility to quinolones (see Table 4).

In situations where tubo-ovarian abscesses (TOAs) are present, emergent surgical therapy may be necessary due to the risk of abscess rupture. Surgical exploration, involving the removal of the affected adnexa and drainage of purulent loculations, is considered a lifesaving intervention [26].

3 Urinary Tract Infections During Pregnancy

During pregnancy, urinary tract infections are quite common. It is recommended that all pregnant women undergo screening for bacteria in their urine and, if needed, receive antibiotic treatment. Recurrent infections are also quite usual during pregnancy and often call for preventive treatment. The occurrence of urinary tract infections in pregnant women can be as high as 8%. It is important to address these issues to ensure the well-being of both the expecting mother and the baby [27].

3.1 Pathogenesis

The likelihood of urinary tract infections (UTIs) tends to rise during pregnancy, typically beginning around week 6 and reaching a peak during 22–24 weeks. Several factors contribute to this increased risk, including heightened bladder volume, reduced bladder tone, decreased ureteral tone, and ureteral dilatation (hydronephrosis). These changes collectively result in increased urinary stasis and ureterovesical reflux.

Around 70% of pregnant women experience glycosuria, a condition that fosters bacterial growth in the urine. Additionally, the increased levels of urinary progestins and estrogens during pregnancy may diminish the lower urinary tract's ability to fend off invading bacteria. It is crucial to recognize these factors as they play a role in the heightened vulnerability to UTIs in pregnant women during specific stages of gestation [28].

3.2 Microbiology

The primary culprit behind most urinary tract infections (UTIs) is *Escherichia coli* (*E. coli*), responsible for 80–90% of these infections. Other commonly encountered Gram-negative rods include Proteus mirabilis and Klebsiella pneumoniae. While less frequent, Gram-positive organisms like group B streptococcus and *Staphylococcus saprophyticus* can also contribute to UTIs. Additionally, less commonly encountered microorganisms that may lead to UTIs encompass *enterococci*, *Gardnerella vaginalis*, and *Ureaplasma ureolyticum*. Understanding these causative agents is vital for effective diagnosis and treatment of UTIs [29].

3.3 Diagnosis of UTIs

There are three types of urinary tract infection (UTI) presentations: asymptomatic bacteriuria, acute cystitis, and pyelonephritis.

1. Asymptomatic Bacteriuria is identified by the isolation of bacteria in amounts exceeding 10^5 (or 100,000) colony-forming units per mL of urine in an individual without any symptoms of a urinary tract infection (UTI). If left untreated during pregnancy, asymptomatic bacteriuria can progress to symptomatic cystitis in about 30% of patients and to pyelonephritis in up to 50%. It is also associated with an increased risk of low-birth-weight infants and intra-uterine growth retardation [30].

Table 5 Treatment of UTIs during pregnancy [31]

Antibiotic	Pregnancy category	Dosage
Cephalexin (Keflex)	B	250 mg two or four times daily
Erythromycin	B	250–500 mg four times daily
Nitrofurantoin (Macrodantin)	B	50–100 mg four times daily
Sulfisoxazole (Gantrisin)	C*	1 g four times daily
Amoxicillin-clavulanic acid (Augmentin)	B	250 mg four times daily
Fosfomycin (Monurol)	B	One 3-g sachet
Trimethoprim-sulfamethoxazole (Bactrim)	C	160/180 mg twice daily

Guyatt, Gordon H.; Oxman, Andrew D.; Vist, Gunn E.; Kunz, Regina; Falck-Ytter, Yngve; Alonso-Coello, Pablo; Schünemann, Holger J.; GRADE Working Group (2008-04-26). “GRADE: an emerging consensus on rating quality of evidence and strength of recommendations”. BMJ (Clinical research ed.). 336 (7650): 924–926

Table 6 Urinary tract infection caused by multidrug-resistant Gram-negative bacteria in patients with any of the following occurrences within the past 3 months

1.	Isolation of a multidrug-resistant Gram-negative urinary strain or a fluoroquinolone-resistant *Pseudomonas aeruginosa* strain.
2.	Recent stay at a healthcare or acute care facility.
3.	Use fluoroquinolones, trimethoprim-sulfamethoxazole, or broad-spectrum beta-lactams.
4.	Travel to regions with high rates of multidrug-resistant organisms.

It is important to note that multidrug resistance defined as a lack of susceptibility to at least one agent in three or more antibiotic classes, and this includes isolates producing an extended-spectrum beta-lactamase (ESBL)

2. Pregnant women should be treated if bacteriuria is isolated during the screening period. The choice of antibiotics should consider the most common isolating organisms in urine, such as Gram-negative gastrointestinal organisms. Moreover, the selected antibiotic should be safe for both the pregnant woman and the fetus. While ampicillin has traditionally been the preferred drug for UTI treatment, it is worth noting that the resistance of *E. coli* to ampicillin has increased in recent years, reaching levels of 20–30%. Therefore, careful consideration of antibiotic choices is crucial for effective and safe treatment of UTIs during pregnancy (Table 5).
3. Multidrug resistance urinary tract infections are defined in Table 6.

4 Acute Cystitis

This form of urinary tract infection (UTI) is frequently observed in women and is distinguishable from asymptomatic bacteriuria by the presence of noticeable symptoms like dysuria, urgency, and frequency, particularly in patients without a fever. If a patient has a history of specific factors within the past 3 months (Table 6), there is a suspicion of a urinary tract infection caused by multidrug-resistant Gram-negative bacteria.

4.1 Duration of Treatment

For non-pregnant patients with acute cystitis, a 3-day treatment course appears to yield a similar cure rate as a longer course of 7–10 days. However, it is essential to note that this finding has not been extensively studied in pregnant individuals. In pregnant patients, opting for shorter treatment periods with a higher rate of recurrence may have serious consequences [31].

5 Pyelonephritis

Acute pyelonephritis, a common bacterial infection affecting the renal pelvis and kidney, poses a substantial risk during pregnancy. It can progress to maternal sepsis, preterm labor, and premature delivery. Symptoms include fever, chills, nausea, vomiting, and flank pain. In pregnant women, pyelonephritis occurs in 2%, and up to 23% of these cases experience a recurrence within the same pregnancy [32].

5.1 Diagnostic Tests

A positive urinalysis and urine culture, alongside a compatible history and physical examination, confirm the diagnosis. Blood culture is recommended for hospitalized patients with acute pyelonephritis showing signs of sepsis. Bacteremia is found in 15–30% of non-pregnant women with acute pyelonephritis [33].

5.2 Imaging Studies

Typically, unnecessary unless symptoms persist or there is a recurrence. Imaging aims to identify structural abnormalities, and renal ultrasonography is preferred for pregnant women.

5.3 Microbiology

Escherichia coli is the predominant pathogen in 80% of acute pyelonephritis cases. Other causative organisms include *Enterobacteriaceae*, *Pseudomonas aeruginosa*, group B *streptococci*, *enterococci*, and *Staphylococcus saprophyticus*.

Table 7 Continuous vs. postcoital antimicrobial prophylaxis for recurrent urinary tract infections during pregnancy [35]

Antimicrobial agent	Continuous prophylaxis (daily dosage)	Postcoital (one-time dose)
Cephalexin (Keflex)	125–250 mg	250 mg
Nitrofurantoin	50–100 mg	50–100 mg

5.4 Treatment

Early treatment is crucial to prevent complications. Hospitalization is recommended for patients exhibiting signs of sepsis, vomiting, dehydration, or contractions.

Group B Streptococcal Infection in Pregnant Patients: Group B Streptococcus (GBS) is a bacteria present in the intestines, vagina, and rectum, known to cause neonatal sepsis and associated with preterm rupture of membranes and preterm labor. GBS can also lead to UTIs in 5% of pregnant patients. Pregnant women with GBS bacteriuria should receive treatment at diagnosis, using amoxicillin or cephalexin, and prophylactic penicillin G during labor [34].

5.5 Antimicrobial Prophylaxis

Despite appropriate treatment, recurrent UTIs may occur, defined as two infections in 6 months or three infections in 1 year. Prophylactic therapy is effective in preventing recurrent UTIs. See Table 7 for details on preventive therapy.

6 Sexual Transmitted Disease (STDs)

6.1 Addressing the Global Challenge of Sexually Transmitted Infections (STIs)

Sexually transmitted infections (STIs) pose a significant and widespread public health concern on a global scale. The World Health Organization (WHO) reports that more than one million STIs are acquired daily worldwide. A concerning aspect is that the majority of these infections are asymptomatic, increasing the likelihood of unknowingly transmitting the infection to others.

In 2016, an alarming estimate revealed that almost one million pregnant women were affected by syphilis, leading to over 350,000 adverse birth outcomes. This underscores the far-reaching consequences of STIs, particularly in vulnerable populations.

The imperative for screening for STIs cannot be overstated. This proactive measure is crucial for early identification and treatment of infected individuals before complications arise. Equally important is the identification, testing, and treatment of the sexual partners of those infected. This comprehensive approach is vital to prevent the transmission of STIs and subsequent reinfections, ultimately contributing to improved public health outcomes [36].

6.2 Understanding Sexually Transmitted Infections (STIs)

Sexually transmitted infections (STIs) can be caused by various pathogens, each presenting unique challenges. Bacterial infections such as chlamydia, gonorrhea, and syphilis are among the culprits. Additionally, viral STIs encompass a range of infections, including human papillomavirus (HPV), Hepatitis B, genital herpes, HIV/AIDS, genital warts, while parasitic STIs include trichomoniasis. It is essential to recognize that these infections, if left untreated, can have serious consequences.

6.3 *Neisseria gonorrhoeae*

Unveiling the Impact Gonorrhea, caused by the Gram-negative coccus *Neisseria gonorrhoeae*, is a prevalent infection affecting sexually active individuals globally. This infection stands out as a major contributor to cervicitis in females, potentially leading to pelvic inflammatory disease (PID), infertility, ectopic pregnancy, and chronic pelvic pain. Despite being uncommon, invasive infections with *N. gonorrhoeae*, such as disseminated gonococcal infection, meningitis, and endocarditis, can result in severe morbidity. However, a concerning trend has emerged with the global spread of Gonococcal resistance to various classes of antimicrobial agents. This resistance poses a significant challenge in effectively managing and treating gonorrhea. Genital infections are particularly common in female patients, highlighting the need for heightened awareness and preventive measures.

Understanding the dynamics of these infections is crucial not only for individual well-being but also for the broader public health landscape. Effective strategies for prevention, screening, and treatment are essential in mitigating the impact of STIs and fostering a healthier, more informed society [36], associated infection caused by gonorrhea:

6.4 Cervicitis

The uterine cervix takes center stage as the most common site of mucosal infection with *Neisseria gonorrhoeae* in females [37]. Astonishingly, almost 70% of female patients may exhibit no symptoms. However, some may experience vaginal pruritus and/or a mucopurulent discharge. A physical examination might reveal a normal cervix appearance or signs of frank discharge with friable cervical mucosa.

6.5 *Urethritis*

In up to 90% of females with gonococcal cervicitis, *Neisseria gonorrhoeae* can be isolated from the urethra. Clinical symptoms may include dysuria, urinary urgency, or frequency [37].

6.6 *Pelvic Inflammatory Disease (PID)*

As discussed earlier, PID can result from untreated infections and is associated with serious complications such as infertility, ectopic pregnancy, and chronic pelvic pain.

6.7 *Bartholinitis*

Inflammation of Bartholin's glands, situated behind the labia, may occur in up to 6% of females with genital gonococcal infection. Symptoms may include perilabial pain and discharge, with signs like edema of the labia and enlargement and tenderness of the gland [38].

6.8 *Complications of Pregnancy*

Urogenital gonococcal infections during pregnancy have been linked to adverse outcomes, including chorioamnionitis, premature rupture of membranes, preterm birth, low birth weight, and spontaneous abortions [39].

6.9 *Other Infections Caused by* N. Gonorrhoeae *in Female Patients*

6.9.1 Pharyngitis

Typically acquired through oral sexual exposure, pharyngeal Gonococcal infection prevalence among females ranges from 0% to 30%.

6.9.2 Disseminated Gonococcal Infection

Bacteremia secondary to *N. gonorrhoeae* infection can occur in 0.5–3% of infected patients, leading to various clinical manifestations, including purulent arthritis, tenosynovitis, dermatitis, and poly-arthralgias [40].

6.9.3 Conjunctivitis

More commonly seen in infants born to untreated mothers, adult cases may result from autoinoculation from an anogenital source.

6.10 Diagnostic Testing

6.10.1 Nucleic Acid Amplification (NAAT)

Recommended for diagnosing *N. gonorrhoeae* infections, providing rapid results with good sensitivity [41].

6.10.2 Testing for Extra Genital Specimens

NAAT is highly sensitive for detecting *N. gonorrhoeae* at extra genital sites like the oropharynx and rectum [42].

6.10.3 Gram Stain (Microscopy)

Limited specificity in females due to the presence of other non-pathogenic Gram-negative diplococci in cervical secretions.

6.10.4 Culture

Necessary for assessing antibiotic susceptibilities, especially in cases of suspected antibiotic-resistant infections.

6.10.5 Antigen Detection

Enzyme immunoassay (EIA) for gonococcal antigens, with acceptable predictive value in populations with a high prevalence of infection.

6.10.6 Evaluation of Co-infection

Recognition of potential coexistence with *Chlamydia trachomatis*, prompting testing for both pathogens. Screening for additional sexually transmitted pathogens such as HIV and syphilis is also indicated [36].

Table 8 Treatment of urogenital and anorectal infections [44]

Antibiotic		Dose
Preferred	High" dose intramuscular ceftriaxone	For those with a weight below 150 kg, administer a single dose of 500 mg of Ceftriaxone intramuscularly (IM) Weighing 150 kg or more, administer a single dose of 1 g of Ceftriaxone IM
Alternative	Ceftazidime	500 mg IM
	Cefoxitin plus Probenecid	2 g IM Cefoxitin Plus Probenecid 1 g orally
	Cefotaxime	500 mg IM
	Cefixime	800 mg orally once
	Azithromycin plus gentamicin	Azithromycin 2 g PO once Plus gentamicin 240 mg IM once
	Spectinomycin	2 g IM

6.10.7 Treatment of *Neisseria Gonorrhoeae* Infections

Gonorrhea has exhibited increasing resistance to antimicrobial therapy over time. The Global Gonococcal Antimicrobial Surveillance Program (GASP), initiated in 1992 by the World Health Organization (WHO), diligently documents the emergence and spread of antimicrobial resistance in gonorrhea globally. Refer to Table 8 for specific details [43].

Treatment of urogenital and anorectal infections is described in Table 8.

7 Pregnant Women

Pregnant women diagnosed with uncomplicated gonorrheal infection can receive high-dose intramuscular ceftriaxone (as mentioned earlier).

For presumptive treatment of chlamydia in pregnant individuals, azithromycin is preferred over doxycycline. In cases where a pregnant patient exhibits a severe mediated allergy to cephalosporins, desensitization procedures should be undertaken before administering treatment. If desensitization is not feasible or the patient has a severe beta-lactam allergy preventing cephalosporin treatment, an alternative regimen involving gentamicin plus azithromycin can be considered [44].

Retesting is necessary for all individuals, including pregnant women, within 3 months after treatment, with pregnant women requiring an additional test during the third trimester.

8 Prevention [45]

Individuals should abstain from all sexual activity for at least 7 days after treatment, and their sexual partners should also undergo appropriate treatment. Providing education on precautions and preventive measures, such as offering condoms and using therapeutic antibiotics immediately before or soon after exposure, can help mitigate the risk of infection.

8.1 Behavioral Counseling

Behavioral counseling in STD clinics has been shown to effectively reduce the incidence of STDs in at-risk adults. Patients should be actively encouraged to inform their sexual partners of the infection and motivate them to seek medical care.

8.2 Maternal Immunization

Ensuring the health and well-being of pregnant women involves incorporating maternal immunization as a crucial component of care. Vaccination plays a vital role in offering maternal protection against infections associated with particular pathogens, including influenza, pneumococcus, hepatitis, and meningococcus. Regular evaluation of the vaccination status of pregnant women is a fundamental aspect of prenatal care and should be carried out by obstetrician and gynecologist providers. According to the American College of Obstetricians and gynecologists committee (ACOG), there is no evidence of adverse fetal effects resulting from maternal vaccination with inactivated or killed bacteria or virus vaccines, as well as toxoids [46].

8.3 Background

Ensuring the health and well-being of pregnant women involves prioritizing influenza vaccination as a crucial measure. This vaccination significantly reduces the risk of maternal morbidity and mortality, along with minimizing fetal complications such as congenital anomalies, spontaneous abortion, and preterm birth. Pregnant women who are at risk for infections like pneumococcus, hepatitis, and meningococcus are also recommended to receive vaccines targeting these specific infections. Vaccines such as tetanus toxoid, diphtheria, and acellular pertussis (Tdap) are administered to pregnant women ideally between the 27th and 36th weeks of gestation. It is essential for all pregnant women to receive influenza vaccination during the influenza season, along with the Tdap vaccine. Certain vaccinations are reserved for use exclusively in the post-partum period, as outlined in Table 9.

Table 9 Maternal vaccination during pregnancy [48]

COVID-19	CDC and ACOG guidance state that COVID-19 vaccination is recommends for pregnant women who haven't received it before. This vaccination is safe during any trimester. The pregnant, recently pregnant individuals up to 6 weeks post-partum are recommended to receive a bivalent mRNA COVID-19 vaccine booster after completing their last primary vaccine dose or monovalent booster. Post-partum and/or lactating women who were not previously vaccinated are also encouraged to get vaccinated.
Inactivated influenza	Influenzas vaccine is safe and can be given in any trimester, recommended during seasonal influenza.
Tetanus, reduce diphtheria toxoid, and acellular pertussis (Tdap)	Tdap vaccine can be given at 27–36 week of pregnancy to support the mother's immune system and enhance the passive antibody to the newborn.
Quadrivalent meningococcal conjugate	The quadrivalent conjugate meningococcal vaccine is advisable for individuals with complement deficiency, HIV, asplenia, and those traveling to endemic areas. Pregnancy should not be a deterrent to vaccination when the vaccine is strongly indicated.
Pneumococcal vaccines	Pregnant women deemed to be at high risk for severe pneumococcal diseases can be vaccinated with 13-valent pneumococcal vaccine.
Hepatitis A	Pregnant women who are at risk of severe Hepatitis A infection, those traveling to endemic areas or with chronic liver diseases and clotting factor disorders, should consider vaccination. The vaccine can be administered either during pregnancy or post-partum.
Hepatitis B	Pregnant women identified as at risk of hepatitis B during pregnancy, those with a hepatitis B surface antigen-positive sex partner, multiple sex partners in the last 6 months, a history of STD evaluation, HIV infection, chronic liver disease, or recent travel to specific countries, should receive counseling.
Human papillomavirus (HPV)	Not recommended during pregnancy, can be given post-partum and breast-feeding women. Women up to the age of 26 who have not received the HPV vaccine previously are advised to consult with an infectious diseases expert before getting vaccinated.
Measles-mumps-Rubella	Live attenuated vaccines, such as Measles-Mumps-Rubella (MMR) and Varicella, are not recommended during pregnancy. However, they can be administered post-partum if deemed necessary.
Varicella	Live attenuated vaccine is contraindicated during pregnancy. Can be give post-partum.

A. A history of severe allergy to eggs or any vaccine ingredients, as well as a history of Guillain-Barré syndrome within 2–3 weeks post-vaccination

B. The CDC recommends pneumococcal vaccination for adults aged 19–64 with specific chronic medical conditions, including chronic heart disease, liver disease, chronic obstructive pulmonary disease (COPD), emphysema, asthma, chronic renal failure, diabetes, HIV, malignancy, etc.

C. The serogroup B vaccine should be postponed in pregnant individuals unless they are at an elevated risk of serogroup B meningococcal disease

D. This applies particularly to seronegative individuals

Obstetricians, gynecologists, and other healthcare providers play a critical role in assessing the vaccination status of their pregnant patients. Studies have demonstrated that when healthcare providers directly recommend vaccinations to their patients, the likelihood of vaccine acceptance increases significantly, with odds ratios ranging from fivefold to 50-fold. Consequently, all healthcare providers should routinely assess the eligibility of their patients for vaccination and promptly administer the necessary vaccines to pregnant individuals [47, 48].

9 Conclusion

Patients undergoing obstetric and gynecologic procedures are increasingly vulnerable to both community- and hospital-acquired infections. One of the most globally impactful conditions affecting patient safety in healthcare is Surgical Site Infection (SSI). It has been associated with significant morbidity, mortality, prolonged hospital stays, and increased hospital costs. Pelvic Inflammatory Disease (PID) is an infection involving the upper female genital system, encompassing the uterus, fallopian tubes, and nearby pelvic tissues. Sexually transmitted infections, particularly chlamydia or gonorrhea, are often implicated. Urinary tract infections are prevalent during pregnancy, emphasizing the importance of screening pregnant women for bacterial presence in the urine and administering antibiotic therapy when necessary. The inclusion of preventive antibiotics in prenatal care is essential due to the recurrence of these infections.

References

1. Gomaa K, Abdelraheim AR. Incidence, risk factors and management of post cesarean section surgical site infection (SSI) in a tertiary hospital in Egypt: a five-year retrospective study. BMC Pregnancy Childbirth. 2021;21:63.
2. Owens CD, Stoessel K. Surgical site infections: epidemiology, microbiology, and prevention. J Hosp Infect. 2008;70(Suppl. 2):3–10.
3. Ekanem EE, et al. Surgical site infection in obstetrics and gynaecology: prevention and management. Obstet Gynaecol. 2021;23:124–37.
4. Weigelt JA, Lipsky BA, Tabak YP, Derby KG, Kim M, Gupta V. Surgical site infections: causative pathogens and associated outcomes. Am J Infect Control. 2010;38:112–20.
5. Lazenby GB, Sober DE. Prevention, diagnosis and treatment of gynaecological surgical site infections. Obstet Gynecol Clin N Am. 2010;37:379–86.
6. Peipert JF, Weitzen S, Cruickshank C, Story E, Etheridge D, Lapane K. Risk factors for febrile morbidity after hysterectomy. Obstet Gynecol. 2004;103:86–91.
7. Kim MH, Park JH, Kim JT. A reliable diagnostic method of surgical site infection after posterior lumbar surgery based on serial C-reactive protein. Int J Surg Glob Health. 2021;4(5):e61.
8. Berrios-Torres SI, Umscheid CA, Bratzler DW, Leas B, Stone EC, Kelz RR, et al. Centers for Disease Control and Prevention guideline for the prevention of surgical site infection, 2017. JAMA Surg. 2017;152:789–91.

9. Kaiser AB, Kemodle DS, Barg NL, Petracek MR. Influence of preoperative showers on staphylococcal skin colonization: a comparative trial of antiseptic skin cleansers. Ann Thorac Surg. 1988;45(35–8):36.
10. Ban KA, Minei JP, Laronga C, Harbrecht BG, Jensen EH, Fry DE, et al. American College of Surgeons and Surgical Site Infection Society; surgical site infection guidelines, 2016 update. J Am Coll Surg. 2017;224:59–74.
11. National Institute for Health and Care Excellence (NICE). Surgical site infections: prevention and treatment. NICE guideline [NG125]. London: NICE; 2019. p. 1–28.
12. Berríos-Torres SI, Umscheid CA, Bratzler DW, Leas B, Stone EC, Kelz RR, Reinke CE, Morgan S, Solomkin JS, Mazuski JE, Dellinger EP. Centers for disease control and prevention guideline for the prevention of surgical site infection. JAMA. 2017;152(8):784–91.
13. Kenyon SL, Taylor DJ, Tarnow-Mordi W, ORACLE Collaborative Group. Broad spectrum antibiotics for preterm, prelabour rupture of fetal membranes. The ORACLE study. Lancet. 2001;357:979–88.
14. Mangram AJ, Horan TC, Pearson ML, Silver LC, Jarvis WR. Hospital Infection Control Practice Advisory CommitteeGuideline for prevention of surgical site infection, 1999. Infect Control Hosp Epidemiol. 1999;20(247):278.
15. [Guideline] Royal College of Obstetricians and Gynaecologists (RCOG). Management of acute pelvic inflammatory disease. London, UK: Royal College of Obstetricians and Gynaecologists (RCOG); 2008.
16. Herzog SA, Althaus CL, Heijne JC, Oakeshott P, Kerry S, Hay P, et al. Timing of progression from Chlamydia trachomatis infection to pelvic inflammatory disease: a mathematical modelling study. BMC Infect Dis. 2012;12:187.
17. Romero R, Espinoza J, Mazor M. Can endometrial infection/inflammation explain implantation failure, spontaneous abortion, and preterm birth after in vitro fertilization? Fertil Steril. 2004;82(4):799–804.
18. Patton DL, Wolner-Hanssen P, Zeng W, Lampe M, Wong K, Stamm WE, et al. The role of spermatozoa in the pathogenesis of Chlamydia trachomatis salpingitis in a primate model. Sex Transm Dis. 1993;20(4):214–9.
19. Westrom L. Effect of acute pelvic inflammatory disease on fertility. Am J Obstet Gynecol. 1975;121:707–13.
20. World Health Organization. Sexually transmitted and other reproductive tract infections: a guide to essential practice; 2005.
21. Eckert LO, Thwin SS, Hillier SL, Kiviat NB, Eschenbach DA. The antimicrobial treatment of subacute endometritis: a proof of concept study. Am J Obstet Gynecol. 2004;190:305–13.
22. Centers for Disease Control and Prevention. Updated treatment recommendations for gonococcal infections and associated conditions. GA, USA: CDC; 2007.
23. Workowski KA, Berman SM, Centers for Disease Control and Prevention. Sexually transmitted diseases treatment guidelines. MMWR Recomm Rep. 2006;55(RR-11):1–94. Erratum in: *MMWR Recomm.* Rep 55, 7 (2006)
24. Reed SD, Landers DV, Sweet RL. Antibiotic treatment of tuboovarian abscess: comparison of broad-spectrum β-lactam agents versus clindamycin-containing regimens. Am J Obstet Gynecol. 1991;164:1556–62.
25. Sivapalasingam S, Steigbigel NH. Macrolides, clindamycin, and ketolides. In: Principles and practice of infectious diseases. 7th ed. Philadelphia, PA: Churchill Livingstone Elsevier; 2010. p. 442.
26. Wiesenfeld HC, Sweet RL. Progress in the management of tuboovarian abscesses. Clin Obstet Gynecol. 1993;36:433–4.
27. Patterson TF, Andriole VT. Bacteriuria in pregnancy. Infect Dis Clin N Am. 1987;1(4):807–22.
28. Lucas MJ, Cunningham FG. Urinary infection in pregnancy. Clin Obstet Gynecol. 1993;36:855–68.
29. Barr JG, Ritchie JW, Henry O, el Sheikh M, el Deeb K. Microaerophilic/anaerobic bacteria as a cause of urinary tract infection in pregnancy. Br J Obstet Gynaecol. 1985;92:506–10.

30. Harris RE, Thomas VL, Shelokov A. Asymptomatic bacteriuria in pregnancy: antibody-coated bacteria, renal function, and intrauterine growth retardation. Am J Obstet Gynecol. 1976;126:20–5.
31. Duff P. Antibiotic selection for infections in obstetric patients. Semin Perinatol. 1993;17:367–78.
32. Gilstrap LC 3rd, Cunningham FG, Whalley PJ. Acute pyelonephritis in pregnancy: an anterospective study. Obstet Gynecol. 1981;57:409–13.
33. Velasco M, Martínez JA, Moreno-Martínez A, et al. Blood cultures for women with uncomplicated acute pyelonephritis: are they necessary? Clin Infect Dis. 2003;37(8):1127–30.
34. Anon. Prevention of perinatal group B streptococcal disease: a public health perspective. Centers for Disease Control and Prevention. MMWR Morb Mortal Wkly Rep. 1996;45:1–24. [published erratum in MMWR Morb Mortal Wkly Rep 1996;45(31): 679]
35. Pfau A, Sacks TG. Effective prophylaxis for recurrent urinary tract infections during pregnancy. Clin Infect Dis. 1992;14:810–4.
36. Ghanem KG. Screening for sexually transmitted infections. UpToDate. 2022;
37. Barlow D, Phillips I. Gonorrhoeae in women. Diagnostic, clinical, and laboratory aspects. Lancet. 1978;1:761.
38. Rees E. Gonococcal bartholinitis. Br J Vener Dis. 1967;43:150.
39. Walker CK, Sweet RL. Gonorrhea infection in women: prevalence, effects, screening, and management. Int J Women's Health. 2011;3:197–206.
40. O'Brien JP, Goldenberg DL, Rice PA. Disseminated gonococcal infection: a prospective analysis of 49 patients and a review of pathophysiology and immune mechanisms. Medicine (Baltimore). 1983;62:395.
41. Centers for Disease Control and Prevention. Recommendations for the laboratory-based detection of Chlamydia trachomatis and Neisseria gonorrhoeae—2014. MMWR Recomm Rep. 2014;63:1.
42. Walsh A, Rourke FO, Crowley B. Molecular detection and confirmation of Neisseria gonorrhoeae in urogenital and extragenital specimens using the Abbott CT/NG RealTime assay and an in-house assay targeting the porA pseudogene. Eur J Clin Microbiol Infect Dis. 2011;30:561.
43. World Health Organization. The Gonococcal Antimicrobial Surveillance Programme (GASP) http://www.who.int/reproductivehealth/topics/rtis/gonococcal_resistance/en/ (Accessed on July 10, 2017).
44. Seña AC, Cohen MS. Treatment of uncomplicated Neisseria gonorrhoeae infections. Up to date to CDC's treatment guidelines for gonococcal infection. 2020;69(50):1911–16.
45. Qureshi S, Chandrasekar PH. Gonorrhea treatment & management. Medscape; 2021.
46. Ault KA, Laura E. Maternal immunization. ACOG committee Opinion. Obstet Gynecol. 2018;131(6):e214–7.
47. CDC. Use of 13-valent pneumococcal conjugate vaccine and 23-valent pneumococcal polysaccharide vaccine for adults with immunocompromising conditions: recommendations of the Advisory Committee on Immunization Practices (ACIP). MMWR Morb Mortal Wkly Rep. 2012;61:816–9.
48. American College of obstetricians and Gynecologists. Update on immunization and pregnancy, tetanus, diphtheria and pertussis vaccination. Committee opinion No.718. Obstet Gynecol. 2017;130:e153–7.

Radiological Imaging in the Intensive Care Management of Obstetric Emergencies: Safety Considerations, Best Practices, and Common Pathologies

Adam Mushtak, Umais Zaid Momin, Zahoor Ahmed, Shaikh Asra Mahemood, and Khulood AbdulHameed

Abstract Radiology and imaging play an important role in the management of critically ill obstetric patients in the intensive care unit (ICU). These patients require specialized imaging techniques to diagnose and monitor their medical conditions, which can be complex and often life-threatening.

One of the key considerations when imaging critically ill ICU obstetric patients is radiation exposure. Pregnant patients are particularly sensitive to radiation, and radiation exposure can pose a risk to the developing fetus. Therefore, imaging protocols must be carefully tailored to minimize radiation exposure while still providing accurate diagnostic information. Techniques such as ultrasound and magnetic resonance imaging (MRI) are preferred over computed tomography (CT) scans, which expose patients to higher levels of radiation.

Imaging is often required for a variety of medical conditions that obstetric patients may experience. One such condition is preeclampsia, a pregnancy-related disorder characterized by high blood pressure and damage to organs such as the liver and kidneys. Ultrasound can be used to assess fetal growth, blood flow, and amniotic fluid levels, while MRI can provide information on the extent of organ damage.

Another condition that may require imaging in critically ill ICU obstetric patients is pulmonary embolism (PE), a blockage in the lungs caused by a blood clot. PE is a leading cause of maternal mortality, and prompt diagnosis and treatment are essential. Imaging techniques such as CT pulmonary angiography and ventilation-perfusion (V/Q) scanning can be used to diagnose PE and assess its severity.

A. Mushtak (✉) · K. AbdulHameed
Clinical Imaging Department, Hamad General Hospital, Doha, Qatar

Weill Cornell Medicine—Qatar, Al-Rayyan, Qatar

U. Z. Momin · Z. Ahmed
Clinical Imaging Department, Hamad General Hospital, Doha, Qatar

S. A. Mahemood
Department of Radiology, Al Ahli Hospital, Doha, Qatar

N. Shaikh et al. (eds.), *Updates in Intensive Care of OBGY Patients*,
https://doi.org/10.1007/978-981-99-9577-6_15

Imaging may also be required for obstetric emergencies such as placental abruption, a condition in which the placenta separates from the uterine wall before delivery. Ultrasound can be used to diagnose placental abruption and assess fetal well-being, while MRI can provide additional information on the extent of placental separation.

Other medical conditions that may require imaging in critically ill ICU obstetric patients include hemorrhage, sepsis, and acute respiratory distress syndrome (ARDS). Hemorrhage can be diagnosed using ultrasound and CT scans, while sepsis can be diagnosed using a combination of blood tests and imaging techniques such as CT scans and chest X-rays. ARDS, which is characterized by severe respiratory failure, can be diagnosed using chest X-rays and CT scans to assess the extent of lung damage.

This chapter focuses on the role of radiology and imaging in the management of critically ill obstetric patients in the ICU, with considerations for radiation exposure and medical conditions that require imaging.

Keywords Radiology · Imaging intensive care unit · Critical illness · Obstetrics · Pregnancy · Radiation exposure · Ultrasound · Magnetic resonance imaging · Computed tomography · Preeclampsia · Pulmonary embolism · Placental abruption · Hemorrhage · Diagnostic imaging · Maternal mortality · Medical imaging techniques

1 Introduction

Radiological imaging remains to be a crucial part of diagnosis, wherein the role of imaging, if anything has been further increasing with further advances in technology and the complexities in management and treatment.

The indications for imaging in pregnant woman can be broadly classified into pathologies as being obstetric related or non-obstetric related (Fig. 1).

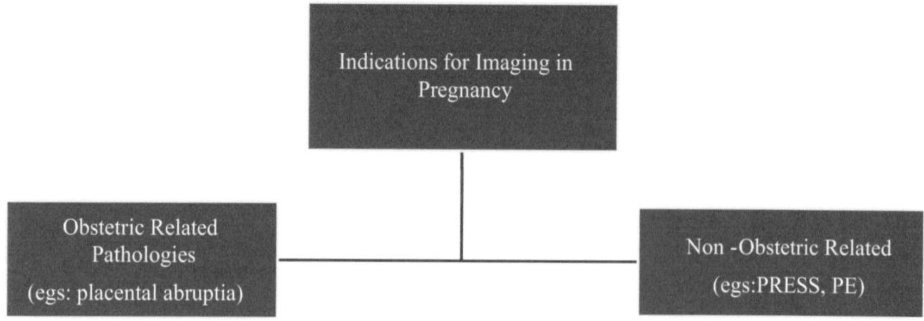

Fig. 1 Flowchart showing the categories of pathologies that require imaging during pregnancy in terms of organ/organ system involvement

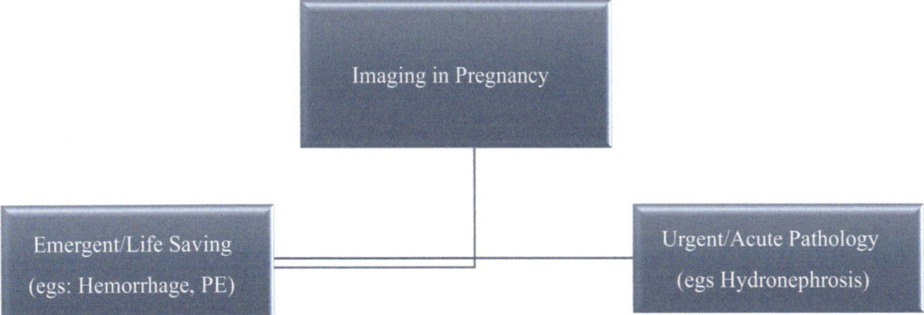

Fig. 2 Flowchart showing the categories of pathologies that require imaging during pregnancy in terms of the severity and acuity

In terms of indications for imaging in pregnant woman, they can also be classified into life-saving/emergent or acute/urgent imaging based on the severity of the pathology (Fig. 2).

A brief discussion/description of the various commonly encountered emergent, urgent both obstetric and non-obstetric complications/pathologies that require imaging are discussed later in this chapter.

1.1 Why a Pregnant Woman Is in the ICU?

Pregnant women make up a small proportion of ICU admissions and may require intensive care for obstetric or non-obstetric reasons. They may be admitted at any stage of pregnancy or in the postpartum period, with pregnancy sometimes being discovered during ICU admission. Therefore, managing the mother optimally is crucial for the fetus as well. Diagnostic imaging that uses ionizing radiation must be considered carefully, along with other factors such as maternal shock, physiological disturbances, and medications, due to the potential harmful effects on the fetus [1].

Hypertensive disorders of pregnancy are the most common reason for ICU admission, with a median of 0.9 cases per 1000 deliveries. The profile of ICU admissions is similar in both developed and developing countries, except for a significantly higher maternal mortality rate in developing countries (median 3.3% vs. 14.0%, $p = 0.002$). Common indications for ICU admission include preeclampsia, sepsis, obstetric hemorrhage, cerebral encephalopathy, amniotic fluid embolism, trauma, and preexisting medical problems [2].

A complete exhaustive list of conditions that could lead to ICU care in a pregnant woman is beyond the scope of this chapter; however, a review of the most commonly encountered etiologies and pathologies in a seriously ill pregnant woman are discussed later in this chapter.

2 Principles of Imaging in Pregnancy and Obstetrics

Radiation hazards are a concern due to their possible negative effects on the fetus. However, some ionizing radiation-based tests must be carried out on pregnant patients when referring doctors are concerned about maternal health. To give the patient the best, safest, and most effective care possible, it is necessary to maintain a balance between the relevance and the overuse of imaging modalities.

Every imaging technique should follow the "as low as reasonably achievable" (ALARA) tenet. This section of the chapter reviews safety concerns as well as potential hazards associated with imaging pregnant and lactating mothers. It also discusses concerns with contrast administration, informed consent and risk management, emotional support, considerations specific to certain modalities, and evidence-based imaging guidelines.

Imaging in pregnant women is more complicated due to the need to factor in the "second patient"—the fetus. Hence, risk stratification of these patients involves considering both maternal and fetal risks.

3 Maternal Risk

Deterministic effects (effects associated with a threshold dose and whose severity increases with dose) are rare in adults at diagnostic exposure levels. However, complications or errors during interventional radiology cases or perfusion CT can still lead to tissue effects such as erythema, epilation, or skin necrosis (Fig. 3). The

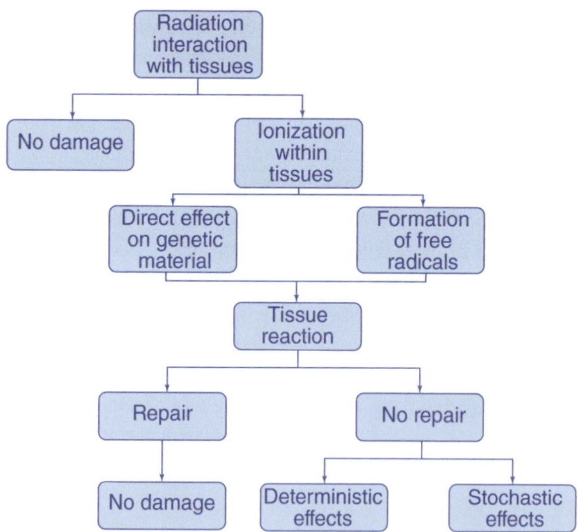

Fig. 3 Flowchart demonstrating the influence/interactions and effects of radiation on tissues

threshold for transient skin effects is approximately 2 Gy single site acute skin dose, while effects that may cause longer term issues do not appear until 5 Gy. At diagnostic imaging doses, the primary risk to adults is from stochastic effects (effects that occur randomly and have no threshold dose), particularly the induction of cancer. The risk of cancer from radiation exposure is influenced by factors such as age, sex, rate of exposure, and genetics. The most commonly used estimate for radiation-induced cancer risk is a 5% risk per 1 Sievert dose for the adult general population although this risk is orders of magnitude smaller than the spontaneous cancer risk [3].

4 Fetal Risk

Fetuses are more sensitive to radiation than adults or children due to their high rate of cellular proliferation. The potential risks include deterministic effects such as microcephaly, mental retardation, organ malformation, fetal death, and stochastic effects such as carcinogenesis (Table 1). The fetal risks at typical diagnostic imaging dose levels are minimal, but careful consideration should be taken to maintain the fetal dose as low as possible while achieving the greatest diagnostic value from the exam [3, 4].

The threshold for fetal death varies with gestational age, ranging from 50 to 250 mGy. The main risk during organogenesis is for teratogenic effects, while during the fetal growth stage, neuro-pathologies such as mental retardation are more likely. The threshold dose for these effects is believed to be 500 mGy [4].

Fetal doses due to diagnostic imaging are rarely high enough to significantly increase the risk to the fetus, and the 50-mGy threshold is considered negligible or nonexistent by regulatory and professional groups [4].

To better understand the imaging safety considerations, we can analyze them under the groups of modality-specific considerations—radiation related and non-radiation related.

Table 1 Effects of radiation on teratogenesis in relation to the postconceptional age[a]

Postconceptional age	Effects	Estimated threshold dose
Post-conception period		
0–2 weeks	Death of embryo or no effects	50–100 mGy
2–8 weeks	Congenital defects in skull, eyes, genital, and skeleton	20–0 mGy
Fetal period		
8–15 weeks	High risk of severe mental retardation	60–10 Gy
16–25 weeks	Low IQ	25 IQ point/Gy
	Microcephaly	200 mGy
	Low risk of severe mental retardation	250–80 mGy

[a]Adapted from Baysinger CL. Imaging during pregnancy. Anesth Analg. 2010 Mar 1;110(3):863-7 doi: 10.1213/ANE.0b013e3181ca767e. PMID: 20185662

Specific considerations apply to modalities that use ionizing radiation (i.e., radiography, CT, nuclear medicine, and fluoroscopy) and those that do not use ionizing radiation (i.e., magnetic resonance imaging [MRI] and ultrasound) (Table 2).

Table 2 Tabulated summary of the fetal and maternal risks and considerations for the various imaging modalities and contrast studies[a]

Radiographs (X-rays), computed tomography (CT) and nuclear medicine)	Potential indications	• *Plain Radiographs*: Radiographs are used for the evaluation of acute respiratory illnesses, i.e., chest XRs and radiographs of extremities are employed in the evaluation of trauma for suspected fractures. • *Computed Tomography (CT)*: CT head is useful in ruling out acute intracranial pathologies. CT pulmonary angiogram (CTPA) is used to rule out pulmonary embolism (PE) and CT abdomen in the setting of trauma. • *Nuclear Medicine Scans:* Ventilation/perfusion (VQ) used in suspected pulmonary embolism (if CTPA is not the first-choice imaging for the patient).
	Potential risk summary (evidence based)	• Diagnostic imaging uses radiation levels that for the most part do not directly cause fetal harm, i.e., malformation, IUGR, IUFD, and intellectual disability (deterministic). • Cancer risk depends on the organ imaged and has no definite threshold (stochastic).
	IV contrast use (iodinated contrast)	Used for assessment of pulmonary embolism, most abdominal CTs and cerebral stroke perfusion/angiography studies. No documented harm to the fetus exists except a theoretical risk of neonatal hypothyroidism.
	Guidelines	1. Follow ALARA principle (as low as reasonably achievable). 2. Low fetal dose procedures like chest/upper abdominal radiography, CT above the diaphragm or below the knees pose negligible risk (less than 1 in 10,000–100,000) of childhood cancer induction and can be justified when clinically indicated. 3. Higher fetal dose procedures like CT pelvis must be considered when information cannot be obtained without ionizing radiation, and if it is seriously detrimental to the patient's health is likely without the scan. If performed, fetal dose should not exceed 50–100 mGy. IV contrast can be used if clinically warranted and must be followed by neonatal hypothyroidism screening in their first week of life.

Table 2 (continued)

MRI	Potential indications	Indicated in maternal brain imaging, fetal imaging, and maternal acute abdomen.
	Potential risk summary (evidence based)	No conclusive evidence for MRI induced fetal harm (routinely used setting). Theoretical risks exist for fetal hyperthermia and inner ear damage (can be avoided by scanner modification).
	IV contrast use (gadolinium-based contrast)	Used sparingly since contrast crosses the blood–placental barrier. Limited evidence exists for MRI contrast associations with several neonatal, rheumatological, inflammatory, and/or infiltrative skin conditions, stillbirth, or neonatal demise.
	Guidelines	MRI is relatively safe in pregnancy. Some health authorities (Medicines and Healthcare Product Regulatory Agency-UK) advise caution in the first trimester (though it is advised this can be done when the benefits outweigh the risks). Others, such as the American College of Radiologists (ACOG), suggest that patients in the first trimester of pregnancy should not be treated differently from those in later stages of pregnancy. Avoid IV gadolinium unless it will change the management during pregnancy or no other modality of imaging is applicable.
Ultrasound	Potential indications	Indicated for obstetric imaging, suspected acute abdominal/pelvic pathology and cardiac imaging, i.e., echocardiography.
	Potential risk summary (evidence based)	No adverse maternal, fetal, perinatal, or childhood effects/outcomes. Theoretical risks of heating and movement effects but no adverse outcomes have been documented in human studies.
	IV contrast use (microbubbles)	Rarely used in the imaging of heart, some hepatic and kidney lesions. Microbubbles used can burst and cause cavitations. They could enter the placenta, and placental damage risk has not been well investigated.
	Guidelines	Safest modality overall, however use as low as reasonably achievable principle (ALARA) principle, i.e., only request if clinically indicated. Refrain from ultrasound contrast use unless benefits clearly outweigh the risks.

[a]Modified from "Wiles, R., Hankinson, B., Benbow, E., & Sharp, A. (2022). Making decisions about radiological imaging in pregnancy. Bmj, 377"

4.1 Ultrasound Imaging

The recommended first imaging test for evaluating suspected maternal intra-abdominal pathology is transabdominal ultrasound as it does not expose the mother or fetus to ionizing radiation. Acute appendicitis is the most common non-obstetric surgical emergency affecting 1 in 1500 pregnancies. Although ultrasonography has been in clinical practice for over 40 years, it has not been shown to cause significant health risks to the fetus or mother. However, most safety data were collected before 1992 when the permissible power output of scanners was lower than that of contemporary scanners. It is unlikely that tissue temperature increases would exceed 0.5 °C even with prolonged examinations using modern scanners, and therefore would not have significant adverse effects. The American College of Obstetricians and Gynecologists (ACOG) states that the casual use of ultrasound without medical indication is inappropriate, and the lowest possible ultrasound exposure setting should be used to obtain the necessary diagnostic information [5].

4.2 Magnetic Resonance Imaging

Fetal teratogenicity and acoustic damage are the primary concerns with MRI use during pregnancy, but studies on rodents [6, 7] and children up to 9 years old exposed to MRI in utero at 1.5 T showed no adverse teratogenic, behavioral, or hearing effects. However, the safety of MRI at 3 T has not been studied [8].

While most radiologists would avoid using MRI in the first trimester of pregnancy, it is preferred over any study involving ionizing radiation. Although there are no studies that demonstrate fetal harm when gadolinium is used for contrast, most radiologists avoid routine use of it during pregnancy as it can be excreted into the amniotic fluid and potentially absorbed by the fetus from the gastrointestinal tract [9].

The fetal half-life of gadolinium is unknown, and prolonged fetal exposure is possible. Fortunately, most maternal pelvic and fetal MRI does not require the use of gadolinium although it may be necessary in cases of suspected placenta accreta to better assess the placental/myometrial interface [5].

4.3 X- Ray Imaging

X-rays play an essential role in imaging obstetric patients in the ICU, particularly in identifying complications such as pulmonary edema, pneumothorax, and pleural effusion. However, the use of X-rays in pregnant women raises concerns due to the potential risk of fetal ionizing radiation exposure. Therefore, the American College of Radiology recommends limiting exposure to the fetus by using appropriate shielding techniques and alternative imaging modalities such as ultrasound or MRI when feasible. Despite these concerns, X-ray imaging remains a valuable tool in the ICU management of obstetric patients [5, 8].

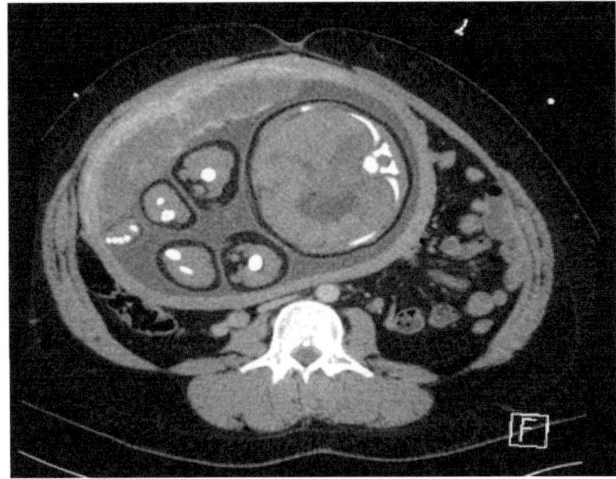

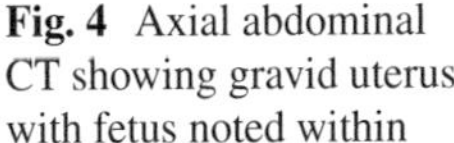

Fig. 4 Axial abdominal CT showing gravid uterus with fetus noted within

4.4 *Commutated Tomography*

CT is commonly used to evaluate pregnant patients with trauma or suspected pulmonary embolism, which are the main causes of maternal mortality [9]. Trauma increases the risk of pregnancy loss, which ranges from 1% to 34%, with penetrating trauma having a higher rate of pregnancy loss, up to 73% [10].

Maternal death almost always leads to fetal loss, but rare cases of emergency cesarean section despite lethal maternal injuries have been reported. Therefore, maternal stabilization is prioritized, followed by imaging with radiography, CT, or angiography as needed. Focused abdominal sonography for trauma is performed at the bedside, and if positive or highly suspicious, CT is preferred for evaluating organ and vascular injury (Fig. 4) [9].

The risk of radiation exposure from imaging pregnant trauma patients is outweighed by the risk of missed or delayed diagnosis, and appropriate techniques and dose settings should be used to minimize radiation exposure. Non-extreme low-dose exams, single-phase exams, and appropriate coverage of the anatomy should be used. Delayed scans are focused on the area of interest and performed at a lower dose. CT cystography may be necessary for suspected bladder rupture and can be performed with low-dose techniques [11].

4.5 *Fluoroscopy/Interventional*

Fluoroscopic and interventional procedures are performed using the same principles as with all radiation-related modalities and are indicated only when there is a dire necessity or strong indication that justifies the cause/life-saving like embolization for hemorrhage.

4.6 Nuclear Medicine/Imaging

Nuclear imaging of pregnant women poses a challenge for nuclear medicine physicians because of the potential risk of radiation exposure to the embryo or fetus. Recent concerns about medical procedures involving radiation have added to the anxiety surrounding nuclear medicine scans, leading some clinicians to be hesitant to order them due to fear of malpractice or uncertainty about fetal radiation dose. However, when used appropriately, the benefits of nuclear imaging procedures usually outweigh the minimal risks associated with low levels of radiation, even in pregnant patients (Fig. 5) [12].

Radiation exposure during pregnancy has been well studied, and the risk of fetal malformation or carcinogenesis is low when the radiation dose is below certain thresholds. The International Commission on Radiological Protection has recommended an annual dose limit of 1 mSv for pregnant women, and most nuclear medicine scans have a fetal radiation dose below this limit [13].

The decision to perform nuclear imaging on a pregnant patient should be made on a case-by-case basis, taking into account the potential benefits and risks. Alternative imaging modalities, such as ultrasound or MRI, should be considered when feasible, but nuclear imaging can provide important diagnostic information that may not be obtainable with other modalities [9].

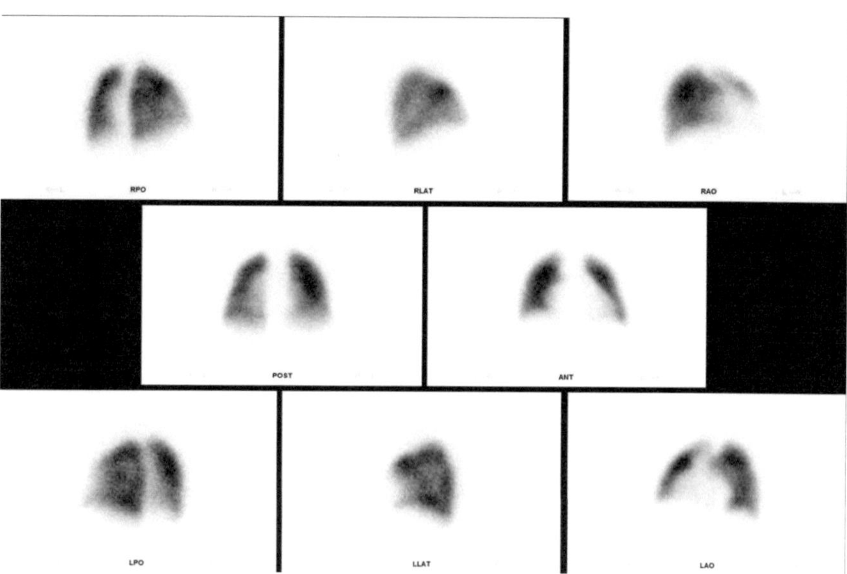

Fig. 5 Ventilation-perfusion (V/Q) nuclear medicine scan used in the diagnosis of pulmonary embolism in pregnancy

5 Imaging Contrast Usage in Pregnancy

The use of contrast media in pregnant presents a challenge for radiologists and physicians, but their use has increased in recent years. While mutagenic and teratogenic effects of gadolinium and iodinated contrast media have not been reported, the presence of free iodide in radiographic contrast media can potentially depress fetal thyroid function. Therefore, neonatal thyroid function should be checked within the first week if iodinated contrast media have been administered during pregnancy. No adverse effects on the fetus have been observed with gadolinium contrast media [9].

When considering the use of contrast media in pregnant or lactating patients, the potential risks and benefits should be carefully weighed. Alternative imaging modalities, such as ultrasound or MRI, should be considered when feasible. However, in some cases, contrast-enhanced imaging may provide important diagnostic information that cannot be obtained with other modalities [14].

Radiologists and other physicians should take appropriate precautions to minimize radiation exposure and ensure patient safety. They should also be aware of the relevant guidelines and recommendations for the use of contrast media in pregnant patients [15].

6 Gastrointestinal and Genitourinary Pathology

6.1 Gastrointestinal Pathologies

Investigation of the acute abdomen in pregnancy presents a complex clinical scenario with unique challenges. Clinical assessment is often difficult as there is a significant overlap between symptoms that occur as part of a normal pregnancy (including nausea and vomiting) and those due to underlying pathological processes, some of which require emergent operative management.

6.1.1 Appendicitis

Appendicitis is the most common non-obstetric surgical problem in pregnancy. US with graded compression is a valuable diagnostic tool for the diagnosis of acute appendicitis in the pregnant patient especially during the first trimester [16, 17] (Fig. 6a); however, sensitivity of US is reduced particularly in the third trimester where the enlarged gravid uterus causes displacement of anatomical structure and can prevent graded compression. Equivocal or even false-positive sonographic assessments along with the clinical decision to expedite surgery and avoid appendiceal perforation, is associated with high rates of miscarriage and leads to increase negative laparotomy rate. MRI has been shown to have increased sensitivity in the diagnosis of appendicitis when compared to US [18] in particular pregnant women who underwent MRI after inconclusive transabdominal US (Fig. 6b).

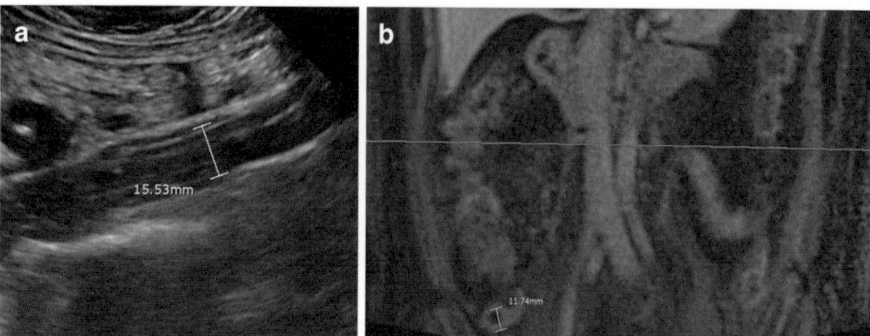

Fig. 6 (**a**) High frequency ultrasound of right iliac fossa demonstrating sonographic appearance of acute appendicitis. (**b**) Coronal T1 image of MRI demonstrating a thick-walled dilated appendix

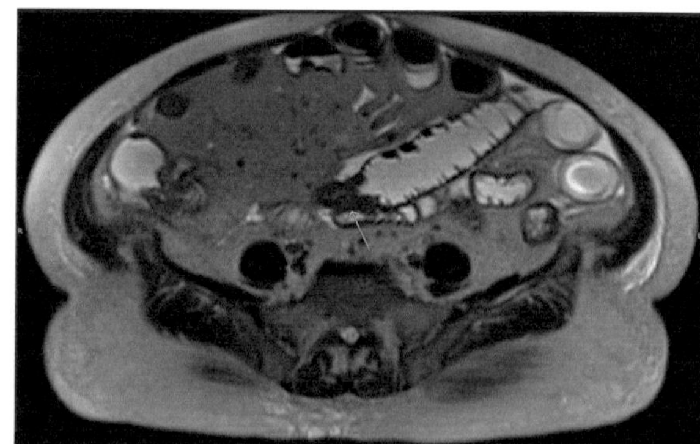

Fig. 7 Axial T2-weighted MRI image demonstrates dilated fluid-filled loops of the ileum with stricture (arrow)

6.1.2 Bowel Obstruction

Bowel obstruction in pregnancy has an incidence of approximately 1 in 1500 to 1 in 66,000 [19]. Causes of obstruction are similar to those in non-pregnant patients, with adhesions being most common [20]. A unique cause of bowel obstruction in pregnancy results from bowel compression by gravid uterus [21]. MRI is excellent for the evaluation of bowel obstruction and can be performed without oral or IV contrast and is the modality of choice (Fig. 7). Role of X-ray for diagnosing bowel obstruction is limited in pregnant patient due to risk of Ionizing radiation to fetus

6.1.3 Inflammatory Bowel Disease

Inflammatory bowel disease (IBD) is a common cause of abdominal pain in pregnancy as the age of presentation for Crohn's disease and ulcerative colitis (UC) overlaps with reproductive age. IBD mimics other surgical condition in pregnancy. Crohn's disease frequently affects the terminal ileum, making it a diagnostic

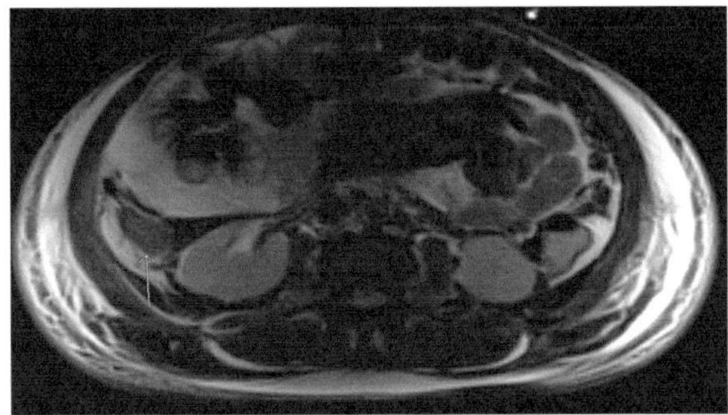

Fig. 8 Axial sections of MRI abdomen showing segments of circumferentially thickened, edematous bowel on T2-weighted images with free fluid

dilemma with acute appendicitis in pregnancy as both conditions have similar clinical presentation [22].

Imaging modality of choice is MRI. Active Crohn's disease appears as segments of circumferentially thickened, edematous bowel on T2-weighted images, free fluid frequently with skip lesions and involvement of the terminal ileum (Fig. 8)

6.2 Genitourinary Pathologies

Common genitourinary pathologies manifesting as abdominal pain in pregnancy includes obstructive urinary tract calculi, ovarian torsion, and degenerating fibroids.

6.2.1 Obstructive Hydronephrosis

Acute obstructive hydronephrosis is the most common cause of non-obstetric hospital admission during pregnancy [22, 23].Imaging plays a vital role in differentiating between physiologic and obstructive hydronephrosis. Typically, patients present in the second and third trimester of pregnancy. Ultrasound is usually the first imaging technique of choice for evaluating hydronephrosis. The absence of the ureteral jet on the suspected side of obstruction is reported to have a sensitivity of 100% and a specificity of 91% for the diagnosis of obstructive hydronephrosis and indicates complete obstruction [24] (Fig. 9a, b). In physiologic hydronephrosis, no filling defect is seen, the ureter is not dilated distal to the sacral promontory and only rarely is there associated renal enlargement or perinephric fluid.

MRI features of obstructive uropathy include an abrupt change in ureteral caliber, renal enlargement, perinephric fluid, and when visible, a low-signal intensity ureteral filling defect on T2-weighted imaging, which reflects the obstructing calculus (Fig. 10).

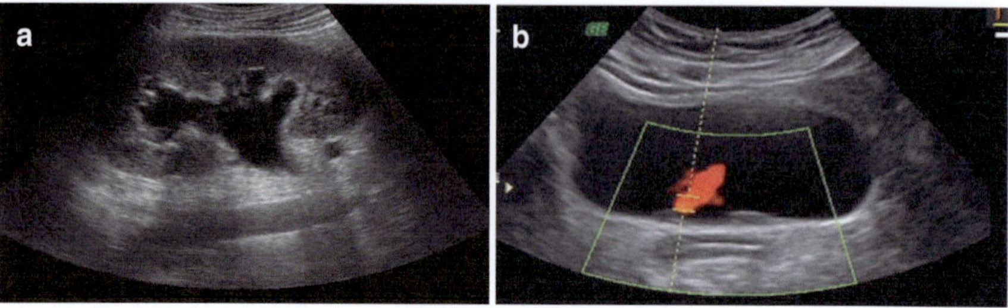

Fig. 9 Obstructive hydronephrosis in 23-year-old pregnant woman who presented with left flank pain. (**a**) Sagittal gray-scale ultrasound image of left kidney shows moderate hydronephrosis. (**b**) Transverse color Doppler ultrasound image through bladder shows right ureteral jet but absence of left ureteral jet. Neither left ureteral calculus nor dilatation of left ureter was seen sonographically

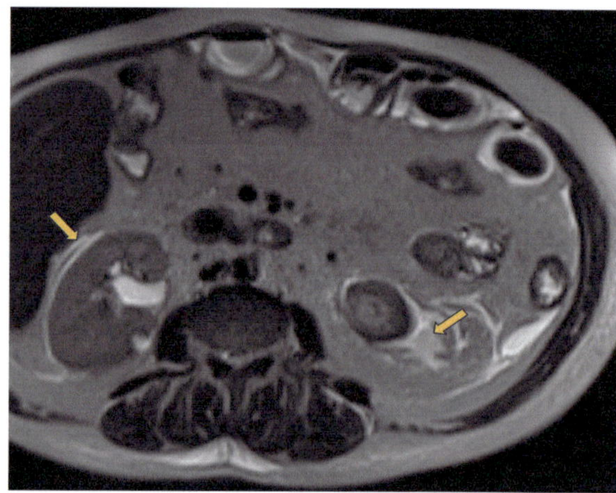

Fig. 10 Axial T2-weighted MRI shows perinephric fluid (arrow) in a case of obstructive uropathy

6.2.2 Ovarian Torsion

Fivefold increase in incidence of ovarian torsion during pregnancy, most frequently occurs during first trimester [25]. MRI is the imaging modality of Choice. MRI features of ovarian torsion include an enlarged abnormally positioned ovary with peripherally arranged follicles with hyper intense, edematous ovaries stroma on T2-weighted imaging. Thickened fallopian tube and swirling of vascular pedicle can also be seen (Fig. 11).

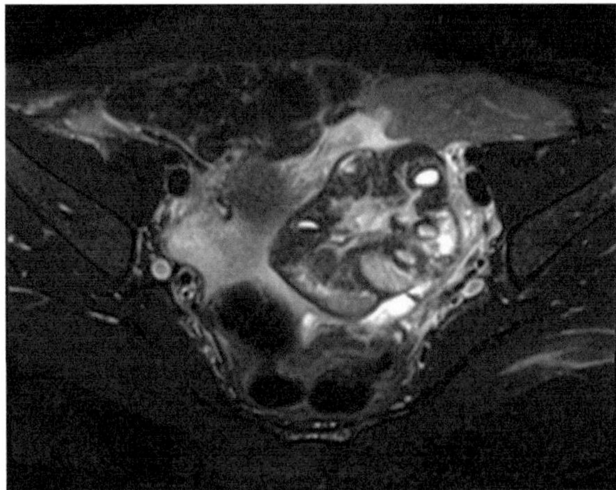

Fig. 11 Axial T2-weighted image shows an enlarged right ovary (abnormally positioned—left adnexa) with multiple peripherally arranged follicles

7 Neuro Imaging in Pregnancy

Neurological evaluation in symptomatic pregnant patients typically commences with non-contrast CT scan which can diagnose hemorrhage with high accuracy. MRI and MR angiography is essentially used in evaluation of ischemic stroke and white matter white matter disease.

The common neurological conditions requiring imaging are discussed in brief as follows:

7.1 Preeclampsia-Eclampsia

Preeclampsia is new onset hypertension in pregnancy and manifests with severe throbbing headache, sometimes associated with visual blurring and blind spots in the visual field [26]. Preeclampsia complicated with seizures is referred to as eclampsia. Common neuroimaging findings include cerebral edema, ischemia, and hemorrhage (Fig. 12) [27].

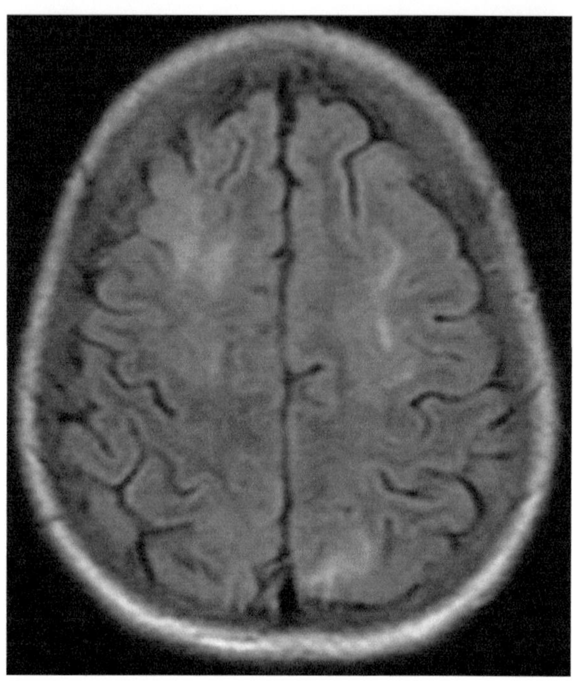

Fig. 12 Brain MRI images (diffusion weighted) demonstrating bilateral frontoparietal lobe edema

7.2 Posterior Reversible Encephalopathy Syndrome (PRES)

Characterized by the inability of posterior circulation to auto regulate in response acute change in the blood pressure. Disruption of blood–brain barrier due to hyper perfusion results in vasogenic edema often without infarction, commonly in the parieto-occipital regions (Figs. 13, 14, and 15). Clinical presentation includes headache, seizures, and visual disturbance. MRI brain shows areas of high signal intensity involving the cortex and subcortical white matter, predominantly in the occipital lobes [28].

DWI typically shows elevated rather than restricted diffusion, allowing confident exclusion of irreversible ischemia and guiding hemodynamic medical management [29, 30].

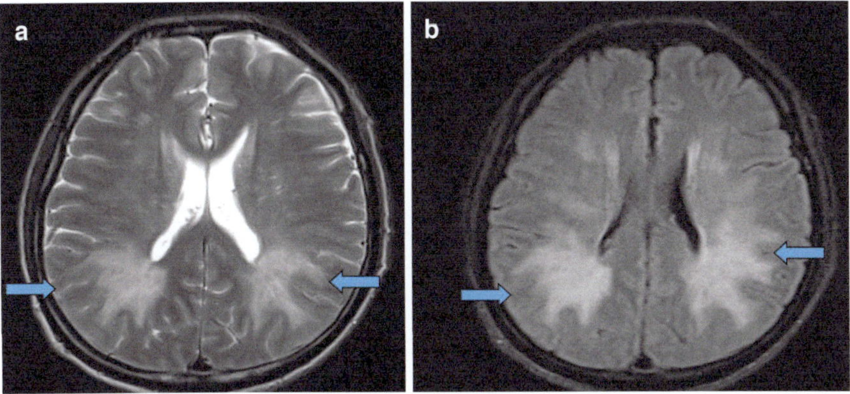

Fig. 13 T2-weighted (**a**) and FLAIR (**b**) images, MRI shows areas of high signal intensity involving the cortex and subcortical white matter, predominantly in the occipital lobes (arrows)

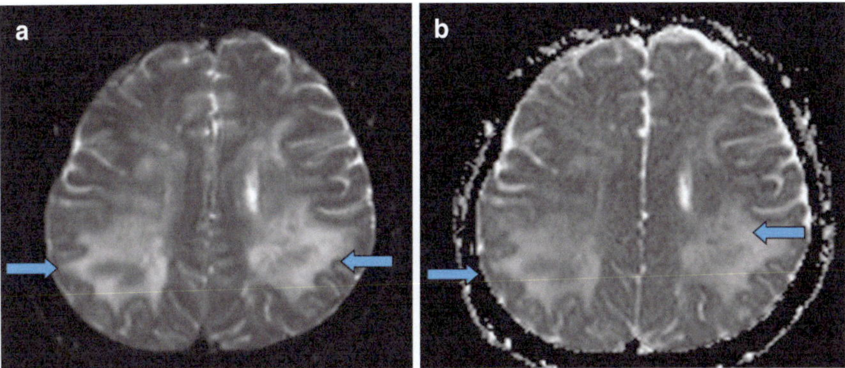

Fig. 14 Diffusion-weighted image (DWI) and corresponding ADC map showing no regions of diffusion restriction, i.e., high signal on DWI and corresponding low-signal regions on ADC

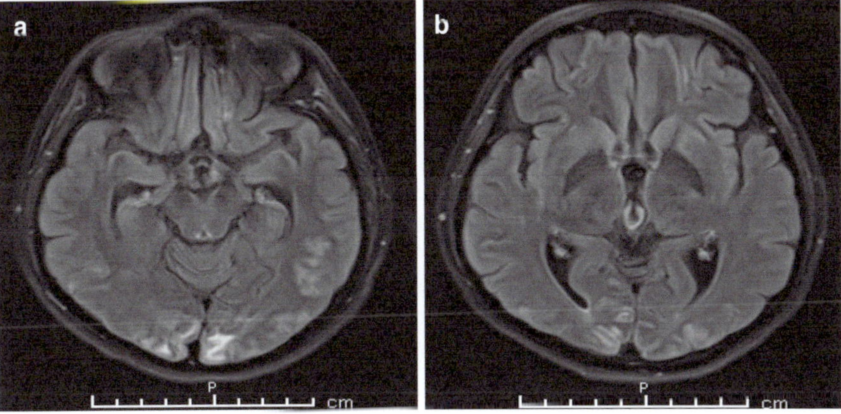

Fig. 15 MRI T2 FLAIR axial sections showing regions of hyperintensities in the bilateral occipital regions classic for PRES syndrome

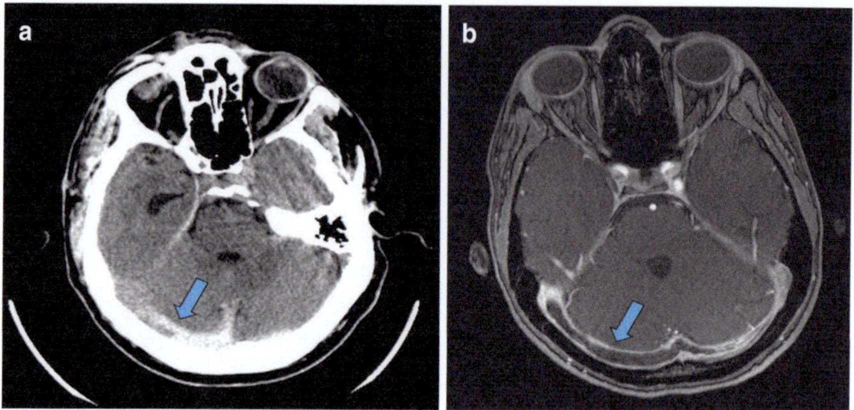

Fig. 16 (**a**) Unenhanced CT Head showing hyperdense right transverse sinus suggestive of right transverse sinus thrombosis. (**b**) Contrast-enhanced MRI with the inclusion of MR venography

7.3 Cerebral Venous Thrombosis

Non-contrast CT scan (Fig. 16a) can depict shows a high-attenuation thrombus within a cerebral dural sinus in only about 30% of cases [27]. More often, the thrombus in the dural sinus causes only a small increase in CT attenuation, making the diagnosis difficult (Fig. 16a) [31].

Contrast-enhanced MRI with the inclusion of MR venography (Fig. 16b) and susceptibility-weighted imaging is the imaging study of choice for diagnosing cerebral venous thrombosis [32]. CT angiogram has a high accuracy in depicting dural sinus and cortical vein thrombosis and the compensatory venous collateral pathways.

Cerebral angiography is generally reserved for cases wherein a neuro-interventional procedure is needed.

7.4 Embolism

This includes amniotic fluid embolism, thromboembolism, and air embolism. The neuroradiological manifestations of amniotic fluid embolism and thromboembolism include findings of generalized cerebral hypoxemia and ischemia due to hypoperfusion or multiple cerebral emboli. Thromboembolism on plain CT scan demonstrates is seen as loss of gray-white matter differentiation and decreased attenuation of basal ganglia (Fig. 17a). Cerebral perfusion imaging demonstrates reduced perfusion in the affected cerebral hemispheres (Fig. 17b) with non-opacification of the involved intracranial vessels most commonly middle cerebral artery (MCA) on CT cerebral angiography (Fig. 17c).

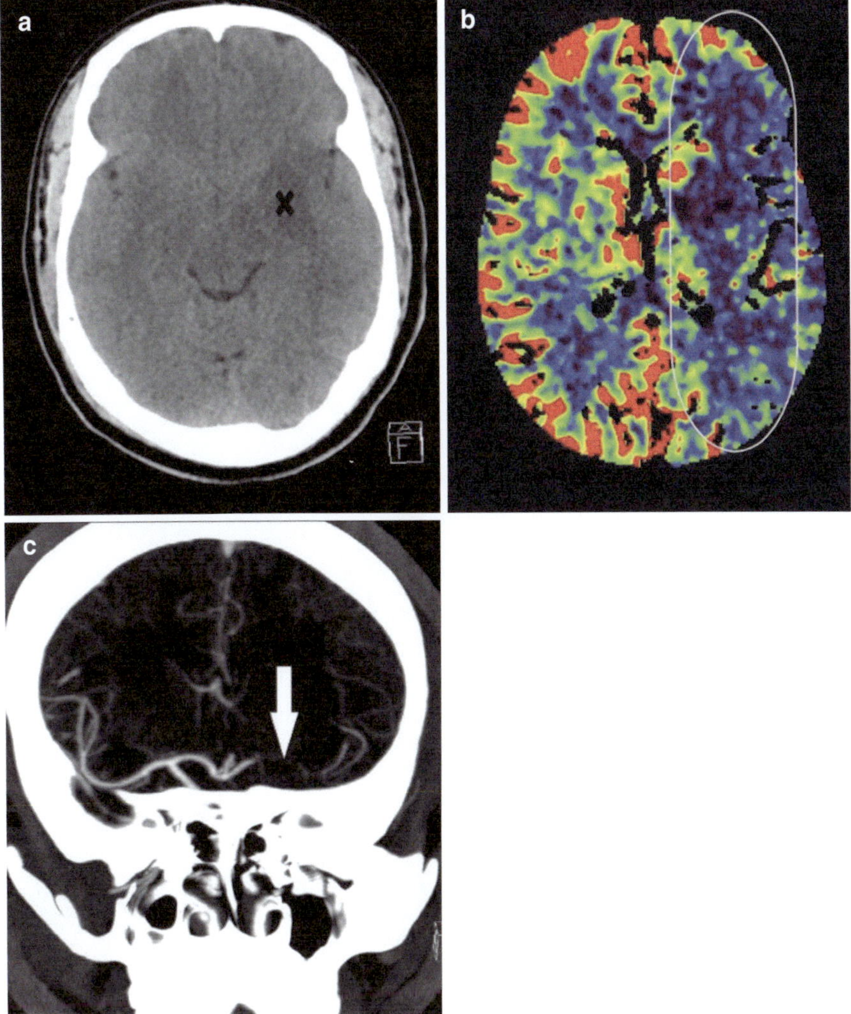

Fig. 17 (**a**) Plain CT scan demonstrates effacement of the left lentiform nucleus, loss of gray-white matter differentiation and decreased attenuation of the basal ganglia. (**b**) Perfusion imaging shows reduced perfusion in the left cerebral hemisphere. (**c**) Non-visualization of the left middle cerebral artery (MCA) on CT cerebral angiography

7.5 Ischemic Stroke

During pregnancy, diffusion-weighted MRI is the mainstay in the radiologic diagnosis of acute ischemic stroke, which demonstrates restricted diffusion in ischemic brain tissue within minutes of stroke onset (Fig. 18) [33].

7.6 *Cerebral Hemorrhage*

Cerebral arteriovenous malformations (AVMs), intracranial aneurysms, and cavernomas are the most common lesions related to cerebral hemorrhage in pregnancy [27]. Ruptured aneurysms, most commonly cause subarachnoid hemorrhage, with intraventricular extension, all easily identified with CT or MRI (Fig. 19a, b).

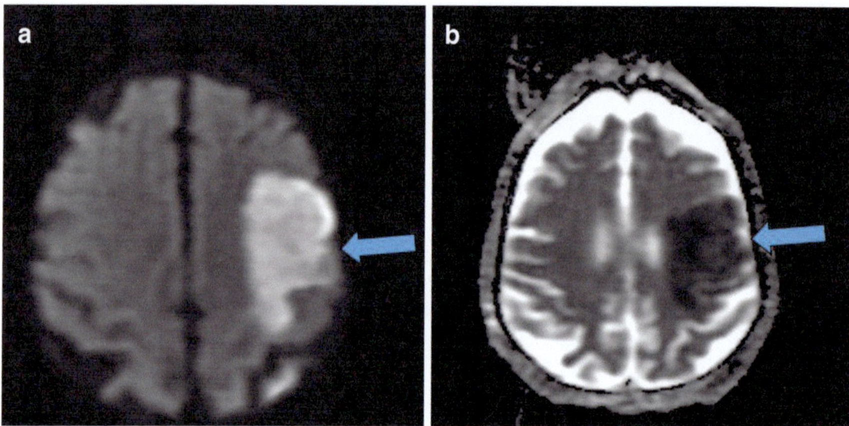

Fig. 18 Diffusion-weighted images (DWI) showing high signal in the left frontoparietal region with corresponding low signal, i.e., diffusion restriction suggestive of ischemic stroke

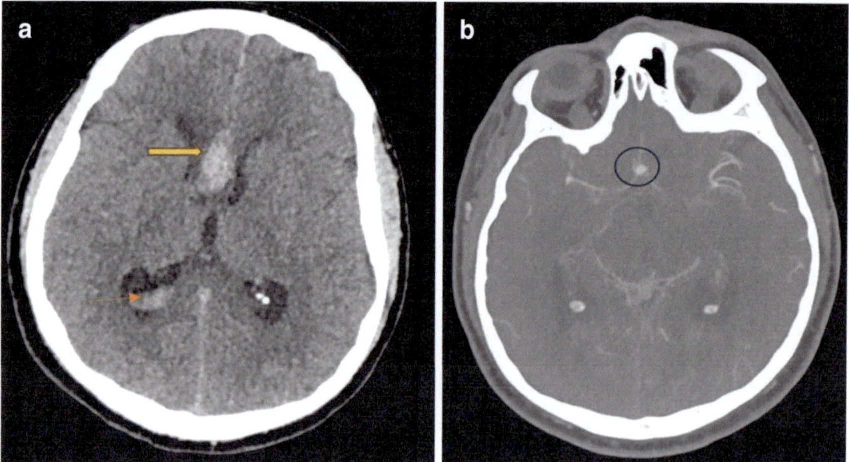

Fig. 19 Plain head CT scan (**a**) demonstrates subarachnoid hemorrhage (⇒) with intraventricular hemorrhagic extension (→). (**b**) Contrast enhanced CT scan demonstrates the anterior communicating artery aneurysm (○)

7.7 *Pulmonary Thromboembolism (PTE)*

The preliminary investigation of choice for the diagnosis of PTE is lower limb venous Doppler, which does not involve the use of contrast agents nor ionizing radiation [34, 35]. If deep venous thrombosis is detected, treatment should be commenced without any further imaging studies. If the Doppler study is inconclusive, it is recommended to proceed with either CT pulmonary angiography (CTPA) or ventilation/perfusion scintigraphy, depending on the availability of the modality and upon the clinical background of the patient (Figs. 20 and 21). Scintigraphy renders lower exposure to radiation and is preferred in patients allergic to iodinated contrast [36] and in those with a normal chest radiograph. CT pulmonary angiography has the advantage of providing an alternative diagnosis [35] and is preferred in patients with an abnormal chest radiograph [37].

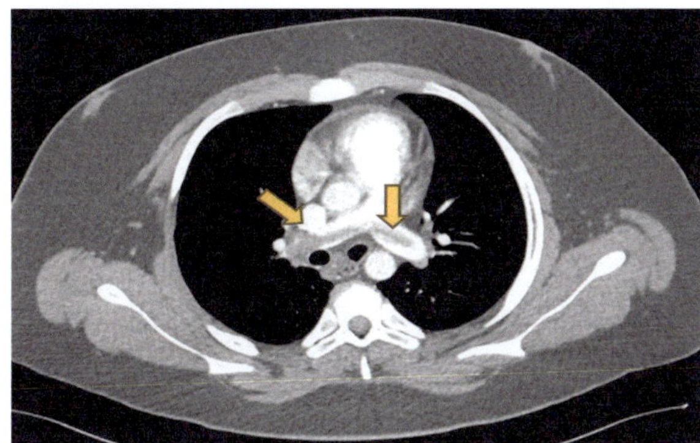

Fig. 20 CTPA demonstrating a "Saddle embolus" at the pulmonary artery bifurcation, extending into the right and left main pulmonary arteries

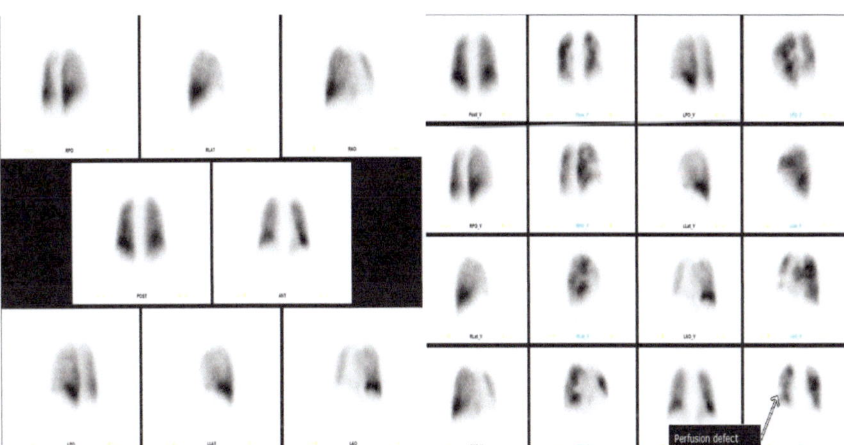

Fig. 21 V/P scan showing large mismatched perfusion defects (arrow) with no ventilation defects, indicating a high probability for pulmonary embolism

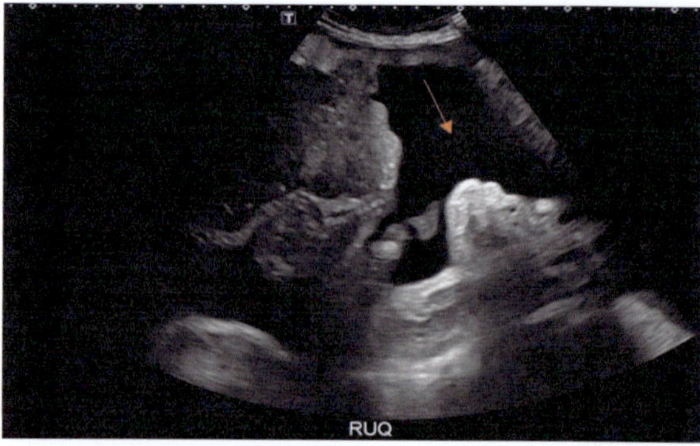

Fig. 22 FAST ultrasound demonstrating hemoperitoneum (arrow)

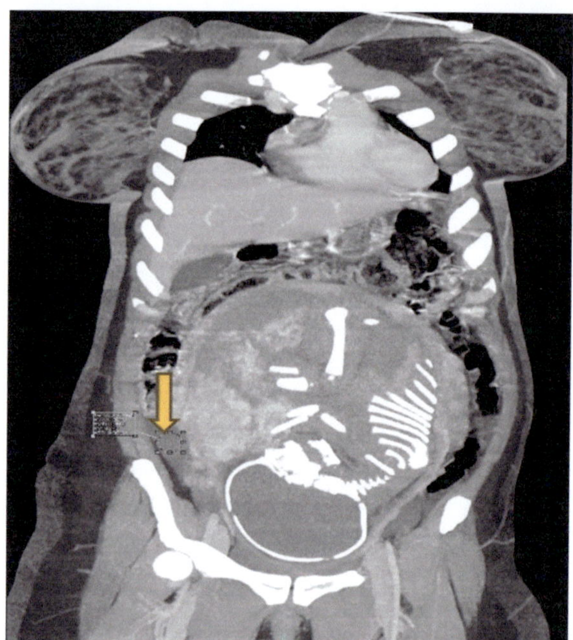

Fig. 23 Contrast enhanced CT abdomen showing hemoperitoneum with gravid uterus (arrow)

8 Trauma in Pregnancy

Trauma is one of the leading non-obstetric causes of maternal mortality [38]. Ultrasonography plays an important role in the initial assessment of the fetal well-being; however, it has a limited role in evaluation of maternal injuries (Fig. 22) [39]. A preliminary chest radiograph and focused assessment with sonography in trauma (FAST) is required to rule in maternal injuries like pneumothorax and hemoperitoneum. However, when potential life-threatening injury is suspected, CT scan with intravenous contrast is the modality of choice as the risks of radiation to the pregnancy are trivial as compared with the risk of missed or delayed diagnosis of maternal injury (Fig. 23).

9 Gynecological Conditions Leading to Intensive Care in a Pregnant Woman

Gynecological disorders can be acute and requiring medical or surgical attention or both. However, it is rather rare for gynecological disorders to lead to severe illness and intensive care requirement especially if the patient receives prompt medical care.

The following conditions however can potentially be life-threatening and require immediate medical intensive care.

9.1 *Hemorrhagic Shock*

Hemorrhage of any kind when in considerable volumes can lead to hypovolemia and cardiovascular failure/collapse. Hence, all causes of hemorrhage be it traumatic, gynecologic like uterine rupture, placental abruption, ruptured ectopic pregnancy, or hemorrhagic ovarian cyst rupture must be treated with caution and appropriate management.

Hemoperitoneum must be evaluated and considered seriously in pregnant patients as unchecked hemoperitoneum is a leading cause of hemorrhagic shock.

On ultrasound-free fluid in the cul-de-sac, peritoneum, and pelvis is suggestive of possible hemoperitoneum given if it is accompanied with the related clinical indicators.

On plain CT, the sentinel clot sign could suggest the site of bleeding in the setting of hemoperitoneum. Fluid density above 20 HU is considered hemorrhagic and 50–60 HU would suggest freshly clotted hemorrhagic blood. Contrast-enhanced CT can demonstrate sign of active bleed or bleeding by showing contrast extravasation or blush, etc.

10 Conclusion

Radiological imaging plays a vital role in the management of critically ill ICU obstetric patients. Medical conditions such as preeclampsia, pulmonary embolism, and placental abruption may require specialized imaging techniques to diagnose and monitor. Radiation exposure is a key consideration when imaging pregnant patients, and imaging protocols must be carefully tailored to minimize radiation exposure while still providing accurate diagnostic information. Through careful use of imaging techniques, clinicians can effectively manage and treat critically ill obstetric patients in the ICU.

References

1. Shehabi K, Chan L, Kadry M. Critical care management of the pregnant patient. Anaesth Intensive Care. 2010;38(4):621–33. https://doi.org/10.1177/0310057X1003800412.
2. Lapinsky JR, Ross RL. Critical illness in pregnancy. Crit Care Med. 2009;37(Suppl. 10):S372–9. https://doi.org/10.1097/CCM.0b013e3181b6e9c5.
3. Brown JK, Potter EJ. Radiation safety in diagnostic imaging. In: Siegel EJ, Brant WA, editors. Radiology Secrets Plus. 4th ed. Philadelphia: Mosby; 2017. p. 26–32.
4. Balter S, Siegel DS. Radiation exposure in the pregnant patient. In: Siegel EJ, Brant WA, editors. Radiology Secrets Plus. 4th ed. Philadelphia: Mosby; 2017. p. 33–7.
5. American College of Obstetricians and Gynecologists. ACOG Committee Opinion No. 723: Guidelines for diagnostic imaging during pregnancy and lactation. Obstet Gynecol. 2017;130(4):e210–6. https://doi.org/10.1097/AOG.0000000000002352.
6. Shellock FG. Safety considerations with MRI. J Magn Reson Imaging. 2004;19(6):885–96. https://doi.org/10.1002/jmri.20072.
7. Kanal E, Barkovich AJ, Bell C, Borgstede JP, Bradley WG Jr, Froelich JW, Gilk T, Gimbel JR, Gosbee JW, Kuhni-Kaminski E, Larson PA, Lester JW Jr, Schaefer DJ, Sebek-Scoumis EA, Weinreb J, Zaremba LA, Wilcox P. ACR guidance document on MR safe practices: 2013. J Magn Reson Imaging. 2013;37(3):501–30. https://doi.org/10.1002/jmri.24011.
8. American College of Radiology. (2015). ACR-SPR practice parameter for the safe and optimal performance of fetal magnetic resonance imaging (MRI). https://www.acr.org/-/media/ACR/Files/Practice-Parameters/mri-fetal.pdf.
9. American College of Radiology. (2017). ACR-SPR practice parameter for imaging pregnant or potentially pregnant adolescents and women with ionizing radiation. https://www.acr.org/-/media/ACR/Files/Practice-Parameters/pregnant-patients.pdf.
10. Rincon TA, Baker CJ. Pregnancy and trauma. In: StatPearls. StatPearls Publishing; 2019. https://www.ncbi.nlm.nih.gov/books/NBK470157/.
11. American College of Radiology. (2014). ACR Appropriateness Criteria® pregnant patient with trauma. https://acsearch.acr.org/docs/69444/Narrative/.
12. Zanotti-Fregonara P, Hindie E, Quinto MA. Radiation exposure of pregnant women in nuclear medicine: a review. Eur J Nucl Med Mol Imaging. 2019;46(12):2517–29. https://doi.org/10.1007/s00259-019-04498-w.
13. International Commission on Radiological Protection. The 2007 Recommendations of the international commission on radiological protection. Ann ICRP. 2007;37(2-4):1–332. https://doi.org/10.1016/j.icrp.2007.10.003.
14. Kim HC, Yang DM. Gadolinium-based contrast agent in pregnancy: fetal harm or not? Korean J Radiol. 2015;16(1):1–4. https://doi.org/10.3348/kjr.2015.16.1.1.
15. European Society of Urogenital Radiology. (2018). ESUR guidelines on contrast media version 10.0. https://www.esur.org/guidelines/
16. Lim HK, Bae SH, G.S. Seo diagnosis of acute appendicitis in pregnant women: value of sonography. AJR Am J Roentgenol. 1992;159(3):539–42.
17. Baruch Y, Canetti M, Blecher Y, et al. The diagnostic accuracy of ultrasound in the diagnosis of acute appendicitis in pregnancy. J Matern-Fetal Neonatal Med. 2020;33(23):3929–34.
18. Incesu L, Coskun A, Selcuk MB, et al. Acute appendicitis: MRI and sonographic correlation. AJR Am J Roentgenol. 1997;168(3):669e74.
19. Perdue PW, Johnson HW, Stafford PW. Intestinal obstruction complicating pregnancy. Am J Surg. 1992;164(4):384–8.
20. Unal A, Sayharman SE, Ozel L, et al. Acute abdomen in pregnancy requiring surgical management: a 20-case series. Eur J Obstet Gynecol Repro Biol. 2011;159(1):87–90.
21. McKenna DA, Meehan CP, Alhajeri AN, et al. The use of MRI to demonstrate small bowel obstruction during pregnancy. Br J Radiol. 2007;80(949):e4–11.

22. Spalluto LB, Woodfield CA, DeBenedictis CM, et al. MR imaging evaluation of abdominal pain during pregnancy: appendicitis and other nonobstetric causes. Radiographics. 2012;32(2):317–34.
23. Cappell MS, Friedel D. Abdominal pain during pregnancy. Gastroenterol Clin N Am. 2003;32(1):1–58.
24. Deyoe LA, Cronan JJ, Breslaw BH, Ridlen MS. New techniques of ultrasound and color Doppler in the prospective evaluation of acute renal obstruction: do they replace the intravenous urogram? Abdom Imaging. 1995;20:58–63.
25. Masselli G, Brunelli R, Monti R, et al. Imaging for acute pelvic pain in pregnancy. Insights Imaging. 2014;5(2):165–1.
26. Fletcher JJ, Kramer AH, Bleck TP, Solenski NJ. Overlapping features of eclampsia and postpartum angiopathy. Neurocrit Care. 2009;11:199–209.
27. Hacecin-Bey L, Varelas PN, Ulmer JL. Imaging of Cerebrovascular disease in Pregnancy and puerperium. AJR Am J Roentgenol. 2016;206(1):26–38.
28. Schwartz RB, Jones KM, Kalina P, et al. Hypertensive encephalopathy: findings on CT, MR imaging, and SPECT imaging in 14 cases. AJR. 1992;159:379–83.
29. Bartynski WS, Boardman JF. Catheter angiography, MR angiography, and MR perfusion in posterior reversible encephalopathy syndrome. AJNR. 2008;29:447–55.
30. Schaefer PW. Diffusion-weighted imaging as a problem-solving tool in the evaluation of patients with acute stroke like syndromes. Top Magn Reson Imaging. 2000;11:300–9.
31. Saposnik G, Barinagarrementeria F, Brown RD Jr, et al. American Heart Association Stroke Council and the Council on Epidemiology and Prevention. Diagnosis and management of cerebral venous thrombosis: a statement for healthcare professionals from the American Heart Association/American Stroke Association. Stroke. 2011;42:1158–92.
32. Ganeshan D, Narlawar R, McCann C, et al. Cerebral venous thrombosis: a pictorial review. Eur J Radiol. 2010;74:110–6.
33. Wintermark M, Sanelli PC, Albers GW, et al. Imaging recommendations for acute stroke and transient ischemic attack patients: a joint statement by the American Society of Neuroradiology, the American College of Radiology and the Society of NeuroInterventional Surgery. J Am Coll Radiol. 2013;10:828–32.
34. Rocha APC, Carmo RL, Melo RFQ, Vilela DN, Leles-Filho OS, Costa-Silva L. Imaging evaluation of nonobstetric conditions during pregnancy: what every radiologist should know. Radiol Bras. 2020;53(3):185–94.
35. Wieseler KM, Bhargava P, Kanal KM, et al. Imaging in pregnant patients: examination appropriateness. Radiographics. 2010;30:1215–29.
36. Malhotra A, Weinberger SE. Pulmonary embolism in pregnancy: epidemiology, pathogenesis, and diagnosis; 2016. [cited 2018 Feb 7]. Available from: http://www.uptodate.com/contents/pulmonary-embolismin-pregnancy-epidemiology-pathogenesis-and-diagnosis.
37. Leung AN, Bull TM, Jaeschke R, Lockwood CJ, Boiselle PM, Hurwitz LM, James AH, McCullough LB, Menda Y, Paidas MJ, Royal HD. An official American Thoracic Society/Society of Thoracic Radiology clinical practice guideline: evaluation of suspected pulmonary embolism in pregnancy. Am J Respir Crit Care Med. 2011;184:1200–8.
38. Sadro C, Bernstein MP, Kanal KM. Imaging of trauma: Part 2, Abdominal trauma and pregnancy—a radiologist's guide to doing what is best for the mother and baby. AJR Am J Roentgenol. 2012;199:1207–19. https://doi.org/10.2214/AJR.12.9091.
39. Raptis CA, Mellnick VM, Raptis DA. Imaging of trauma in the pregnant patient. Radiographics. 2014;34(3):748–63.

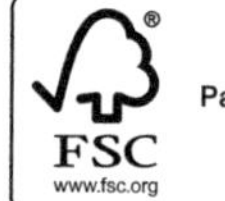

MIX
Papier aus verantwortungsvollen Quellen
Paper from responsible sources
FSC® C105338

If you have any concerns about our products,
you can contact us on
ProductSafety@springernature.com

In case Publisher is established outside the EU,
the EU authorized representative is:
Springer Nature Customer Service Center GmbH
Europaplatz 3, 69115 Heidelberg, Germany

Printed by Libri Plureos GmbH
in Hamburg, Germany